CLINICAL PRACTICE
OF THE
DENTAL HYGIENIST

By

ESTHER M. WILKINS, B.S., R.D.H., D.M.D.

*Formerly Associate Professor and Director, Department of Dental Hygiene,
School of Dentistry, University of Washington*

AND

PATRICIA A. McCULLOUGH, B.S., R.D.H., M.Ed.

*Associate Professor and Head, Department of Dental Hygiene,
Medical Arts Division, Idaho State University, Pocatello, Idaho*

Second Edition, Thoroughly Revised
76 Illustrations

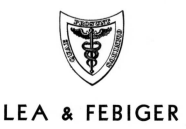

LEA & FEBIGER

PHILADELPHIA

1964

PREFACE TO THE SECOND EDITION

THE aim of this book is to include the fundamental knowledge from which the dental hygienist can understand, evaluate, and apply clinical procedures for the care and instruction of individual patients. Periodic revision is essential since scientific research continually is providing new or improved concepts and techniques. In this edition, material has been brought up to date, the original text has been improved, and new technical data and bibliographic contributions have been added.

With the addition of the chapter on radiography, the material of this book includes the fundamental clinical procedures which have made up the basic services performed by the dental hygienist. Current discussion, analysis, and research to evaluate the effective utilization of dental auxiliary personnel, provide realistic emphasis on the role of the dental hygienist. Whatever the future may find added to the responsibilities of the dental hygienist, the specific contribution to service and instruction focused on the prevention of oral diseases and the maintenance of oral health will remain of primary importance.

Acknowledgment is sincerely given to the many friends and colleagues, who have contributed unselfishly of their time and specialized knowledge to offer constructive suggestions for the improvement of the text. Their critical evaluation has resulted in the correction of errors or misinterpretations, in clarification of specific areas, and in supplementation for more thorough coverage. It is hoped that such critical evaluation will continue in order to provide a text which includes the most generally accepted concepts of the clinical practice of the dental hygienist.

ESTHER M. WILKINS
PATRICIA A. McCULLOUGH

SEATTLE, WASHINGTON

PREFACE TO THE FIRST EDITION

THE major purpose of this book is to provide the dental hygienist with a comprehensive outline of the principles and techniques of dental hygiene care and instruction for the individual patient. It is hoped that through greater understanding of the patient's oral and general health needs, more complete and effective service may be rendered. It is expected that the book will be useful as a textbook for preclinical and clinical theory and practice courses for students, as a reference and guide for practicing dental hygienists, and as a source of review material for temporarily retired dental hygienists with plans for returning to practice.

The content of the book is based on the premise that the dental hygienist has a specific role in the preventive care and instruction program for the patient. If the dental hygienist is to apply her specialized education and carry out legally assigned responsibilities effectively, a majority of her time must be utilized for the direct services and instruction required in the prevention of oral diseases and maintenance of oral health.

The plan of the book is first to describe the fundamental techniques and instruction of the dental hygiene appointment and then to consider applications required for patients with special oral or general health problems. In the first five parts of the book the sequence of chapters follows, insofar as possible, the procedures as they would be carried out in the dental hygiene appointment. It is emphasized that through understanding the patient as a person and applying information gained from the patient history and oral inspection, complete dental hygiene care and instruction can be visualized and planned in terms of present and future appointments. The integrated parts of the appointment are described in detail except for oral radiographic techniques. The authors believe that an entire book could be devoted to the knowledge and skill required for this service. Applications for use of radiographs in the dental hygiene appointment are included. Each chapter contains references and suggested readings for those who wish to supplement the material presented.

The role of the dental hygienist as a health teacher is stressed throughout the book. Because the public has increased awareness of oral health, more specific instruction is necessary. In addition to the detailed chapters devoted to oral physical therapy, other chapters contain a section listing "Factors to Teach the Patient." The suggested "Factors" are selected from the many possibilities which may be used to develop an educated, appreciative patient who will maintain attitudes and habits conducive to the success of dental and dental hygiene care. While the dental hygienist needs to exercise judgment in counseling patients, she must assume responsibility for interpretation of phases of dental care in accord with the policies of the dentist with whom she practices. Knowledge of principles and procedures of dental diagnosis and treatment is basic. Since this book is devoted to details of dental hygiene care, the dental hygienist is referred to dental texts, periodicals and lectures for information on dental care.

This book could never have been completed without the encouragement and help of many people. It evolved from a syllabus for the preclinical and clinical courses for dental hygiene students at the University of Washington. The preparation of the original syllabus was the result of the combined efforts of the entire faculty, past and present, of the Department of Dental Hygiene. Particular appreciation goes to Mrs. Beverly Leggett and Mrs. Jean McCann Quam who wrote a number of sections. From the syllabus came the preliminary mimeographed edition of the present book of which Miss Claudette Stickels was a coauthor. Sincere gratitude is expressed for her assistance in planning the over-all organization of the book as well as writing several chapters. Miss Margaret Ryan's many practical suggestions relating to dental hygiene techniques are greatly appreciated. Mrs. Alice Tronquet and Mrs. Jean McCann Quam, faculty coworkers during the final months of manuscript preparation, are given deep-felt thanks, not only for their suggestions for the many chapters which they reviewed, but also for their patience in assuming added departmental responsibilities.

Sections of the book were critically reviewed by faculty members of many dental hygiene programs and the suggested applications to the techniques used in their clinical courses have been of invaluable assistance. Others offered encouragement after use of the mimeographed text in their student courses and provided additional suggestions for the revision. Particular thanks are due Miss Evelyn Hannon, University of Oregon; Miss Helen Newell and Mrs. Janet Burnham, State University of Iowa; Miss Alberta Beat and Miss Eleanor Forbes, University of North Carolina; Miss Gertrude Sinnett, University of Alabama; Mrs. Lorna Bruning Long, formerly of the University of Texas; Dr. Dorothy Hard, University of Michigan; Miss Evelyn Maas, Northwestern University; Mrs. Frances Dolan, University of Bridgeport; Miss Louise Hord, Forsyth School for Dental Hygienists; Miss Phyllis Quinby, University of Vermont; Dr. Frances Stoll, Columbia University; Mrs. Hazel Koga, University of Hawaii; Miss Victoria Krohr, University of California; Miss A. Rebekah Fisk, Indiana University; Miss Margaret Bailey, Temple University; Mrs. Ruth Vaughn, University of Southern California; and Miss M. Freeman Wallis, Eastman Dental Hospital, London.

Consultants were sought in the preparation of specialized areas. Appreciation is extended to Dr. Alton Moore and Dr. Richard Riedel for their contributions to the text and illustrations for the chapter on Inspection of the Occlusion; Dr. Bernard Zeldow for reviewing Prevention of Disease Transmission; Dr. Frank Everett and Dr. Leo Sreebny, Dental Calculus; Dr. Basil Bibby, Topical Application of Fluorides; Dr.

John Gehrig, Oral and General Surgery Patients; Dr. Oscar Beder, Cleft Lip and Palate Patients; Dr. Robert Deisher, Mentally Retarded Patients; Dr. Louise Wiegenstein, Patients with Circulatory Diseases; and Dr. Ralph Swenson, First Aid.

Special thanks is expressed to Dean Maurice J. Hickey for his encouragement and understanding.

The clear-cut illustrations are chiefly the result of the skill and experience of a talented artist, Miss Virginia Brooks. Her care in interpreting ideas for the preparation of drawings with exacting detail is deeply appreciated. The authors wish to thank Mr. Clifford Freehe, whose mastery of the illustrative medium is displayed in the photographs in this book.

All past and present University of Washington dental hygiene students have helped make this book possible. Their interest and patience in the use of sections of the original syllabus and, more recently the mimeographed edition, have provided a continued stimulus and challenge to modify and improve materials. The authors will feel amply rewarded if *Clinical Practice of the Dental Hygienist* helps dental hygienists better to understand and meet the oral health needs of their patients.

ESTHER M. WILKINS
PATRICIA A. McCULLOUGH

SEATTLE, WASHINGTON

CONTENTS

(9)

10   Contents

PART IV. AUXILIARY PROCEDURES OF THE DENTAL
HYGIENE APPOINTMENT

PART V. PATIENT INSTRUCTION

12   Contents

PART I

Orientation to Clinical Dental Hygiene Practice

Chapter 1

THE PROFESSIONAL DENTAL HYGIENIST

THE dental hygienist is a licensed, professional, oral health educator and clinical operator who, as an auxiliary to the dentist, uses scientific methods of control and prevention of oral disease to aid individuals and groups in attaining and maintaining optimum oral health. The services of the dental hygienist are utilized in programs of public health, school health, industrial health and institutional care, and in private dental practice, research, and teaching in schools of dental hygiene.

The term *dental hygiene care* is used to denote all integrated preventive services administered to the patient by the dental hygienist. This term is parallel to the commonly used term *dental care* which refers to the services performed by the dentist. Clinical services, both dental and dental hygiene, have limited long range probability of success if the patient does not understand the need for cooperation in daily procedures of personal care and diet, and for regular appointments for professional care. Educational and clinical services are, therefore, mutually dependent and inseparable in the total dental hygiene care of the patient.

Dr. Alfred C. Fones who initiated the active use of the dental hygienist and founded the first formal course of professional study, emphasized the important role of education. He wrote:

> "It is primarily to this important work of public education that the dental hygienist is called. She must regard herself as the channel through which dentistry's knowledge of mouth hygiene is to be disseminated. The greatest service she can perform is the persistent education of the public in mouth hygiene and the allied branches of general hygiene."[1]

Dental hygiene has been studied and the scope of practice has developed from Dr. Fones' original concept. Scientific information about the prevention of oral diseases is accumulating steadily. The need for dental hygiene care and oral health instruction is being emphasized. The clinical practice of the dental hygienist integrates specific care and instructional services required by the individual patient.

I. ROLE IN CLINICAL PRACTICE

A. Clinical Services

The clinical services of the dental hygienist provide preventive care for the patient. Data are obtained from the patient's medical history, record of the oral inspection, radiographic survey, and charting of existing conditions in the oral cavity, all of which are prepared by the dental hygienist for approval by the dentist. This information is used by the dental hygienist in planning the dental hygiene care for the patient. The information then becomes a part of the patient's permanent record and is used by the dentist in diagnosis and treatment planning.

Specific services are the oral prophylaxis, primarily for the prevention of periodontal diseases which may be caused by local factors, and the topical application of fluoride solution for the prevention of dental caries.

B. Scope of Practice

The dental hygienist's clinical services are entirely preventive in scope since the treatment of pathological conditions is the legal responsibility of the dentist. The American Dental Association in 1949 reinforced the clinical role of the dental hygienist in the definition of function adopted by the House of Delegates as follows:

"The prime function of the dental hygienist is to assist the members of the dental profession in providing oral health care to the public.

"The intra-oral operations performed by the dental hygienist shall be limited to the natural and restored surfaces of the crowns of the teeth, beginning at the epithelial attachment; in no circumstances shall she attempt to treat pathological involvements of the crowns of the teeth or of the supporting and adjacent tissues."[2]

II. FACTORS INFLUENCING CLINICAL PRACTICE

A. Legal Factors

The law of a state must be studied and respected by the dental hygienist practicing within that state. Although the various laws have basic similarities, there are specific differences which need careful review.

All states are consistent in the provision that a dental hygienist may practice only under the direction and supervision of a licensed dentist. Terminology varies, but each law defines the scaling and polishing of the teeth as an accepted responsibility of the dental hygienist. Not all states permit the dental hygienist to make topical applications of fluoride solution.

B. Ethical Factors

Professional people in the health services are set apart from others by virtue of the dignity, worthiness, and responsibility of their work. Service to mankind is the primary objective of the dental hygienist and is the reason for the existence of the profession.

Others look to the professional person for leadership and expect more than ordinary demonstration of good human relations. Being professional requires interpersonal, professional, interprofessional and community relationships of a high standard.

The American Dental Hygienists' Association has defined the principles of ethics for the professional dental hygienist. Understanding of and loyalty to these principles is essential to the successful practice of dental hygiene.

PRINCIPLES OF ETHICS OF THE AMERICAN DENTAL HYGIENISTS' ASSOCIATION[3]

The maintenance and enrichment of this heritage of professional status place on everyone who practices Dental Hygiene an obligation which should be willingly accepted and willingly fulfilled. This obligation cannot be reduced to a changeless series of urgings and prohibitions for, while the basic obligation is constant, its fulfillment may vary with the changing needs of a society composed of human beings that a profession is dedicated to serve. The spirit and not the letter of the obligation, therefore, must be the guide of conduct for the professional woman. In its essence this obligation has been summarized for all times and for all men in the golden rule which asks only that "whatsoever ye would that men should do to you, do ye even so to them."

The following statements constitute the *Principles of Ethics* of the American Dental Hygienists' Association. The constituent and component societies are urged to adopt additional provisions or interpretations not in conflict with these *Principles of Ethics* which would enable them to serve more faithfully the traditions, customs and desires of these societies.

Section 1.   Basic Deportment

If and when a member of this Association is employed, she shall be associated with a member of the American Dental Association or with a dentist whose practice is in accord with the *Principles of Ethics* of the American Dental Association.

Section 2.   Education Beyond Usual Level

The right of a dental hygienist to professional status rests in the knowledge, skill and experience with which she serves her patients and society. Every dental hygienist has the obligation to keep her knowledge and skill freshened by continuing education throughout her professional life.

Section 3.   Service to the Public

The dental hygienist has a right to win for herself of those things which give her the ability to take her proper place in the community which she serves, but there is no alternative for the professional woman in that she must place first her service to the public.

The dental hygienist's primary duty of serving the public is discharged by giving the highest type of service of which she is capable and by avoiding any conduct which leads to a lowering of esteem of the profession to which she belongs.

Section 4.   Government of a Profession

Every profession receives from society the right to regulate itself, to determine and judge its own members. Such regulation is achieved largely through the influence of the professional societies, and every dental hygienist has the dual obligation of making herself a part of a professional society and of observing its rules of ethics as defined by statute and ordinance in various states, territories and dependencies.

Section 5. Leadership

The dental hygienist has the obligation of providing freely of her skills, knowledge and experience to society in those fields in which her qualifications entitle her to speak with professional competence. The dental hygienist should be active in and available to her community, especially in all efforts leading to the improvement of the dental health of the public.

Section 6. Limited Practice

The dental hygienist has an obligation to protect the health of her patient by not taking upon herself any service or operation which requires the professional competence of a dentist. The dental hygienist has a further obligation to the patient of placing herself under the supervision of a dentist at all times, as prescribed by law.

Section 7. Consultation

The dental hygienist has the obligation of referring for consultation and diagnosis to her supervisor all patients, whose welfare should be safe-guarded or advanced by having recourse to those who have special skills, knowledge and experience.

Section 8. Unjust Criticism

The dental hygienist has the obligation of not referring disparagingly to the services of another dental hygienist or dentist in the presence of a patient. A lack of knowledge of conditions under which the services are afforded may lead to unjust criticism and to a lessening of the patient's confidence in the dental profession.

Section 9. Advertising

Advertising reflects adversely on the dental hygienist who employs it and lowers the public's esteem of the dental hygiene profession. The dental hygienist has the obligation of advancing her reputation for fidelity, judgement and skill solely through her professional service to her patients and to society. The use of advertising, in any form, to solicit patients is inconsistent with this obligation.

Section 10. Cards, Letterheads and Announcements

A dental hygienist may not utilize professional cards, announcement cards, recall notices to patients of record, or letterheads other than as an adjunct to that of her supervisor.

Section 11. Office Door Lettering and Signs

A dental hygienist may properly utilize office door lettering and signs, providing that they are utilized as an adjunct to those of her supervisor.

Section 12. Use of Professional Titles

A dental hygienist may use the title of dental hygienist or letters of R.D.H. in connection with her name on cards, letterheads, office door signs and announcements, but only as an adjunct to those of her supervisor.

Section 13. Directories

A dental hygienist may not permit the listing of her name in other than professional directories.

Section 14. Health Education of the Public

A dental hygienist may properly participate in a program of health education of the public involving such media as the press, radio, television and lecture, provided that such programs are in keeping with the dignity of the profession and the custom of the dental profession of the community.

Section 15. **Judicial Procedure**

Problems involving questions of ethics should be solved at the state level within the broad boundaries established in these *Principles of Ethics* and within the interpretation of the code of ethics of the constituent society. If a satisfactory decision cannot be reached, the question should be referred to the Judicial Committee of the American Dental Hygienists' Association.

C. **Personal Factors**

Each dental hygienist represents the entire profession to the patient whom she serves. Her attitude toward her profession, health, appearance and associates is very apt to be reflected in the subsequent attitude of the patient toward other dental hygienists, and dental and dental hygiene care in general.

Members of health professions need to exemplify the traits which they hold as objectives for others if response and cooperation is to be expected. There are many personal factors of general physical health, oral health, cleanliness, appearance, and mental health to be considered. A few of these are mentioned below.

1. *General physical health*

A routine plan for complete physical examination is important since the maintenance of personal health is a necessity to continued service. Optimum physical health depends primarily upon a well planned diet, a sufficient amount of sleep, and an adequate amount of exercise.

2. *Oral health*

The maintenance of a clean, healthy mouth demonstrates by example that the dental hygienist practices what she teaches. The dental hygienist, particularly one who smokes, must attend to keeping her mouth free from offensive odors since she works in such close proximity to her patients.

3. *General cleanliness and appearance*

A professional appearance includes the spotless, fresh uniform, cap, hose and shoes, moderation in make-up, and no jewelry except the professional pin and plain wedding ring. Hair should be worn in a neat arrangement which prevents it from falling below the collar of the uniform.

From the point of view of avoiding infection for both the operator and the patient, daily care of the hands and the fingernails is required. The nails are trimmed short and the hands protected by lotions to keep them soft and smooth.

The skin should be clear and impressively clean. Frequent baths and hair shampoos prevent bodily odors and aid in maintaining cleanliness.

4. *Mental health*

The mental health of the dental hygienist reflects in all phases of her work, particularly in interpersonal relations. It is her responsibility to inspire confidence through a display of professional and emotional maturity. The degree of emotional maturity is related in part to the satisfaction derived from her work.

Adequate physical health, recreation and participation in professional and community activities contribute to optimum mental health.

III. **OBJECTIVES FOR CLINICAL PRACTICE**

Self-analysis is essential to the attainment of goals of perfection in service to the patient and assistance to the dentist in the total dental and dental hygiene care program. Personal objectives need to be outlined and reviewed frequently in a plan for continued self-improvement. The goal for patients was included in the definition of the dental hygienist at the beginning of this chapter: *to aid individuals and groups in attaining and maintaining optimum oral health.* Other objectives are related to this primary one.

The professional dental hygienist will:
A. Strive toward the highest degree of professional ethics and conduct.
B. Identify continuously and carry out effectively the role in the integrated services of a total dental care program for the individual patient.
C. Apply knowledge and understanding of the basic and clinical sciences in the intelligent recognition of oral conditions and prevention of oral diseases during clinical practice.
D. Apply scientific knowledge and skill to all clinical techniques and instructional procedures.
E. Recognize each patient as an individual and adapt techniques and procedures accordingly.
F. Identify and care for the needs of patients who have unusual general health problems affecting dental hygiene procedures.
G. Demonstrate interpersonal relationships which permit attending the patient with assurance and presenting dental health information effectively.
H. Provide a complete and individualized instructional service for each patient.
I. Practice efficient procedures pertaining to sterilization of instruments, care of equipment, record keeping and general clinical routines.
J. Apply a continuing process of self-evaluation in clinical practice throughout professional life.
   1. Be objective and critical of procedures used in order to perform the ideal service.
   2. Appreciate the need for expanding acquired knowledge and skill in keeping with current advancements.

IV. **FACTORS TO TEACH THE PATIENT**

A. The role of the dental hygienist as an auxiliary in the dental profession.
B. The scope of service of the dental hygienist as defined by state laws.
C. The interrelationship of instructional and clinical services in dental hygiene care.

REFERENCES

1. FONES, A. C.: *Mouth Hygiene*, 4th ed. Philadelphia, Lea & Febiger, 1934, p. 248.
2. American Dental Association, Council on Dental Education: Definition of the Function of Dental Hygiene Education, (adopted July 2, 1949) reported in News of Dentistry, Am. Dent. A. J., *39*, 216, August, 1949.
3. American Dental Hygienists' Association: Principles of Ethics of the American Dental Hygienists' Association, adopted in 1957, Revised 1961.

Chapter 2

INTRODUCTION TO THE DENTAL HYGIENE APPOINTMENT

FREQUENTLY in dental practice the first appointment for the patient is with the dental hygienist. Through her the patient should gain a specific impression of the working relationship in the office, the attitude of the dental personnel toward the patient and his needs, and what is expected of the patient himself in the total care program for his own mouth. This impression is essentially the same for new as well as recall patients. The recall patient needs former impressions renewed or enhanced.

The dental assistant or the secretary usually receives the new patient in the waiting room. Information is obtained for the office records necessary to handling the business aspects of the appointment.

It is important for the dentist to participate in this first appointment. When the new patient is not familiar with the work of a dental hygienist, the dentist should take the responsibility for introducing the services which he is delegating, and proposing the objectives for these services in terms of their relationship to the continued oral care by the dentist, the patient, and the dental hygienist.

The dentist's schedule does not always permit him to meet the patient at the beginning of the appointment with the dental hygienist, and frequently this has to be accomplished at the completion of the appointment. The dentist routinely inspects the patient's mouth at that time. When this procedure is followed, the dental hygienist has more responsibility in helping to orient the new patient, and reestablishing rapport with the recall patient.

The "Dental Hygiene Appointment" is used to accomplish the group of services performed by the dental hygienist. In dental hygiene practice, the oral prophylaxis becomes a part of the total appointment in addition to patient instruction, preparation of radiographs, topical fluoride application, and charting of existing dental conditions. These services may be completed in a single appointment for certain patients, whereas others may require a series of appointments.

I. OBJECTIVES OF THE DENTAL HYGIENE APPOINTMENT

Each part of the appointment has specific objectives which are listed and described in the chapters devoted to the particular technique or service. The dental hygienist's over-all purposes in caring for the patient and assisting the dentist are to:

A. Gain rapport.
  1. Help the patient develop appreciation for the need for continued professional dental and dental hygiene care.

2. Motivate the patient to be receptive to instruction relative to his individual needs.
3. Influence the patient in accepting responsibility for his share in the total care program through routine personal oral care procedures.

B. Prepare the patient's medical history, record of the oral inspection, radiographs, and chart of oral conditions.
1. Plan dental hygiene care.
2. Provide information for the dentist for use in diagnosis and treatment planning.

C. Accomplish the preventive clinical services of the oral prophylaxis and topical application of fluoride solution.

D. Assist the patient in learning adequate methods for obtaining and maintaining optimum oral health.

II. SUGGESTED PROCEDURE FOR THE DENTAL HYGIENE APPOINTMENT

When a recall appointment is arranged, the patient's permanent record must be examined in advance to determine whether premedication is required. For example, if the use of an antibiotic is indicated as for the patient with a history of rheumatic fever or diabetes, arrangements are made to accomplish the premedication in ample time before the dental hygiene appointment. With a patient who has not previously had an appointment, the necessity for premedication may not be revealed until the medical history has been taken. A reappointment may be required for instrumentation and the first appointment used to complete the history and oral inspection records and to make the radiographic survey.

The dental hygienist plans the appointment for the best interests of the patient's oral health in accord with the objectives and customs of the dentist by whom she is employed. A suggested order for procedure follows. Each step will be discussed in the section following.

A. Preparation

1. Preparation of the operating room and instruments.
2. Reception and preparation of the patient.

B. Obtaining Data

1. The patient's personal, medical and dental history.
2. Inspection of the oral cavity.
3. Bite-wing radiographic survey for use during the appointment.

C. Introduction to Patient Instruction

D. The Oral Prophylaxis

1. Scaling procedures.
2. Polishing procedures.

E. Auxiliary Procedures

1. Topical application of fluoride solution.
2. Complete oral radiographic survey.
3. Charting of the existing oral conditions.

F. Patient Instruction Continued and Summarized

  1. Demonstration by the patient.
  2. Summary of points discussed throughout the appointment.
  3. The need for routine recall appointments.

G. Inspection of the Patient by the Dentist

H. Postoperative Procedures for the Patient

I. Planning for the Next Appointment

J. Dismissal of the Patient

K. Postoperative Care of Instruments and Equipment

III. INTERRELATIONSHIP OF THE PARTS OF THE APPOINTMENT

When performing the techniques of the dental hygiene appointment, the dental hygienist needs to formulate her objectives for the patient in terms of the anticipated outcome of the preventive care which she provides.   Definition and eventual realization of these objectives depends upon her ability to interpret to the patient applications of the basic and clinical dental hygiene sciences involved.   The individual dental hygiene care program is presented tactfully, yet firmly, to assure patient understanding and cooperation.

The routine procedures of the appointment need clarification and integration for the patient.   Here is an important learning situation during which the dental hygienist helps the patient to become more than a passive recipient of services.

Courtesy and respect demonstrated by complete attention to the patient are fundamental.   The dental hygienist must recognize each patient as an individual if the patient is, in turn, to respect dental personnel and follow the suggestions which they offer.

The discussion of the parts of the dental hygiene appointment reviewed in this section is introductory to all of the chapters following. This brief overview of the steps attempts to show the patient relationships during the appointment and to explain reasons for the recommended sequence of events.

A. Preparation

  1. *Preparation of the Operating Room and Instruments*
  A neat, clean, shining operating room contributes a great deal to the development of confidence and appreciation on the part of the patient.   Clean sanitized equipment and sterile instruments are prerequisite to the patient's safety.   Dental personnel must never be responsible for the transmission of disease.

  Whenever possible, instruments are not removed from the dental cabinet until after the patient has been seated in the dental chair in order to show the patient that each instrument has been prepared for him.

  2. *Reception and Preparation of the Patient*
  First impressions are important.   A warm, friendly reception sets the pace for the establishment of good rapport.   Observation

of the patient's physical characteristics and general health begins as the patient enters the room.

Immediate attention to the patient's comfort through chair and light adjustment is followed by the routine preparation of the bracket table. Frequent handwashing throughout the appointment demonstrates to the patient the dental hygienist's attempt to maintain hygienically clean surroundings.

B. Obtaining Data

1. *The Medical, Dental and Personal History*

   The manner in which information is obtained varies. The patient may be interviewed in the consultation room or at the dental chair, or may be requested to complete a questionnaire prior to being seated. For the recall patient the previous history is reviewed. Rapport is important if accurate information is to be obtained. The dental hygienist begins to formulate her plan for patient care while the history is being prepared.

2. *The Oral Inspection*

   As the oral inspection is made and recorded, reservation in commenting on observations is important. The patient must never be made to feel alarmed or ashamed of his oral condition.

   Analysis of patient inspection provides the basis for both clinical and instructional techniques. All observations up to this point are used to outline a tentative plan for the patient's dental hygiene care. When more than one appointment is indicated, the reasons should be carefully explained.

3. *Bite-wing Radiographic Survey for use During the Appointment*

   The dental hygienist will use bite-wing radiographs to guide her oral prophylactic techniques as well as for charting of existing restorations and carious lesions. Many dentists prefer that the charting be made from radiographs taken after the oral prophylaxis. All radiographs become part of the patient's permanent record for comparison with future radiographic surveys.

   Radiographs are particularly useful as a visual aid for patient instruction. It is essential that the patient understand the need for radiographs. When the dental hygienist must leave to process the films, the patient should be made comfortable and offered reading material. This may be an opportunity to present a pamphlet which concerns oral health, and may aid in motivating further discussion of the patient's needs.

C. Introduction to Patient Instruction

Instruction should be a continuing process from the beginning of the appointment to the end, and adapted to the individual needs of the patient. When only one appointment is required, it is particularly important that the demonstration of personal oral care procedures be given early to provide an opportunity for review before the patient leaves.

It is frequently advisable to demonstrate toothbrushing and have the patient practice in his mouth before performing the oral prophylaxis. One reason is that the gingival tissue may be sensitive after scaling and polishing if extensive calculus deposits were present.   Another reason is that the patient can see the effects of thorough brushing more clearly before the teeth are polished professionally.

Learning involves a change of behavior. New ideas are presented carefully and slowly with respect for the patient's present knowledge.

"Awareness of the situation" is of primary importance. The patient first needs motivation for learning. The dental hygienist begins by identifying the patient's concept of his own oral health. The patient can be helped to develop new interests in personal oral care as his knowledge and understanding increases.

D. The Oral Prophylaxis

Scaling procedures precede polishing of the teeth. Dental floss is used as the final step. When calculus deposits are heavy and difficult to remove, scaling is continued in more than one appointment rather than subjecting the patient to a single, long, tiring period. Patient instruction and review of personal daily care procedures accompany each appointment, as the patient's cooperation is essential to the success of the oral prophylaxis.

E. Auxiliary Procedures

The oral prophylaxis is completed first because a clean mouth is prerequisite to performing the auxiliary services.

1. *Topical Application of Fluoride Solution*
   This service may be performed routinely for children and young people. A series of applications provides an excellent opportunity to review personal oral care procedures at succeeding appointments. When a single application technique is employed, alternate plans must be made for continuing personal care instruction.

2. *Complete Oral Radiographic Survey*
   Frequently a separate appointment is arranged to make the complete survey. This depends on the length of time reserved for the appointment, the extensiveness of the oral prophylaxis procedures, and the stamina of the patient.

   Universally, a new patient will be required to have a complete survey. The recall patient, on the other hand, will be required to have a complete survey every 2 or 3 years depending on the dentist's plan for routine care, and on the special conditions in a patient's mouth which need regular check-up. At each recall appointment between complete surveys, the bite-wing survey is used for the detection of proximal dental caries and as a guide during the oral prophylaxis.

3. *Charting of the Teeth*
   Essentially this is the continuation of the oral inspection made prior to the oral prophylaxis. The patient's questions concerning the charting are directed to the dentist, since the dental hygienist's role is to provide a diagram of observations, rather than to diagnose their meaning. It is important to explain this to the patient.

F. **Patient Instruction Continued and Summarized**

If the toothbrushing procedure which has been selected for the individual patient has not been demonstrated earlier in the appointment, it is done at this time. The patient participates by practicing the procedure in his mouth, and is guided by suggestions from the dental hygienist. The purposes of toothbrushing, the care of the brush, and all related factors are discussed.

The patient whose principal oral problem is dental caries needs information on the cause and prevention of this disease. When periodontal disease prevention is the main concern, special personal oral care procedures are emphasized.

The patient may not understand the reasons for the frequency of recall dental hygiene appointments. The development of understanding is the responsibility of the dental hygienist.

Instruction is planned to prepare the patient for appointments with the dentist. After the dentist has outlined the treatment plan, the dental hygienist assists in interpreting the plan to the patient. Familiarity with the policies of the dentist is essential. The dental hygienist may be required to describe the various dental operations, combat misconceptions and dispel fears.

G. **Inspection of the Patient by the Dentist**

Procedures for this step vary in different dental practices. Certain dentists prefer to do the inspection for dental caries and dictate their observations to the dental hygienist or assistant for recording. When this procedure is followed, the dentist combines his over-all observation of the completed oral prophylaxis with the specific one for dental caries. In other offices, the dentist checks the completed oral prophylaxis but his inspection for dental caries is reserved for a future appointment.

The participation of the dentist is important to the dental hygienist and she should help the dentist to make this interruption from his other work meaningful to the patient. Having instruments and patient ready contributes much to the efficient routine of the office.

H. **Postoperative Procedures**

Digital massage of the gingiva and the application of a soothing antiseptic as directed by the dentist promotes postoperative comfort. Explanation of the reasons for these procedures results in an appreciative patient.

I. **Planning for the Next Appointment**

The next appointment may be a continuation of the oral prophylaxis since many cases require two or more appointments, or it may be with the dentist for restorative dentistry. Certain patients will not require another appointment until their oral prophylaxis recall. The patient is provided with an appointment card with the date and time of the next appointment specified in ink.

J. **Dismissal of the Patient**

As the patient leaves, he is treated as courteously and warmly as a guest leaving a private home.

PART II

Preliminary Procedures of the Dental Hygiene Appointment

Chapter 3

PREPARATION OF THE OPERATING ROOM AND INSTRUMENTS

THE details for the preparation of the operating room and instruments are divided between duties which must be accomplished immediately following the completion of an appointment and those which are performed just prior to reception of the patient for the next appointment. Instruments are cleaned, sharpened and sterilized at the completion of each appointment in anticipation of the next. Operating room and equipment care is a continuing process.

The cleanliness and neatness of the operating room reflect the character and conscientiousness of the dental personnel. The patient, with his limited knowledge of dental science, may judge the ability of the dental personnel by the appearance of the office.

The significance of the attitude of the patient is appreciated, but the most important consideration is the relationship of cleanliness to the occurrence of microorganisms and the need for performing techniques in a hygienic situation. It is also recognized that when equipment receives adequate care it will operate more efficiently and maintain its attractive appearance longer.

Fastidiousness in housekeeping duties defines efficiency and appreciably increases the value of a dentist's auxiliary. Meticulous attention to the details of general office cleanliness and care of the equipment and instruments is essential.

A schedule for housekeeping needs to be maintained since certain duties must be carried out at the completion of each patient appointment, some once daily, and others weekly or biweekly.

I. OBJECTIVES IN THE CARE OF INSTRUMENTS AND EQUIPMENT

Effective care of instruments and equipment contributes to the following:

A. Prevention or control of the spread of pathogenic microorganisms.
B. An increase in the operating efficiency of the office personnel.

C. An atmosphere of cleanliness and orderliness which will contribute to the patient's mental well-being.

D. An increase in the patient's confidence in the ability of dental personnel.

E. The maintenance of the working efficiency of office equipment and instruments which will prolong their span of usefulness.

F. A decrease in the occurrence of unpleasant odors in the dental office.

II. CARE OF MOTOR-DRIVEN INSTRUMENTS

Because the prophylaxis angle and handpiece contain intricate moving parts, they require regular cleaning and lubrication. They are constantly exposed to dust, polishing agents and friction from movement. The original cost and the cost for maintenance and repairs are high, and it is inconvenient to be without the instruments while repairs are made.

Manufacturers of the instruments enclose instructions for their care. These should always be followed carefully with attention to the directions which refer to a specific product.

Experience will prove that any attempt to disassemble a prophylaxis angle or a handpiece in the effort to "fix" it is futile. Such procedures should be avoided, particularly because it is possible to do more harm than good to the instrument, and the eventual repairs may be more extensive as a result.

A. Care of the Prophylaxis Angle

It cannot be overemphasized that the prophylaxis angle must be cleaned and lubricated soon after each oral prophylaxis. This is important first for the patient's safety as related to the transmission of microorganisms, and second because polishing agents and debris become lodged within the instrument and damage the parts. Since each prophylaxis angle is different from the others available commercially, only a general procedure for care is included here.

1. Manual cleaning
   a. Attach prophylaxis angle to handpiece.
   b. Separate rubber cup attachment and removable gears in accord with manufacturer's specifications, using the wrench or screw driver provided for the specific instrument.
   c. Run forward and backward in cleaning fluid.
   d. Scrub inside of head (opening into main body of angle) with end of pipe cleaner.
   e. Again, run forward and backward in cleaning fluid.
   f. Clean the parts which were separated: use a small soft brush dipped in the cleaning agent.
   g. Wipe off cleaning fluid.
   h. Reassemble for sterilization.
2. Ultrasonic cleaning[1-3]
   a. Disassemble rubber cup attachment and removable gears.
   b. Place in ultrasonic tank solutions in sequence specified by manufacturer's directions.
   c. Time: approximately 1 minute immediately after use; 3 to 5 minutes when postponed.

3. Sterilization
   a. Autoclave or hot oil. Autoclaving procedure is outlined on page 45 and hot oil on page 50.
   b. Use a corrosion-preventive agent to coat the prophylaxis angle prior to autoclaving (see page 46).
4. Lubrication[4]
   a. Lubricate prophylaxis angle after sterilization by autoclave.
   b. Apply sterile oil with sterile swab.
   c. Place a drop of oil under cap (rubber cup attachment).
   d. Fill head with petroleum jelly.
   e. Reassemble parts carefully, allowing gears to mesh so that the shaft turns easily.

B. Care of the Handpiece

1. Cleaning
   a. Remove outer sheath (Figure 1).
   b. Wipe spindle (covering of inner part) with a clean dry cloth.
   c. Ultrasonic cleaning may be used.
2. Sterilization
   a. Autoclave or hot oil (see pages 45 and 50).
   b. Use corrosion preventive agent to coat the handpiece prior to autoclaving (see page 46).
3. Lubrication
   Ordinarily the handpiece should be lubricated each morning as the oil will drip out while it hangs overnight. When the handpiece is laid flat, it may be lubricated at the end of the day. Caution should be used when applying oil as an excessive amount causes increased heat production and unnecessary wear.
   a. Lubricate handpiece after sterilization by autoclave.
   b. Apply sterile oil with sterile swab or pipe cleaner.
   c. Oil chuck opening (at working end of spindle) with pipe cleaner dipped in oil. Insert pipe cleaner into the opening as far as it will go.

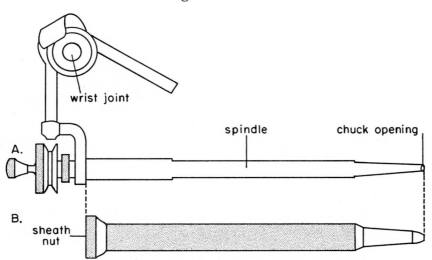

FIGURE 1.—Parts of a dental handpiece. *A.* Handpiece with sheath removed. *B.* Sheath.

> d. Hold handpiece with chuck opening up, and apply 2 drops of oil to tip of spindle. Draw the oil moistened pipe cleaner across the back of the spindle once.
>
> e. Apply a small amount of oil to wrist joint of handpiece attachment with cotton pliers; press ball of joint as oil is applied.
>
> f. Replace sheath slowly to avoid splashing oil.

III. CARE OF MANUAL INSTRUMENTS

A. Handling

During cleaning and sterilization, careless handling of instruments with delicate working ends such as scalers and explorers may lead to fracture of their tips. Bending will distort such instruments as cotton roll holders. Careful handling of glassware such as dappen dishes is necessary to prevent chipping or breakage. Contact of sharp blades or tips with other instruments will dull them.

Consideration must be given the potential for transfer of microorganisms by means of cake soap or the brushes used to scrub instruments. Equipment used for instrument cleaning should be kept apart from handwashing brushes and soap.

B. Postappointment Care

1. Manual cleaning
   a. Dismantle all instruments having detachable parts, for example the mouth mirror and porte polisher.
   b. Scrub with soap and water using stiff brush reserved for this purpose. Particular attention must be paid to scrubbing grooves and joints where debris may collect and harden. Examples of this are the mouth mirror since there are grooves at the attachment of the handle as well as around the mirror rim, and the cotton roll holders with their flexible joints.
   c. Clean saliva ejector
      (1) Wide opening: slide pipe cleaner through tube back and forth; rinse thoroughly with running water.
      (2) Narrow opening
         (a) Clean small metal tip by passing point of broken explorer through each of the small openings.
         (b) Clean curved metal standard by doubling and twisting a fine wire and passing it back and forth through tubes; rinse thoroughly with running water.
   d. Stain or tarnish removal from metal instruments: a paste made of strong ammonia solution and pumice is applied with a cloth. Scrub well with soap and water following application.
3. Ultrasonic cleaning[1-3]
   a. Used instruments may be transferred directly from the tray cover to the ultrasonic cleaning solution.
   b. Time: 1 to 2 minutes according to manufacturer's specifications.
   c. Change solutions and clean ultrasonic unit regularly.
4. Scaler sharpening: prior to sterilization (see pages 34–43).
5. Sterilization: autoclave (see pages 45–47).

IV. CARE OF THE OPERATING ROOM FURNITURE AND EQUIPMENT

Neatness and orderliness accompanied by immaculate cleanliness is all important. An excellent test is to sit in the dental chair occasionally and look around at what the patient sees from that vantage point.

All exterior surfaces of the dental cabinet, unit, including rheostat and light, chair, waste receiver, operating stool and x-ray unit should be thoroughly cleaned once each week, wiped daily and following each appointment as needed. The weekly cleaning includes washing with a mild soap and water (abrasive cleaning agents should be avoided), drying the surfaces and applying furniture polish to protect the finish. Use metal polish on metal parts. Attention should be given to spots on walls near sinks, door knobs and window sills.

A. The Cabinet

1. Cleanliness

The drawers of the cabinet should be washed and relined with fresh paper at least every two weeks. The trays in the drawers may receive the instruments as they are taken from the sterilizer which points to the need for unusual care (pages 56–57).

2. Arrangement

Convenient, consistent arrangement of instruments and supplies in the cabinet promotes efficiency. In general, items which are used together are placed in the same drawer with respect to their requirements for sterilization and disinfection.

3. Appearance

Clutter in the dental operatory decreases efficiency as well as lessens the patient's impression of the quality of service performed. The top of the dental cabinet tends to be a particularly vulnerable place for the collection of many items which rightfully belong elsewhere. The cabinet top is used during the dental hygiene appointment to hold equipment such as the toothbrushing model and patient's permanent record, but should be clear at other times.

B. The Dental Unit

1. Dental motor and arm
   a. Daily care: dust arm, including pulleys.
   b. Weekly care: oil pulley wheels with end of pipe cleaner saturated in oil.
   c. Monthly care: place *one* drop of oil in each oil hole of motor.
2. Engine belt
   a. Wash occasionally with mild soap and water to remove grease and oil. Grease and oil cause loss of traction and attract dust.
   b. Replace belt while still wet after washing.
   c. Adjust tension of belt so that it runs smoothly.
   d. Replace belt when it begins to fray to avoid its breaking during an appointment.

C. **Cuspidor**

1. Purposes of care
   a. Maintain clean, shining appearance.
   b. Prevent odors from debris accumulations in receptacle.
2. Procedure for care
   a. Following each appointment: wipe thoroughly to remove all spots.
   b. Daily: remove receptacle and clean thoroughly. Polish metal parts with appropriate agent. Use special cleaning agent for removal of rust stains from porcelain.
   c. Weekly or biweekly: pour down a strong solution of bicarbonate of soda or disinfectant to dispel odors and clean drain.

D. **Saliva Ejector Attachment**

1. Purpose of care: to maintain maximum function of suction.
2. Procedure for care (at end of day): run water through tubing for several minutes to clear accumulated saliva and debris. Tube may be attached to small outlet used to fill drinking cup.

E. **Waste Receiver**

The waste receiver requires a fresh liner daily. The inside of the waste receiver should be thoroughly washed and a disinfecting rinse applied at least biweekly to dispel possibility of odors.

V. **END OF DAY APPEARANCE OF OPERATORY**

A. All electric switches turned off.
B. X-ray machine wall plug disconnected.
C. Main water switch to unit turned off.
D. Furniture in orderly arrangement.
E. Used towels in laundry receiver.
F. No evidence of previous patients.

REFERENCES

1. CHARBENEAU, G. T.: Use of Ultrasonic Techniques for Cleaning Instruments and Appliances, J. Pros. Dent., *11*, 573, May–June, 1961.
2. SHANER, E. O.: Cleaning of Dental Instruments. Time-saving Considerations, D. Surv., *37*, 1289, October, 1961.
3. SHANER, E. O.: Cleaning Dental Instruments with Ultrasonic Equipment, D. Assistant, *30*, 20, November, 1961.
4. CHARBENEAU, G. T. and PEYTON, F. A.: Evaluation of Lubricants for Dental Handpieces and Contra-angles, J. Dent. Res., *36*, 479, June, 1957.

SUGGESTED READINGS

BARTON, R. E.: Housekeeping Duties in Office, Operatory, and Laboratory, in Peterson, Shailer: *The Dentist and His Assistant.* St. Louis, Mosby, 1961, pp. 141–157.
BRAUER, J. C. and RICHARDSON, R. E.: *The Dental Assistant*, 3rd ed. New York, Blakiston Division, McGraw-Hill, 1964, pp. 376–414, 521–529.
LEVY, I. R.: *A Textbook for Dental Assistants*, 4th ed. Philadelphia, Lea & Febiger, 1955, pp. 61–72.

Chapter 4

INSTRUMENT SHARPENING

SHARP blades and tips are essential for safe, effective instrumentation (see pages 79 and 150). Instruments should be checked after scrubbing, and dulled blades and tips sharpened before sterilization. Adherence to this routine prevents the necessity for stopping work in the middle of an appointment.

SHARPENING STONES

I. TYPES

Sharpening devices for dental instruments may be classified according to their source, abrasiveness, or method of use. Table 1 provides a comparison of the characteristics, use and care of natural and artificial sharpening stones.

II. SOURCE

A. **Natural Abrasive Stones:** quarried from mineral deposits. The hard Arkansas oilstone is preferred for sharpening dental instruments because of its fine abrasive particle size.

B. **Artificial Materials**

1. Manufactured stones: hard, nonmetallic substances impregnated with aluminum oxide, silicon carbide or diamond particles, which are larger or coarser than particles of the Arkansas stone. Example: Ruby stone, a variety of corundum (aluminum oxide), second to diamond in hardness.
2. Steel alloys: metals which are harder than most dental instrument steel, therefore will abrade the surface of the instrument. Example: tungsten carbide steel.

III. ABRASIVENESS

Generally, a smaller particle size results in a slower rate of abrasion and a finer edge on the blade being sharpened. Abrasives and their properties are described on pages 167 to 171.

IV. METHOD OF USE

Dental instruments can be sharpened manually or with motor-driven sharpeners. Manual sharpening is preferred because the rate of abrasion, or reduction of the instrument blade, is slower, less frictional heat is generated, and the operator is better able to control the sharpener and instrument positions.

A. **Manual Sharpening**

1. *Unmounted flat stones:* rectangular stones which may have all surfaces flat with square or rounded edges, or one surface grooved lengthwise to permit adaption of curved instrument blades. The stone is placed flat on a table top and the instrument blade is moved across the abrasive surface.
2. *Unmounted hand (slip) stones:* rectangular square or rounded edge, cylindrical, or tapered stones. The stone is held in the hand and moved across the instrument blade.
3. *Stones or knives mounted on a handle:* thin, rectangular, cylindrical or tapered stones, or carbide steel mounted on a wooden or metallic handle. The sharpener handle is held in the hand and the abrasive portion is moved across the instrument blade.

TABLE 1.—COMPARISON OF NATURAL AND ARTIFICIAL
SHARPENING STONES

	Natural Stones	*Artificial Stones*
EXAMPLE	Arkansas Stone	Ruby Stone
TEXTURE	Hard: fine grit; grinds slowly. Soft: coarser grit; not for sharpening dental instruments because it produces rough edges.	Coarser grit than Arkansas stone. Grinds faster than Arkansas stone.
USES	To complete entire sharpening process for slightly dulled instruments. To complete sharpening process after excessively dulled edge has been recontoured on coarser stone.	To sharpen instruments which have been excessively dulled. To recontour surfaces which have undergone extensive grinding.
CARE Before use	*Unmounted stone:* Spread thin film of machine oil over surface of stone to facilitate movement of instrument over surface and to keep in suspension the metallic particles removed from blade during sharpening. *Mounted stone:* Dip in clean, thin oil to prevent drying out of stone and to reduce heat produced during sharpening.	*Mounted stone:* Dip in clean water to reduce heat produced during sharpening.
After use	*Unmounted stone:* Clean with cloth soaked in gasoline to remove excess oil and metallic particles. *Mounted stone:* Dip in oil or gasoline and wipe away metallic particles. Leave thin film of oil on clean stone prepared for sterilization.	*Mounted stone:* Scrub with brush, soap and water to remove metallic particles and prepare for sterilization.
STERILIZATION	Autoclave or hot oil.	Autoclave or chemical disinfection.
STORAGE	Leave oil film on stone surface, or if stone has absorbed cover film, apply additional sterilized oil. Stone must not be allowed to dry out. Place in protective box to keep clean and to prevent breakage.	Leave stone in autoclave bag; place in clean tray in instrument cabinet or in clean protective box.

B. **Motor-Driven Sharpening**

    1. *Mandrel mounted stones:* cylindrical flat-end or tapered stones available in various diameters. The cylindrical flat-end stone with a diameter of $\frac{3}{8}$ inch is preferred because the side of the cylinder can be adapted to the blade with greater control of the resultant contour.

    2. *Use with handpiece:* The instrument is braced while the rotating stone is brought along the blade. Only very fine abrasive stones should be used because of the rapid rate of abrasion.

    3. *Use with dental lathe:* not recommended because the rate of abrasion is rapid and control of the blade against the sharpening stone is difficult.

SHARPENING EXPLORERS

Working ends of explorers are constructed of thin, relatively nonresilient wire tapered to a fine, sharp point to permit tactile inspection of tooth surfaces. The tip must be sharp to gain access to minute defects in the tooth and tapered so it will flex readily when tooth surface irregularities are encountered.

Explorer tips are subjected to dulling and loss of taper when pressed against a hard surface. Pointed wire tips may be bent if the instruments are dropped accidentally or packed carelessly in the cabinet drawer or sterilizer. Explorer tips are inspected for sharpness and adequate taper prior to use and before sterilization.

I. **TEST FOR SHARPNESS AND TAPER**

    A. Place point of tip on fingernail at 90° angle, and without exerting pressure, attempt to move tip across nail; sharp point will catch, not slide along nail.

    B. Place side of tip on fingernail at 15° angle, and without exerting pressure, draw side of tip along nail; correct taper will transmit vibrations through shank and handle as tip strikes nail irregularities.

II. **SHARPENING PROCEDURE**

A. **Preparation**

    1. Inspect tip under concentrated light; if tip is bent, straighten with small-nosed pliers.

    2. Lubricate surface of unmounted flat Arkansas stone with light oil.

B. **Sharpening and Tapering**

    1. Hold instrument in pen grasp with fulcrum established on stone.

    2. Place side of tip on stone with a 15° angle between wire and stone, and with tip directed toward operator.

    3. Slowly pull tip across stone while rotating handle to reduce circumference of wire evenly.

    4. *Angled or curved-end explorers:* place side of tip on end surface of stone with a 15° angle between inner curvature of wire and

stone.   Slowly draw tip against stone, and rotate handle to taper tip evenly.

5. *Precautions*
   a. Maintain control of tip against stone; use light pressure.
   b. Maintain 15° angle between side of wire and stone to assure even taper.
   c. Never draw the point across stone at a 90° angle because this will mar the stone and dull the point.

SHARPENING SCALERS

Scalers are made of steel alloys, which, although hard, retain sharp edges for relatively short periods of time with normal use.   The actual working part of the scaler is the cutting edge formed by the junction of two surfaces of the blade.   When the cutting edge is pressed against a hard surface, the edge becomes rounded or dulled, and if the edge is drawn along an irregular hard surface, it becomes nicked.   Dulling is directly proportional to the degree of pressure and the number of applications of the edge against a hard surface.

Sharpening is accomplished by reducing both surfaces that converge to form an edge, which decreases the proportionate size of the blade.   If only one surface is reduced until the rounded edge becomes sharp, that dimension, the height or width, is reduced twice as much as the opposite dimension and the blade's original contour is lost.   To recontour the blade, the larger dimension must be reduced until the original contour is regained.   The useful condition of scalers will be prolonged if they are sharpened at the first signs of dullness before extensive grinding becomes necessary.

I. GENERAL PRINCIPLES

A. Preparation of Instruments for Sharpening
1. Scrub scalers with brush, soap and water to remove debris.
2. Remove tarnished spots from blades (see page 28).
3. Dry instruments.

B. Tests for Scaler Sharpness
1. Inspect cutting edge under concentrated light.   Sharp edge is a fine line and will not reflect light.
2. Without pressure, place blade on fingernail at angle for which it was designed to be used on tooth. Sharp edge will catch on nail; dull edge will slide or require pressure to catch nail.

C. Tests for Scaler Contour (Figure 38, page 148).
1. *Curets:* viewed from tip, the blade forms a half moon, the convex curve represents the underside of blade, and edges are equidistant from center of long axis of shank; viewed from top, surface between cutting edges is rounded at the tip of blade.
2. *Sickles:* viewed from tip, the blade forms an isosceles triangle, the short side of which is formed by the surface between the cutting edges, the edges are equidistant from center of long axis of shank, the apex at the junction of the equilateral sides is rounded.

3. *Hoes:* viewed from side, the blade is perpendicular to the shank, the cutting edge at a 45° angle formed by the inner shank surface and angled outer surface of the blade; viewed from end, the cutting edge is perpendicular to shank, with outer angles of edge slightly rounded.

D. **General Sharpening Procedures**

1. Use concentrated illumination on working area: spotlight over laboratory bench or unit light over bracket table.
2. Inspect contours of blade against light background.
3. Use magnifying lens to determine exact linear relationship of surfaces forming the cutting edge with each other and with the shank.
4. Hold instrument with firm grasp: use fulcrums to stabilize instrument and sharpening stone.
5. Stabilize arms and hands.
   a. Rest elbows and/or arms on solid surface such as laboratory bench, bracket table or dental cabinet.
   b. Hold upper arms against body.
   c. When possible, assume seated position which provides opportunity to rest lower limbs and to stabilize arms and hands.
6. Obtain maximum contact of blade against stone at correct angle to maintain original contour of surface next to cutting edge.
7. Grind surfaces forming the cutting edge: pull blade across flat stone toward the cutting edge, or draw hand or mounted stone across blade surface from shank toward tip.
8. Use light pressure; excessive pressure abrades too quickly, works metallic particles into the stone, glazing it, and reduces control of the blade and stone positions.
9. Vary the areas used on stone when sharpening to prevent the formation of grooves.
10. Test edge(s) for sharpness and contour against fingernail; note angle of shank to nail; recontour blade if necessary.
11. Test cutting edge(s) under light for sharpness; no metallic particles should project from sharp edge. Sickles: round the edge formed by junction of lateral surfaces. Hoes: round the outer angles of edge.
12. Scrub scalers thoroughly with brush, soap and warm water to remove oily film and/or metallic particles before sterilization.

II. **MANUAL SHARPENING PROCEDURES**

A. **Sickle Scalers**

1. Method: grind surface between the cutting edges, then lateral surfaces of the blade.
2. Grind surface between the cutting edges (Figure 2).
   a. Firmly grasp instrument.
   b. Rest surface to be ground on side of stone, shank perpendicular to edge of stone.
   c. Maintain maximum contact of blade and fulcrum finger against stone while applying gentle pressure on instrument during strokes.

> *d.* With secure grasp on instrument, draw blade back and forth over one inch of side of stone; blade may be drawn up and down over side of stone to achieve same result.
>
> *e.* Repeat several times: slightly dulled edges need few strokes; very dull edges require more strokes, but not more pressure.

3. Grind lateral surfaces (Figures 3 and 4).

> *a.* Firmly grasp instrument.
>
> *b.* Rest lateral surface on top or side of stone and note angle of

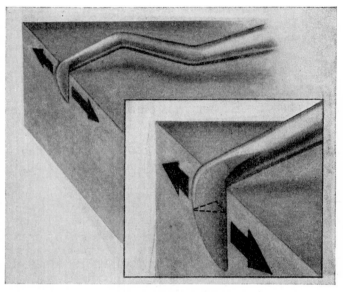

FIGURE 2.—Sickle scaler: Manual grinding of surface between the cutting edges. Surface between cutting edges is held flat against side of stone (see insert) while blade is drawn back and forth or up and down along stone. Shank of instrument must be perpendicular to edge of stone to maintain surface between cutting edges at right angle to shank.

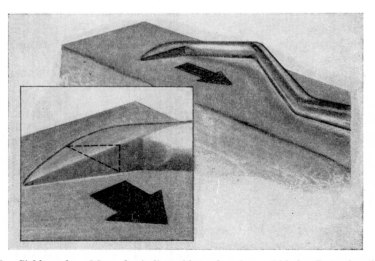

FIGURE 3.—Sickle scaler: Manual grinding of lateral surfaces of blade. Lateral surface is held flat against stone with 20° angle between shank and stone while blade is drawn toward the cutting edge.

lateral surface with shank; obtain and maintain 20° angle between shank and stone; exert gentle pressure.

    c. Pull blade toward cutting edge and maintain maximum contact of blade and fulcrum finger against stone: fulcrum finger moves along stone as blade is pulled across stone.

    d. Repeat several times until sharp edge is obtained.

    e. Grind other lateral surface.

    f. Round the tip and back of sickle by drawing these areas across stone in rolling motion (Figure 5).

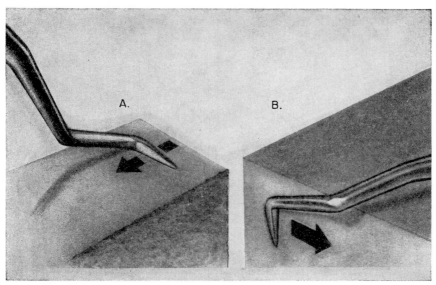

FIGURE 4.—Modified sickle scaler: Manual grinding of lateral surfaces of blade. A. Lateral surface is held flat against top of stone with 20° angle between shank and top of stone while blade is drawn toward the cutting edge. B. Other lateral surface is held flat against side of stone with 20° angle between shank and side of stone while blade is drawn toward the cutting edge.

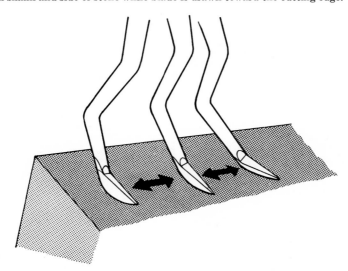

FIGURE 5.—Sickle scaler: Manual rounding of back of blade. Back of blade (where lateral surfaces converge) is drawn back and forth across top of stone until edge produced during sharpening process is rounded.

B. Hoe Scalers

1. Method: grind surface next to shank, then angled outer surface of blade.
2. Grind surface next to shank (Figure 6).
   a. Firmly grasp instrument.
   b. Rest inner shank surface of blade on edge of side of stone; maintain handle close to top of stone with gentle pressure.
   c. With secure grasp on instrument, draw blade back and forth over one-half inch of side of stone; blade may be drawn up over side of stone to achieve same result.
   d. Repeat one or two times: blade contour must not be changed.
3. Grind angled outer surface of blade (Figure 7).
   a. Use firm pen grasp.

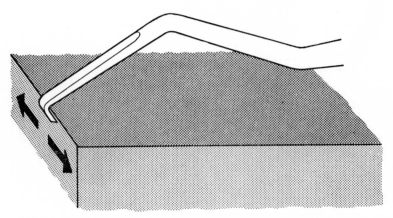

FIGURE 6.—Hoe scaler: Manual grinding of surface next to shank. Surface next to shank is held flat against side of stone while blade is drawn back and forth along stone. Keep shank of instrument perpendicular to edge of stone to maintain correct bevel of blade.

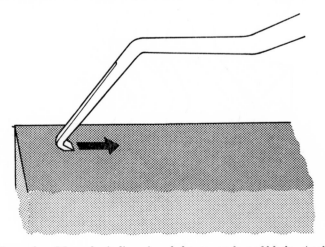

FIGURE 7.—Hoe scaler: Manual grinding of angled outer surface of blade. Angled outer surface of blade is held flat against top of stone with side of shank at 45° angle to stone, and long axis of shank parallel with side of stone.

    b. Rest angled outer surface of blade on top of stone with side of shank at 45° angle to stone, and long axis of shank parallel with side of stone.

    c. Apply gentle pressure and maintain shank position as described in *b,* above.

    d. Maintain maximum contact of blade and fulcrum finger against stone; pull blade toward cutting edge across two-inch-length of stone.

    e. Repeat several times until sharp edge is obtained.

    f. Round angles of cutting edge (Figure 8).

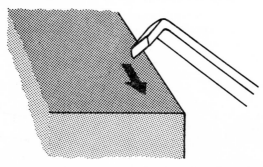

FIGURE 8.—Hoe scaler: Manual rounding of angles of cutting edge. Angle of cutting edge is held against top of stone while blade is gently drawn along stone.

C. Curet Scalers

    1. Method: grind surface between the cutting edges, then lateral surfaces and curved tip of blade.

    2. Grind surface between the cutting edges (Figure 9).

        a. Use firm pen grasp.

        b. Rest shank end of surface to be ground on edge of stone, with shank perpendicular to edge of stone.

        c. Apply gentle pressure; with steady fulcrum rest maintain shank perpendicular to end of stone.

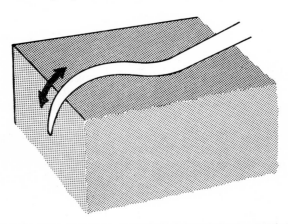

FIGURE 9.—Curet: Manual grinding of surface between the cutting edges. Shank end of surface between the cutting edges is held flat against edge of stone with shank perpendicular to edge of stone. Full length of blade is drawn up and down over edge of stone.

      d. With secure grasp of instrument, push and pull full **length** of blade up and down across edge of stone.

      e. Repeat several times.

  3. Grind lateral surfaces (Figure 10).

      a. Use firm pen grasp.

      b. Rest lateral surface on top of stone; hold surface between cutting edges at slightly less than 90° angle away from stone.

      c. Apply gentle pressure with firm fulcrum rest.

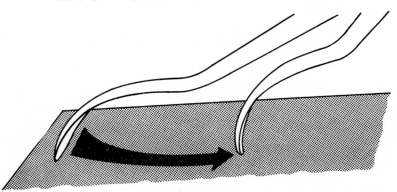

FIGURE 10.—Curet: Manual grinding of lateral surfaces of blade. Lateral surface is placed against stone with length of blade perpendicular to side of stone and surface between cutting edges at less than 90° angle away from stone. As blade is drawn toward cutting edge describing an arc, the tip is pointed in the direction of the stroke and the shank is raised.

      d. Pull blade toward cutting edge with an arcuate motion across 1½ inch length of stone; rotate fulcrum rest to maintain surface between cutting edges at less than 90° angle away from stone. Blade position, beginning of stroke: lateral surface perpendicular to side of stone; during stroke: tip turned in direction of stroke; end of stroke: lateral surface parallel to side of stone.

      e. Repeat several times until sharp edge is obtained.

      f. Grind other lateral surface.

      g. Check to assure original curved contour of tip is maintained.

  4. Grind lateral surfaces: with unmounted, grooved, flat stone.

      a. Use firm pen grasp.

      b. Rest outer lateral surface in groove of suitable contour with shank perpendicular to groove and surface between cutting edges at slightly less than 90° angle away from stone surface.

      c. Apply gentle pressure and pull blade along groove toward cutting edge; maintain surface between cutting edges in position described in *b*, above.

      d. Repeat several times until sharp edge is obtained, then grind other lateral surface.

III. **MOTOR-DRIVEN SHARPENING OF SICKLE AND CURET SCALERS**

Conservative sharpening will prolong the useful life of the delicate scaler blade. A blade that has been reduced to one-half its original dimensions should be discarded, since even moderate pressure applied during use may cause the tip to fracture. Necessary recontouring may be accomplished rapidly with motor-driven stones, but their routine use for sharpening is contraindicated because of the disadvantages listed below.

A. General Principles

1. Use mounted stone of small diameter.
2. Stabilize arms and hands.
   a. Hold upper arms against body.
   b. Stabilize lower arms or wrists against laboratory bench or bracket table.
   c. Stabilize fingers or thumb of one hand against fingers or thumb of other hand as fulcrums.
3. Rotate stone slowly to prevent excessive frictional heat and rapid grinding.

B. Disadvantages of Motor-Driven Sharpening Procedures

1. Blades are reduced rapidly.
2. Frictional heat generated may disturb temper of steel.
3. Hoes cannot be sharpened with motor-driven stones.
4. Uneven cutting edges produced on sickles because cylindrical stone cannot be adapted close to shank on surface between cutting edges.
5. Angle between shank and top surface is altered as stone is stroked across blade and over tip.
6. Blade contour usually altered because stone and instrument are hand-held, thus difficult to stabilize.

C. Sickle Scalers

1. Grind surface between cutting edges.
   a. Place nonrotating stone on surface between cutting edges, with side of stone adjacent and perpendicular to shank (Figure 11A).

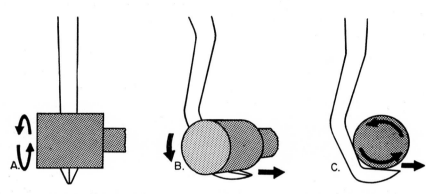

FIGURE 11.—Sickle scaler: Motor-driven grinding of surface between cutting edges. A. Stone is held on surface between cutting edges at right angle to shank to maintain correct bevel of blade. B. Stone is moved from shank end toward and off tip of blade. C. Light, even pressure must be used to maintain flat, straight surface.

    b. Apply very light pressure; maintain steady fulcrum and firm grasp of instruments.

    c. Move rotating stone from shank end toward and off tip of blade; maintain right angle between side of stone and shank (Figures 11 *B* and 11 *C*).

    d. Repeat one or two times: rate of abrasion is rapid.

2. Grind lateral surfaces.

    a. Place nonrotating stone on surface to be ground; note angle between lateral surface and shank (Figure 13 *A*).

    b. Move rotating stone from shank end toward and off tip of blade.

3. Round the back of blade: move rotating stone back and forth over back of blade until sharp edge is dulled.

D. Curets

1. Grind surface between cutting edges.

    a. Place nonrotating stone on surface between cutting edges, with side of stone adjacent and perpendicular to shank (Figure 12 *A*).

    b. Move rotating stone from shank end toward and off tip of blade.

    c. Maintain right angle between side of stone and shank;

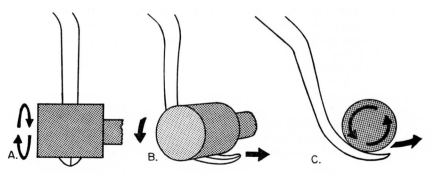

FIGURE 12.—Curet: Motor-driven grinding of surface between cutting edges. *A.* Stone is held on surface between cutting edges at right angle to shank to maintain correct bevel of blade. *B.* Stone is moved from shank end toward and off tip of blade. *C.* Light, even pressure must be used to maintain curved contour of surface from shank to tip.

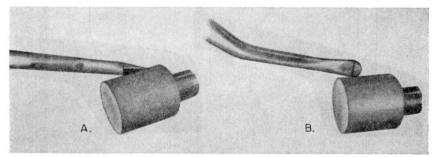

FIGURE 13.—Sickle and curet: Motor-driven grinding of lateral surfaces. Stone is held against lateral surface to maintain original angle of blade. Rotating stone is moved from shank end toward and off tip of blade. *A.* Sickle: back of blade (where lateral surfaces converge) must be rounded after grinding of lateral surfaces. *B.* Curet: care must be taken to maintain original curved contour of tip.

avoid excessive pressure to maintain contour of surface (Figures 12 *B* and 12 *C*).

   2. Grind lateral surfaces.

     a. Place nonrotating stone on surface to be ground, with surface between cutting edges at slightly greater than 90° angle away from side of stone (Figure 13 *B*).

     b. Move rotating stone from shank end toward and off curved end of blade; maintain stone position on lateral surface and follow original curved contour of blade.

TECHNICAL HINTS

I. EXPLORERS

   A. Place explorer tips downward in cabinet instrument tray to avoid pressure on tips when drawer is opened or closed.

   B. Discard ineffective explorers: when tip of sickle explorer has been reduced until it no longer extends past center of long axis of handle; when tip has been sharpened to one-half its original length, has lost its flexibility, or cannot be adapted to tooth surfaces it was designed to explore.

II. SCALERS

   A. If scaler must be sharpened during scaling procedures, clean all debris off blade with hydrogen peroxide or chemical disinfectant before applying blade to stone; clean blade again after sharpening to remove metallic particles.

   B. Round sharp backs of new sickle scaler blades and outer angles of new hoe blades.

   C. Sharpen tungsten-carbide scaler blades with diamond sharpening stone.

   D. Avoid use of boiling water disinfection which will dull sharp edges.

III. STONES

   A. Keep a sterilized mounted sharpening stone on the bracket table for use during extensive scaling procedures.

   B. Resurface glazed stones.

     1. Unmounted flat stones: place emery paper on flat, hard surface and rub stone gently over emery paper.

     2. Mounted stones: place emery paper over soft material, such as foam rubber or thick felt, and gently move rotating stone over emery paper.

SUGGESTED READINGS

Foss, C. L. and Orban, T. R.: Sharpening Periodontal Instruments, J. Periodont., *27*, 135, April, 1956.

Glickman, Irving: *Clinical Periodontology,* 2nd ed. Philadelphia, Saunders, 1958, pp. 619–630.

Graitcer, D. L.: New Sharpening Technic for Cutting Instruments, Dent. Survey, *36*, 1307, October, 1960.

McGehee, W. H. O., True, H. A., and Inskipp, E. F.: *A Textbook of Operative Dentistry,* 4th ed. New York, McGraw-Hill, 1956, pp. 73–76.

Sorrin, Sidney: *The Practice of Periodontia.* New York, McGraw-Hill, Blakiston Div., 1960, pp. 219–221.

Swenson, H. M.: The Sharpening of Prophylactic Instruments, Am. Dent. Hygienists' A. J., *31*, 6, January, 1957.

Chapter 5

PREVENTION OF DISEASE TRANSMISSION
DURING THE APPOINTMENT

TRANSMISSION of disease is an insidious process. When a patient is known to have a condition involving pathogenic microorganisms which can be communicable, special precautions must be taken before instruments and other nondisposable equipment can be used for another patient. The presence of disease-producing organisms is not generally known which defines the need for application of protective, preventive techniques prior to and during *all* patient appointments.

Pathogenic and nonpathogenic or potentially pathogenic microorganisms are present in the oral cavity. The number of nondisease-producing organisms can be minimized by procedures of general cleanliness. Pathogenic organisms of communicable diseases may be transient, and patients may be carriers of certain diseases. Careless procedures of handwashing and inadequate sterilization or handling of instruments permit inadvertent transmission to susceptible patients or to dental personnel. The potentially pathogenic organisms may likewise be transmitted. The intact mucous membrane of the oral cavity is protective against infection to a degree, but when the gingival tissues are manipulated as during an oral prophylaxis, microorganisms are introduced. Trauma from scaling, particularly submarginal, can force organisms into the underlying gingival blood vessels and effect an inoculation.

The marked increase in the incidence of viral hepatitis, and the possible transfer during dental procedures, has brought emphasis on the need for continuous attention to details of sterilization.[1-3] Procedures in dental offices and clinics should be carefully analyzed for each instrument and material used during operation and for the equipment surrounding the patient. Methods used must be specific and carefully executed in a routine manner and therefore must be thoroughly understood by the persons responsible.

I. PROCEDURE

The objective should be to provide the most complete degree of sterile technique possible and practical in order to break any chain of infection. To attain this in the preparation for and procedure during the appointment involves the factors listed below.

A. Proper sterilization and storage of instruments.
B. Adequate sanitization of equipment.
C. Careful handwashing prior to and during the appointment.
D. Utmost care in handling the oral tissues during operation to keep trauma to a minimum.
E. Careful handling of equipment and instruments during operation to prevent transfer of microorganisms to subsequent patients.

II. TERMINOLOGY

Clarification of terms is important to understanding the objective to be attained in the use of the various methods directed at prevention of disease transmission. The action against bacterial spores defines whether or not sterilization has been accomplished since spores are considered to be the most resistant form of bacteria.

- A. **Sterilization:** the process by which all forms of life, including bacterial spores, are destroyed.
- B. **Disinfection:** the process by which most microorganisms, but not ordinarily bacterial spores, are destroyed. Disinfectants are applied to inanimate objects in contrast to antiseptics which are are applied to living tissues.
- C. **Sanitization:** the process by which the number of organisms on inanimate objects are reduced to a safe level. It does not imply freedom from microorganisms and generally refers to a cleaning process.

METHODS OF STERILIZATION

The process of sterilization must provide quick and complete destruction of all microorganisms and bacterial spores, must not damage instruments and other materials, and must be easily and efficiently carried out.

Two agents are capable of producing sterility: moist heat and dry heat. Destruction of microorganisms by heat takes place as a result of inactivation of essential cellular proteins or enzymes. Moist heat causes coagulation of protein whereas with dry heat the action is one of oxidation.

I. MOIST HEAT: STEAM UNDER PRESSURE[4-6]

A. **Use:** for all materials except oils, greases, powders, and solutions affected by heat.

B. Principles for Action

1. Sterilization is achieved by combined action of heat and moisture.
2. Pressure serves as a means of attaining high temperature.
3. Sterilization depends on the penetrating ability of steam.
   - a. Air must be excluded, otherwise steam penetration and heat transfer to the objects being sterilized is prevented.
   - b. Space must be provided between objects being sterilized to insure free access of steam to all parts.
   - c. Materials being sterilized must be thoroughly cleaned since adherent material can provide a barrier to the steam.
   - d. Air discharge occurs in a downward direction: load must be arranged to give steam freedom to pass from top of autoclave chamber toward bottom.

C. Procedures

1. Equipment
   - a. Autoclave: performance is gauged by *temperature*.
   - b. Pressure cooker: limited use for instruments only; no automatic control; articles left wet after sterilization.
2. Preparation of materials
   - a. Cleaning

    (1) Instruments: scrub with stiff brush using soap and water; rinse thoroughly, do not dry; or use ultrasonic cleaner (see page 28).

    (2) Linens: launder.

   b. Protection of metal instruments from corrosion[7-10]

    (1) Immerse cleaned and dried instruments and disassembled handpieces in corrosion-inhibiting solution or oil and water emulsion.

    (2) Drain off excess emulsion.

   c. Wrapping

    (1) Materials are loosely packed and wrapped in small bundles: jointed instruments are opened.

    (2) Muslin, paper or cheesecloth are used since steam cannot penetrate heavy cloth, plastic, cellophane or metal containers; double thickness muslin used when instruments are to be stored.

    (3) Bundle corners are firmly clipped or bundle is tied to prevent contamination during transporting or storage.

    (4) Instruments for direct use: muslin is placed in bottom of tray and instruments are arranged out of contact with each other; muslin covering placed loosely over them.

   d. Packing autoclave with bundles

    (1) Use trays with wire mesh bottoms.

    (2) Separate the articles; pack loosely.

    (3) Place jars or tall vessels on their sides to permit extrusion of air as steam enters.

  3. Time-temperature ratio for operation of autoclave

   An autoclave should be operated according to the manufacturer's specifications and in accord with thorough understanding of the principles and procedures previously listed. Temperature and average time and pressure listed below are accepted for routine use in a dental office. Variations are required under certain circumstances as, for example, when materials are to be wrapped for storage, the time should be increased. Descriptions of the factors requiring variation are recommended for study.[4-6]

   The temperature at 250° F. (121° C.) is considered critical for most materials. Use of higher temperatures which would lower the time required for exposure to steam is destructive to certain materials such as fabrics and rubber goods.

   a. Temperature: 250° F. (121° C.) which is usually attained at 15 to 20 pounds pressure.

   b. Minimum time: 15 to 20 minutes.

   c. Factors affecting time, pressure and temperature.

    (1) Nature or composition of materials.

    (2) Size of items.

    (3) Manner of packaging.

    (4) Packing of sterilizer: size of load.

  4. Cooling process

   a. Dry materials

    (1) Release steam pressure; turn operating valve to produce vacuum for drying; open door.

    (2) Time required for drying: approximately 15 minutes.

      b. Liquids
- (1) Reduce chamber pressure slowly at an even rate over 10 to 12 minutes to prevent boiling, stoppers from blowing out, and escape of solution into chamber.
- (2) When time permits: turn off autoclave and permit cooling to atmospheric pressure before opening door. Check heat sensitivity of solutions and avoid prolonged exposure to high temperatures as indicated.

  5. Care of autoclave
      a. Daily
- (1) Maintain proper level of distilled water.
- (2) Wash trays and interior surfaces of chamber with water and a mild detergent.
- (3) Clean removable plug screen or strainer.

      b. Weekly: flush chamber discharge system with an appropriate cleaning solution such as hot trisodium phosphate.

D. Evaluation

  1. Advantages
      a. All forms of life are destroyed quickly and efficiently, hence it is the most reliable method of sterilization.
      b. Wide variety of materials may be treated because control is possible.
      c. Preserves life of instruments.

  2. Disadvantages
      a. Not suitable for oils, greases or powders.
      b. May cause protein coagulation.
      c. May corrode metal instruments if precautions are not taken.
      d. Tends to reduce sharpness of cutting edges of instruments slightly.
      e. Requires time for preparation of materials.

II. DRY HEAT[10–12]

Dry heat is used primarily when direct contact of the material with moist heat under pressure is impractical or impossible.

A. Use

  1. For all metal and glass instruments and equipment.
  2. For objects and substances which cannot be sterilized by moist heat: oils, waxes, greases and powders when they are heat stabile at required temperatures.
  3. For small metal instruments enclosed in special containers or which might be corroded or rusted by moisture: endodontic instruments, injection needles.
  4. For instruments whose absolute sharpness must be maintained.

B. Principles for Action

  1. Sterilization is achieved by heat.
      a. Heat is conducted from the exterior surface to interior of object or substance.

　　　　b. Time required to heat a quantity of one material to the sterilizing temperature may differ markedly from that required to heat another material.

　　2. Sterilization depends on penetration of heat throughout the material.

　　　　a. Heat penetrates slowly and unevenly.

　　　　b. Long exposure time is required for heat penetration and maintenance at required temperature.

　　　　c. Presence of oil, grease or organic debris insulates or protects microorganisms from the action of dry heat.

　　　　d. Ample air spaces must be left between objects being sterilized to insure access of heat.

　　3. Entire material must be treated for a sufficient length of time at a specified temperature.

C. **Procedures**

　　1. Equipment

　　　　a. Oven or electric roaster which will maintain a temperature of 320° F. (160° C.) for at least 1½ hours may be used.

　　　　b. Commercially manufactured dry heat sterilizer has most effective means for heat distribution and temperature control.

　　2. Preparation of materials

　　　　a. Cleaning: scrub instruments and glassware with soap and water, rinse and dry thoroughly; or use ultrasonic cleaner (see page 28).

　　　　b. Packaging

　　　　　　(1) When practical, quantity should be limited to that required for a single operation.

　　　　　　　　(*a*) Small packages permit greatest area possible to be exposed to direct heating.

　　　　　　　　(*b*) Small packages decrease possibility of contamination when used and therefore prevent need for repeating sterilization.

　　　　　　(2) Use small containers and amounts of solid substances, preferably 1 or 2 ounces, to insure access of heat and lessen sterilizing time.

　　　　c. Packing the sterilizer: allow sufficient space for access of heat to all items.

　　3. Time-temperature ratio for operation of dry heat sterilizer.

　　　　a. Routine: Hold at 320° to 355° F. (160° to 180° C.) for 1 hour, preferably 2 hours. Time does not include the time it takes to bring to this temperature.

　　　　b. Factors affecting time and temperature.

　　　　　　(1) Nature and properties of items or materials: heat stabile substances withstand higher temperatures.

　　　　　　(2) Manner of packaging.

　　　　　　(3) Packing of sterilizer; size of load.

D. **Evaluation**

　　1. Advantages

　　　　a. Only method for sterilizing oils, greases and powders.

　　　　b. Does not harm cutting edges.

c. Does not cause corrosion of metal.
d. Does not erode ground glass surfaces.
2. Disadvantages
   a. Penetrates materials slowly and unevenly.
   b. Long exposure times required for sterilization.
   c. Not useful for fabrics or rubber goods.

METHODS OF DISINFECTION

Disinfection should not be substituted for sterilization but should be considered a supplement to it. For example, chemical disinfectants are used for holding sterilized instruments for short periods of time until needed, at which time they are handled with sterile transfer forceps and dried in a sterile towel.

Physical or chemical means are used for disinfection. The effect produced is one of coagulation, precipitation or other reaction with the protein, particularly the enzymes, of microorganisms.

I. BOILING WATER[13,14]

A. Use

1. For all metal instruments and glassware that can be completely submerged.
2. Not useful for materials which cannot be subjected to water such as fabrics, cotton goods, oils and powders.

B. Principles for Action

1. Disinfection is accomplished by heat.
2. Objects must be completely submerged and water must have access to all parts for a sufficient length of time.
3. Bactericidal effect is increased by the addition of an alkali such as sodium carbonate in 2 per cent solution.

C. Procedure

1. Equipment
   a. Covered pan on hot plate or other means of heat.
   b. Commercially available unit most efficient.
2. Preparation of materials
   a. Cleaning: scrub instruments with stiff brush using soap and water, rinse thoroughly; or use ultrasonic cleaner (see page 28).
   b. Open or disassemble jointed instruments.
   c. Arrange items carefully in unit to protect sharp edges from damage and to permit access of water.
   d. Submerge all parts in water.
3. Time-temperature ratio
   a. Time: a minimum of 10 to 15 minutes should be adequate since it is not expected that bacterial spores will be destroyed. Time must be calculated from the addition of the last item.

   b. Temperature: boiling; varies with altitude: time is increased
      with higher altitudes where boiling temperature is lower.
   c. Increase of heat applied to the water container does not
      raise the temperature: rate of evaporation is increased and
      more violent boiling results.
4. Removal of instruments: remove while still hot and dry immediately with a sterile towel to prevent rusting.
5. Care of equipment
   a. To decrease corrosive action on instruments and formation
      of scaly deposit on sides of unit.
      (1) Use distilled water for filling unit.
      (2) Add alkali such as trisodium phosphate (1 per cent),
         sodium carbonate or borax to the water during boiling.
   b. Cleaning unit
      (1) Daily draining and cleaning is required for units used
         continuously.
      (2) Add a small amount of acetic acid or vinegar and boil for
         10 minutes to loosen scaly deposit; drain and use
         brush with water to clean; rinse thoroughly.

D. Evaluation

1. Advantages
   a. Relatively short time required for disinfection.
   b. Preparation of materials and operation of equipment simple.
2. Disadvantages
   a. Reduces sharpness of cutting instruments.
   b. Tendency for corrosion of instruments if care is not taken.

II. HOT OIL[14–15]

A. Use

1. For metal instruments only.
2. Primarily for jointed or geared instruments, particularly handpieces.

B. Principles for Action

1. Disinfection is achieved by heat.
2. Objects must be completely submerged and hot oil must have
   access to all parts for a sufficient length of time.

C. Procedures

1. Equipment
   a. Commercially available unit.
   b. Oil
      (1) Qualifications[16]
         (*a*) Nonirritating to tissues.
         (*b*) Chemically inert; remains odorless when heated.
         (*c*) Good lubricant.
         (*d*) Clear so immersed instruments can be seen.
         (*e*) Flash point high as possible to reduce chances of
            ignition.

(2) Kinds in current use

    (a) Hydrocarbon oils: effective as lubricants but have low flash point; may break down and produce unpleasant odor on heating.

    (b) Silicone oils: high flash point, do not break down at high temperatures, but are poor lubricants.

2. Preparation of materials

    a. Instruments other than handpieces: scrub with stiff brush using water and soap, dry thoroughly; or use ultrasonic cleaner (see page 28).

    b. Handpieces: for method of cleaning see pages 26–28.

    c. Submerge all parts in oil.

3. Time-temperature ratio

Although hot oil is usually classified as a disinfecting agent, sterilization can be effected with an increase in temperature and time.

    a. 300° F. (150° C.) for 10 minutes or 250° F. (121° C.) for 15 minutes for disinfection.

    b. 300° F. (150° C.) for 1½ hours for sterilization.

4. Removal of instruments

    a. Drain.

    b. Wipe away all oil with sterile towel before use.

    c. Run handpiece or prophylaxis angle in sterile towel to remove oil from inside parts to prevent splashing on patient.

D. Evaluation

1. Advantages

    a. Sharp edges are not dulled.

    b. Provides lubrication at same time as disinfection.

    c. Does not rust or corrode metal.

2. Disadvantages

    a. Long exposure period required.

    b. Oils may produce unpleasant odors.

    c. Cleaning of unit inconvenient and unpleasant.

    d. Dangerous element introduced if oil with low flash point is used.

III. CHEMICAL SOLUTIONS[17–20]

The wide variety of chemical agents which have been tried in the past or are in current use for disinfection are not effective in killing the resistant tubercle bacilli, hepatitis viruses, or bacterial spores. Many of the chemical solutions are only bacteriostatic, a factor which may depend on concentration since some agents are bactericidal at one concentration and bacteriostatic at another. Since chemical solutions do not destroy certain pathogenic microorganisms and spores, it is important to recognize that the solution itself can become contaminated and thus contaminate instruments added to it.[1]

Claims by manufacturers have not always been supported by adequate research. Chemicals to be used should be selected from those recommended by the American Dental Association, Council on Dental Therapeutics.[19] Even then disinfecting solutions should be used only for instruments which cannot be sterilized.

The principles and procedures outlined in this section are important for effective use of chemical disinfectants in general. Before adopting a specific solution for routine use its properties and characteristics should be studied thoroughly and its limitations understood.

A. **Characteristics of an Ideal Solution**[21]

The perfect germicide has not been discovered but ideal characteristics should be kept in mind when analyzing available agents for practical use. The safety of the solution should be the primary consideration.

1. Produces rapid *sterilization* of instruments which have been mechanically cleansed but still carry a few tubercle bacilli, spores or viruses.
2. Retains its activity in the presence of human tissue but does not coagulate it.
3. The quantity of agent remaining on instruments after immersion and drying does not irritate tissues.
4. Does not produce irritating fumes or an unpleasant odor.
5. Does not corrode metal, damage rubber goods or harm other materials.
6. Is economical.

B. **Uses**

1. For disinfection of delicate, expensive instruments which cannot be sterilized by other means because of their sensitivity to heat.
2. For sanitization of operating room furniture and equipment.
3. For use during handwashing as an aid to the removal of microorganisms of the skin.
4. For short-term storage of previously sterilized instruments, including the container for transfer forceps.
5. For disinfection of dental appliances prior to insertion into the mouth.

C. **Principles for Action Related to Procedures**

1. Equipment
   a. Covered pan of material compatible with solution to be used.
   b. Commercially available container fitted with perforated tray for holding and draining instruments.
   c. Concentration of solution: maintained at optimum for disinfection within convenient period of time.
2. Preparation of materials
   a. Scrub thoroughly with stiff brush using soap and water; dismantle instruments with detachable parts and open jointed instruments; or use ultrasonic cleaner.
      (1) To permit direct contact of solution with instrument.
      (2) To eliminate organic matter (blood, debris, oil, grease) which interferes with action of the chemical.
   b. Rinse thoroughly: certain disinfecting chemicals are not compatible with soap.
   c. Dry thoroughly: water left on instruments will dilute the solution and thus lower its effectiveness.
   d. Place in tray and immerse completely: to permit direct contact of solution with all parts.

3. Time-temperature ratio
   a. Temperature: usually applied at room temperature.
   b. Time: varies with chemical being used.
      (1) Minimum of 10 to 20 minutes in accord with manufac-
          turer's specifications.
      (2) Recommended: 20 to 30 minutes for safety.
4. Removal of instruments
   a. Allow to drain briefly.
   b. Remove instruments with sterile forceps and dry carefully
      with a sterile towel.
   c. When solution is known to be irritating to tissue or to be
      distasteful, rinse instruments in sterile water to assure
      removal of all chemical.
5. Care of equipment
   a. Keep container covered.
      (1) To prevent entrance of dust or air-borne microorganisms.
      (2) To prevent evaporation from causing change in dilution.
   b. Place and remove instruments with sterile forceps to prevent
      contamination from hands.
   c. Clean container and change solution frequently.
      (1) To renew disinfecting agent.
      (2) To assure cleanliness and maintain proper concentration.

D. **Types of Chemical Agents for Disinfection**

The value of chemical solutions for disinfection is directly related
to the knowledge of the operator and the care taken in the use of
the agents.   No attempt can be made here to outline the specific
properties of the many types of chemical agents which have been
tested and employed for disinfection.   The major classifications are
listed below with notes concerning the features of each.   A few of
the commercial preparations in current use will be identified with
their group.

1. *Quaternary Ammonium Compounds*
   a. Characteristics
      (1) Surface tension depressants: permit better penetration
          of microorganisms.
      (2) Have mildly detergent action.
      (3) Incompatible with soap.
      (4) Require addition of antirust agent.
      (5) Relatively nonirritating to tissue.
   b. Commercial preparations for dental office disinfection and
      sterile storage of instruments
      (1) Benzalkonium chloride (Zephiran)
      (2) Dynaltone chloride
      (3) Benzethonium chloride (Phemerol)
2. *Organic Mercurials*
   a. Characteristics
      (1) Relatively poor disinfectants; will not kill spores even
          after many hours of exposure.
      (2) Precipitate protein.
      (3) Irritating to tissues; general toxic effects.
   b. Commercial preparation: Nitromersal (metaphen)
      (1) Bacteriostatic only.
      (2) Useful for metals except aluminum.

3. *Phenolic Derivatives*
   a. Characteristics
      (1) Good disinfectants; no effect on spores or viruses.
      (2) Irritating to tissue; react with protoplasm.
      (3) May be injurious to instruments depending on concentration.
   b. Commercial preparations
      (1) Hexachlorophene
          (a) Useful during surgical scrub.
          (b) Retains antibacterial potency in presence of soap.
      (2) Saponated cresol solution
          (a) Antiseptic and detergent.
          (b) Has been used in 3 to 5 per cent solution for instrument disinfection.
      (3) Phenol
          (a) Extremely toxic; highly destructive to tissues.
          (b) Sometimes used in boiling water for disinfection of contaminated instruments from a septic case prior to routine sterilization.
      (4) Lysol: useful as utility disinfectant.
4. *Iodine Solutions*
   a. Characteristics
      (1) Bactericidal.
      (2) Rapid action at low concentrations.
      (3) Produce staining and are caustic to skin and mucous membranes.
   b. Commercial preparations
      (1) Wescodyne: general purpose disinfectant.
      (2) Virac[22,23]
          (a) Composed of iodine with quaternary ammonium base.
          (b) Does not stain; is not caustic.
          (c) Effective use during surgical scrub.
5. *Chlorine Compounds* (hypochlorites)
   a. Characteristics
      (1) Effective disinfectants.
      (2) Will corrode metal instruments and deteriorate rubber goods.
      (3) Destroy tissue; irritating to skin.
      (4) Solutions deteriorate upon aging.
   b. Commercial preparations
      (1) Dakin's Solution: useful for disinfection of toilets and floors.
      (2) Clorox: laundry bleach.
6. *Formaldehyde*
   a. Effective disinfectant.
   b. Produces irritating fumes.
   c. Toxic to tissue: produces dermatitis.
7. *Alcohols*
   a. Characteristics
      (1) Limited disinfecting ability.
      (2) Coagulate protein.
      (3) Volatile: solution concentration changes occur.

      b. Commercial preparations
         (1) Ethyl alcohol: 70 per cent; limited usefulness.
         (2) Isopropyl alcohol: 30 to 50 per cent; more effective and
            less volatile than ethyl alcohol.
  8. *Combination germicides*
      Certain combinations of chemicals have been shown to be more
effective than any one alone. Most of those used contain two or
more of the following: formaldehyde, alcohol, hexachlorophene,
iodine, a quaternary ammonium compound or a phenolic.

PROCEDURES FOR PREVENTION OF DISEASE TRANSMISSION DURING THE APPOINTMENT

After the effort is made to prepare sterilized or disinfected instruments,
equipment and other materials, the procedures of the appointment must be
planned for the prevention of contamination. A strict aseptic technique is
rarely accomplished except in a hospital or institutional situation where
care is given the patient with a recognized communicable disease. The
minimum objective in routine practice should be that instruments applied
to the oral tissues remain uncontaminated by microorganisms from other
patients or dental personnel. In addition, a safe, hygienic environment
should be maintained to minimize transmission of microorganisms.

I. PERSONAL PREPARATION

A. Handwashing[24-27]

    Handwashing properly carried out in accordance with scientific
principles is a safety technique in personal hygiene and patient care.
Hands should be washed before and after care of patients and at
intervals during the appointment as required to prevent direct or
indirect spread of organisms.
  1. *Principles for adequate handwashing*
      a. Use sink with foot pedal for water flow control to avoid con-
         tamination from faucet handles.
      b. Use liquid soap dispenser with foot pedal control to avoid
         contamination from dispenser or bar of soap.
      c. Use cool or lukewarm water: it is less drying to the skin.
      d. Use a germicidal cleansing agent such as a hexachlorophene
         preparation.
      e. Avoid contact with inside of wash basin: it is contaminated.
      f. Wear no jewelry except plain wedding band: microorganisms
         can become lodged in crevices of rings, watches, or watch
         bands.
      g. Maintain clean, smoothly trimmed fingernails with well cared
         for cuticles.
      h. Avoid vigorous use of brush; utilize mechanical motion,
         friction and rinsing to minimize skin irritation.
      i. Use only a clean brush reserved for handwashing.
  2. *Recommended procedure for handwashing*
      It is recommended that at least 3 minutes be used for the first
handwashing of the day and 1 to 2 minutes for subsequent wash-

ings.   Hospital time requirements for the surgical scrub are at least 5 and in some hospitals 10 minutes.

   a. Wet hands and forearms.

   b. Apply germicidal soap and wash well using rotary motion and friction.

    (1) Rub systematically the palmar and dorsal sides of each hand and all four sides of each finger and thumb.

    (2) Interlace fingers and rub back and forth to cleanse the interdigital areas.

    (3) Apply frictional motions to wrists and forearms.

    (4) Add water for additional suds when indicated.

   c. Rinse hands under running water, holding them so water flow is from fingers toward wrists.

   d. Clean under fingernails with an orangewood stick.

   e. Repeat washing and rinsing 3 times.

   f. Dry thoroughly: fingers first, then the rest of the hand, wrists and forearms last.

    (1) Do not reapply towel to hands after drying arms.

    (2) Do not touch towel to unwashed areas.

    (3) Paper towels: use a separate one for each hand and arm.

    (4) Cloth towels: use one end for one hand and the other end for the other or use a separate towel for each.

3. *Adaptations for use of regular sink and bar soap.*

   a. Turn on water faucets at beginning of procedure; leave on during entire washing.

   b. Keep soap in hands until procedure is completed; transfer from one hand to the other as necessary during frictional motions and rinsing.

   c. Follow procedure for handwashing outlined above.

   d. Return soap without touching soap dish.

   e. Turn off faucet with paper towel, not the towel used for drying hands unless it is applied after hands are completely dried and no contact is made with clean hands.

B. Use of Face Mask[28,29]

A suitable form of face mask is recommended for protection of patient and operator particularly when either is known to have a respiratory infection. Although the conventional mask consisting of layers of gauze provides an imperfect barrier against the entrance or escape of respiratory droplets, it is definitely better than no mask at all. The exception to this was shown in one research study where silence, or keeping the mouth closed was found more valuable than wearing a mask.[30]

Not only are gauze masks uncomfortable to wear but they may have a bad psychological effect on child patients. Clear plastic deflector masks are available which cannot be penetrated by droplets and provide comfort since they are made to stand away from the face.

II. STORAGE OF INSTRUMENTS[14,16]

A. Sterilized Instruments

1. Keep in the packages prepared for sterilization.

2. Leave the packages in the autoclave for temporary storage.
3. Place sterile metal instruments in a chemical disinfecting solution until ready to use.
    a. Pay particular attention to prevent contamination of the disinfecting solution.
        (1) Avoid placing nonsterile instruments in the solution.
        (2) Keep solution covered.
    b. Transfer instruments into and from the solution with sterile forceps.
4. Keep sterile items between sterile towels in dust free dental cabinet.
    a. Fold towels over items on all sides.
    b. Remove and resterilize infrequently used items at regular intervals or just prior to use.

B. Disinfected Instruments

1. Place in clean, dust free dental cabinet.
2. Wash and disinfect cabinet trays at frequent intervals.

III. SANITIZATION OF PATIENT SURROUNDINGS

A. General Cleanliness of Furniture and Equipment
(see pages 29–30)

B. Preparation for Patient

1. Method of sanitization: wipe surfaces vigorously with large gauze wipe or towel moistened with appropriate chemical disinfecting solution.
2. Fixtures to be sanitized: all equipment which may be contacted during the appointment including items listed below.
    a. Bracket table top.
    b. Air and water syringes.
    c. Handle and rim of unit light.
    d. Cabinet drawer handles.
    e. Bottles containing materials used during appointment.
    f. Dental chair arms; headrests.
    g. Hand mirror.
    h. X-ray machine cone, timer, handles of tube housing.

C. Preservation of Sanitary Surroundings During Appointment

1. Wash hands before taking clean instruments from cabinet or continuing appointment procedures after touching anything other than equipment which has been sterilized or sanitized.
2. Wipe debris from instruments as soon as they are taken from the patient's mouth to minimize contamination of all instruments and materials on the bracket table: use gauze or cotton and dip in cleansing agent such as 3 per cent hydrogen peroxide.

IV. TECHNIQUES IN HANDLING STERILE SUPPLIES[31]

A. Open sterile packages in such a way that only the outside portion of outer wrapper is touched.

B. Remove contents of sterile package with sterile transfer forceps.
　　1. Keep sterile transfer forceps in container of disinfecting solution.
　　2. Keep ends of forceps sterile during use.
　　　　a. Avoid touching sides and rim of container when removing forceps or returning them.
　　　　b. Handle forceps with ends pointed down to prevent solution on sterile ends from passing over upper unclean portion. When the forceps are again turned down the contaminated solution will run down and make the ends unsuitable for handling sterile articles.
　　　　c. Handle only sterile articles with the forceps.
　　3. Place sterile articles on sterile towel or in sterile container.

REFERENCES

1. American Dental Association, Council on Dental Therapeutics: *Accepted Dental Remedies*, 29th ed. Chicago, American Dental Association, 1964, p. 98.
2. Expert Committee on Hepatitis. World Health Organization, Technical Report Series, No. 62, March, 1953.
3. KNIGHTON, H. T.:　Viral Hepatitis in Relation to Dentistry, Am. Dent. A. J., *63*, 21, July, 1961.
4. REDDISH, G. F.:　*Antiseptics, Disinfectants, Fungicides, and Chemical and Physical Sterilization* 2nd ed.　Philadelphia, Lea & Febiger, 1957, pp. 774–810.
5. PERKINS, J. J.:　*Principles and Methods of Sterilization.*　Springfield, Illinois, Thomas, 1956, pp. 46–146.
6. SYKES, G.:　*Disinfection and Sterilization.*　Princeton, Van Nostrand, 1958, pp. 101–112.
7. NOLTE, W. A. and ARNIM, S. S.:　Sterilization, Lubrication and Rustproofing of Dental Instruments and Handpieces with a Water-oil Emulsion: Laboratory and Clinical Study, Am. Dent. A. J., *50*, 133, February, 1955.
8. CROWLEY, M. C., CHARBENEAU, G. T., and APONTE, A. J.:　Preliminary Investigation of Some Basic Problems of Instrument Sterilization, Am. Dent. A. J., *58*, 45, January, 1959.
9. CHARBENEAU, G. T. and BERRY, G. C.:　A Simple and Effective Autoclave Method of Handpiece and Instrument Sterilization Without Corrosion, Am. Dent. A. J., *59*, 732, October, 1959.
10. REDDISH:　op. cit., pp. 810–828.
11. PERKINS:　op. cit., pp. 160–176.
12. SYKES:　op. cit., pp. 112–114.
13. PERKINS:　op. cit., pp. 196–212.
14. CROWLEY, M. C.:　Obtaining and Maintaining Surgical Cleanliness, *Dental Clinics of North America.*　Philadelphia, Saunders, November, 1957, pp. 835–844.
15. KNIGHTON, H. T.:　Value of Hot Oil as a Means of Disinfecting Instruments, Am. Dent. A. J., *38*, 309, March, 1949.
16. HOLLAND, M. R.:　A Review of Sterilization and Disinfection in Dentistry, Oral Surg., Oral Med., & Oral Path., *8*, 788, August, 1955.
17. REDDISH:　op. cit., pp. 619–646.
18. PERKINS:　op. cit., pp. 213–219.
19. American Dental Association, Council on Dental Therapeutics: op. cit., pp. 97–102.
20. MAURICE, C. G.:　A Critical Survey of the Methods of Instrument Disinfection and Sterilization, Am. Dent. A. J., *55*, 527, October, 1957.
21. REDDISH:　op. cit., pp. 642–643.
22. HARRIS, J. E., ROWELL, P. P., and BEAUDREAU, OLIVE: The Adaptation of Virac, a New Iodophore, to Clinical Use, A.M.A. Arch. Ophthal., *60*, 206, August, 1958.
23. FRISCH, A. W., DAVIES, G. H., and KRIPPAEHNE, William:　Skin Degerming Agents with Special Reference to a New Cationic Iodophore, Surg., Gynec., & Obst., *107*, 442, October, 1958.
24. BENSON, M. E.:　Handwashing—An Important Part of Medical Asepsis, Am. J. Nursing, *57*, 1136, September, 1957.
25. HOFFMAN, HEINER:　Hygiene of the Hands in Dental Practice, Oral Surg., Oral Med., & Oral Path., *11*, 216, February, 1958.
26. THOMA, K. H.:　*Oral Surgery,* 4th ed. St. Louis, Mosby, 1963, pp. 95–96 (Vol. I).

27. ATTERBURY, R. A. and VAZIRANI, S. J.:   Scrubbing for Oral Surgery, D. Surv., *37*, 873, July, 1961.
28. HOFFMAN, HEINER: Air Hygiene in Dental Practice, Oral Surg., Oral Med., & Oral Path., *11*, 1048, September, 1958.
29. DOCKING, A. R. and AMIES, A. P. B.:   The Efficacy of Dental and Surgical Face Masks, Australian J. Dent., *52*, 93, March, 1948.
30. BYRNE, J. J. and OKEKE, N. E.:   Surgical Wound Infections, Am. J. Surg., *94*, 398, September, 1957.
31. PRICE, A. L.:   *The Art, Science and Spirit of Nursing*, 2nd ed.   Philadelphia, Saunders, 1959, pp. 187–189.

SUGGESTED READINGS

Hepatitis

BLACK, S. A.:   Hepatitis—A Menace in the Dental Office, Am. Dent. Hygienists' A. J., *36*, 73, 2nd Quarter, 1962.
ROWLAND, R. T.:   Hepatitis, So. Calif. State Dent. Hygienists' A. J., *5*, 8, January, 1963.

Face Masks

CONDY, K. J.:   Face Masks—Types, Uses and Effectiveness, Dent. Assistant, *30*, 8, September-October, 1961.
ROCKWOOD, C. A. and O'DONOGHUE, D. H.:   The Surgical Mask: Its Development, Usage, and Efficiency, Arch. Surg., *80*, 963, June, 1960.

Sterilization

American Dental Association, Council on Dental Therapeutics: *Accepted Dental Remedies*, 29th ed. Chicago, American Dental Association, 1964, pp. 93–105.
CROWLEY, M. C. and CHARBENEAU, G. T.:   Bacteriological Study of Salivary Contamination of the Dental Contra-angle and Handpiece, Am. Dent. A. J., *55*, 775, December, 1957.
DOBBS, E. C.:   *Pharmacology and Oral Therapeutics*, 12th ed. St. Louis, Mosby, 1961, pp. 420–426, 547–550.
HABERMAN, Sol: Disinfection, Antibiosis, and Sterilization in Modern Dentistry, J. Oral Surg., Anes., & Hosp. D. Serv., *17*, 33, November, 1959.
HUNTER, H. A. and MADLENER, E. M.:   Disinfection of Dental Instruments, Internat. D. J., *11*, 312, September, 1961.
LANNING, B. R., DRABKOWSKI, A. J. and BRITT, E. M.:   Practical Method of Disinfecting Contra-angles, D. Progress, *2*, 274, July, 1962.
MAAS, E. E. and FOSDICK, L. S.:   Methods of Sterilization, in Peterson, Shailer, *Clinical Dental Hygiene*, 2nd ed. St. Louis, Mosby, 1963, pp. 278–301.
MAURICE, C. G. and REMEIKIS, N. A.:   Sterilization of Dental Instruments, D. Progress, *3*, 180, April, 1963.
SCIAKY, I. and SULITZEANU, A.:   Importance of Dental Units in the Mechanical Transfer of Oral Bacteria, J. Dent. Res., *41*, 714, May–June, 1962.

Chapter 6

PATIENT RECEPTION AND POSITIONING AT THE DENTAL CHAIR

The patient's welfare is the most important consideration throughout the appointment. The physical arrangements and interpersonal relations provide the setting for the specific operations to be performed. The patient's presence in the office is an expression of his or his parent's confidence in the dentist and the auxiliary personnel. This confidence is related to the reputation for professional knowledge and skill, the appearance of the office, and the actions of the workers in it.

Preparation for the appointment, then, is directed toward the appearance of the office, the preparation of the instruments and other equipment, and the comfort of the patient. The dental hygienist prepares herself both mentally and physically, if she is to maintain a friendly manner, exhibit self-confidence, and allow the patient to appreciate her sincere concern for his well-being.

I. ARRANGEMENT OF INSTRUMENTS AND EQUIPMENT PRIOR TO PATIENT RECEPTION

A. Instruments

The bracket table, handpiece, air syringe tip and patient's rinsing cup are readied in the presence of the patient whenever possible. When a need for saving time arises and instruments are placed on the bracket table in advance, they should be covered with a clean towel.

B. Positioning of Equipment

The chair is positioned in accord with the general requirements suggested below. For the very large or very small patient, the chair should be repositioned to provide convenience and comfort for both patient and operator.

1. General position of dental chair
   a. Adjacent to cuspidor to allow patient accessibility for rinsing.
   b. Adjacent to unit to allow operator to reach equipment and bracket table conveniently from operating position.
2. Position of equipment for patient reception
   a. Remove from patient's pathway
      (1) Bracket table.
      (2) Motor arm.
      (3) Rheostat.
      (4) Operating stool.
      (5) Operating light.
   b. Lower chair until platform is at lowest level.

II. **RECEPTION OF THE PATIENT**

A. **Introductions**

1. The dental assistant or dentist may introduce the new patient to the dental hygienist, but frequently the dental hygienist introduces herself. She greets the patient by his name and clearly pronounces her own name: "Good morning Mr. Smith. I am Miss Jones, the dental hygienist."
2. Procedure for introducing the patient to others
   a. A lady's name always precedes a gentleman's.
   b. An older person's name precedes the younger person's (when of same sex and when difference in ages is obvious).
   c. In general, the patient's name precedes that of a member of the office personnel.

B. **Procedures**

1. Assist in hanging patient's coat and placing hat if this has not been done previously.
2. Invite patient into the operatory, and precede him to guide the way.
3. Seat patient.
   a. Invite patient to be seated.
   b. Average patient: stand behind chair prepared to adjust it immediately.
   c. Exceptional patient (elderly, infirm, or small child): help into chair by guiding and supporting patient's arm.
   d. Wheel chair patient: remove or lower dental chair arm and assist patient from wheel chair into dental chair.
4. Place female patient's handbag within her view.
5. Care of patient's eyeglasses.
   a. When possible, have patient place glasses in case, and in handbag or pocket.
   b. Never place glasses in line of possible accident.

POSITIONING AT THE DENTAL CHAIR

Proper positioning of the patient in the dental chair will aid both the patient and the operator during the performance of clinical procedures. If the field of operation is readily visible and accessible to the operator, she can perform her services efficiently. Firm support of the patient will help prevent fatigue and restlessness, and allow greater cooperation.

I. **OBJECTIVES**

Correct patient and operator position and observation of the principles of good body mechanics will assist in the achievement of results listed below.

A. Operator has optimum visibility of and accessibility to the patient's oral cavity.
B. Operative procedures can be accomplished in an efficient, accurate and thorough manner.

    C. Operator's physical comfort and health are maintained, and stamina for performance of professional duties is prolonged.

    D. Operator is able to maintain concentration on work at hand over a prolonged period.

    E. Operator and patient are less fatigued, and emotional stability of both is enhanced.

    F. Patient is cooperative during operative procedures.

    G. Patient is responsive to professional counsel.

II. GENERAL PROCEDURES FOR CHAIR POSITIONING

The order of procedures for seating the patient and obtaining proper positioning of the operator and field of operation is listed below. Detailed instructions for these procedures are given under major topics in the sections that follow.

    A. **Seat Patient; Adjust Backrest and Headrests.**

    B. **Incline Chair Backward.**

    C. **Obtain Correct Working Position.**

        1. Operator standing: raise chair until field of operation is at or slightly below operator's elbow level.

        2. Operator sitting: adjust operating stool to correct height.

    D. **Check Backrest and Headrests:** readjust if necessary.

    E. **Check Accessibility to Unit Equipment;** readjust if necessary, then adjust dental light.

III. CHAIR ADJUSTMENT FOR AVERAGE-SIZED PATIENTS
(Figure 14A)

When the dental chair is adjusted as suggested below, the patient will be reasonably comfortable during the appointment. Contoured dental chairs differ from conventional chairs in that contoured seats and backrests are continuous and their positions are controlled as a unit. The entire chair may be adjusted upward or downward, forward or backward within a limited range, and the headrests are adjusted in the same manner as those of the conventional chair.

Dental chairs will accommodate patients within an average range of height, but taller-than-average patients must be placed in a semi-reclining position, with the backrest-seat angulation straightened to avoid undue strain of the lumbar region. All dental chair adjustments can be accomplished with ease if patients are asked to lean forward slightly.

If the patient becomes tired or restless as a result of lack of motion in a reclining position, the operator needs to be understanding and sympathetic. The chair may have to be readjusted or the patient may be placed in an erect position for a few minutes' rest. During the rest period, dental health instruction can be continued to permit efficient use of scheduled time.

    A. **Backrest**

        1. Position

            a. Top of backrest at upper border of patient's scapulæ.

       b. Curvature of backrest against lumbar region (small of back) to provide support.

  2. Effects of incorrect position
       a. Pressure and resultant muscle tension on neck and lumbar region.
       b. Patient becomes restless and slides forward on seat in attempt to relieve tension.

B. Headrest

  1. Position headrests under occipital protuberances, supporting head not more than one-half inch behind normal erect position, with neck straight.
  2. Effects of headrest too far forward (Figure 14*B*)
       a. Operator's visibility of lingual surfaces of maxillary teeth is obscured.
       b. Maxillary teeth block light to mandibular posterior teeth.
       c. Saliva collects around mandibular anterior teeth.
       d. Patient has difficulty opening mouth.
       e. Patient has difficulty swallowing.
       f. Patient's sublingual muscles are tensed, which hinders retraction for instrumentation on lingual surfaces.
  3. Effects of headrest too far back (Figure 14*C*)
       a. Positioning of instruments on mandibular teeth is difficult.
       b. Mandibular anterior teeth block visibility to posterior teeth.
       c. Patient may swallow debris or gag on saliva.
       d. Patient's breathing and swallowing more difficult.
       e. Neck muscles fatigue, causing restlessness.

C. Chair Seat

  1. Incline chair seat backward.
  2. Effects of seat parallel to floor (Figure 14 *B*).
       a. Patient slides forward, which brings head forward and chin downward.
       b. Patient readjusts position after he leans forward to rinse.
  3. Effects of prolonged backward inclination.
       a. Patient's lumbar muscles become fatigued; discomfort and restlessness result.
       b. Upon rising, patient may lose equilibrium momentarily.

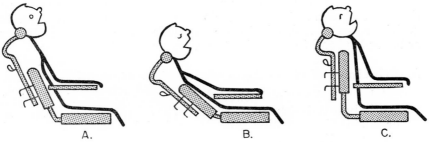

        A.   B.   C.

FIGURE 14.—Chair adjustment for patient comfort. *A.* Correct position, backrest top at upper border of patient's scapulæ, headrest under occipital protuberances supporting weight of patient's head. *B.* Incorrect, headrest too far forward. *C.* Incorrect, headrest too far back and backrest too high. See text for description of difficulties resulting from improper positioning of patient in dental chair.

IV. CHAIR ADJUSTMENT FOR THE VERY SMALL CHILD
(Figure 15)

The normal child has a short attention span and a high energy level, thus operative procedures should be accomplished with maximum efficiency in minimum time. The child must be positioned comfortably yet securely since he could fall from the chair. Either a portable seat attached to the arms of the dental chair, or a large firm cushion can be used to raise the child so his head will reach the headrests. The regular chair seat should be covered if it is used as a footrest by the child. Another simple device used to provide comfortable, firm support for the small child's head is the detachable ring-shaped head cushion, which is placed against the backrest cushion and adjusted to the proper height. When accessory devices are unavailable, the standard dental chair can be adjusted to accommodate the child as suggested below.

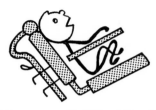

FIGURE 15.—Chair adjustment for very small child. Adjust backrest to lowest position and at right angle to seat pad. Incline chair backward and have child cross legs and place feet on chair seat to prevent child from slipping forward.

A. **Backrest:** Adjust to lowest position and at right angle to seat pad.

B. **Headrest:** Adjust in lowest position adjacent to top of backrest.

C. **Chair:** Incline backward.

D. **Patient Position**
   1. Legs crossed with feet on chair seat when necessary for support.
   2. Buttocks adjacent to backrest.
   3. Head resting on or as close to headrests as possible.

V. WORKING POSITION FOR THE DENTAL HYGIENIST

The principles of good body mechanics should be applied throughout the day to preserve the operator's energy and mental alertness. When positioned comfortably in the dental chair, the patient may turn, raise or lower his head temporarily to accommodate the operator.

A. Principles of Good Body Mechanics: General

The relationship between the operator and the patient essentially remains the same whether the operator works from a seated or a standing position, and the principles listed below apply to either position.
   1. *Back* (vertebral column) vertically positioned to balance torso weight against gravity pull.

2. *Head*
    a. Erect position, balanced directly over vertebral column.
    b. Forward position, relatively balanced with minimum amount of muscle tension.
3. *Shoulders* back, in relaxed position, not slumped.
4. *Upper extremities*
    a. Elbows in toward body.
    b. Wrists straight with forearm.
    c. Hands at or slightly above elbow level.
5. *Abdomen* firm, flat; muscles in good tone.
6. *Pelvic bones* balancing torso weight with lower border of pelvis "tucked in" under torso.

B. **Standing Position** (Figure 16)

1. *Knees* slightly flexed to balance body weight.
2. *Feet* spaced slightly apart with weight evenly distributed and toes pointed outward and forward.

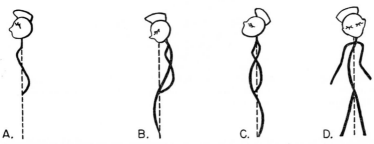

FIGURE 16.—Working position, standing. *A.* Correct: back straight, head balanced over vertebral column, shoulders back and relaxed, abdomen flat, pelvic bones balancing torso weight, knees slightly flexed, feet evenly balancing body weight. *B.* Incorrect: head forward, shoulders slumped; may result in kyphosis (round shoulders). *C.* Incorrect: head and shoulders too far back, pelvic bones forward; may result in lordosis (sway-back). *D.* Incorrect: head tipped to side, shoulders uneven, vertebral column curved; may result in scoliosis (lateral curvature of the spine).

C. **Sitting Position** (Figure 17)

The dental hygienist should operate from a sitting position to avoid fatigue and the development of varicose veins.

1. *Thighs* firmly positioned on chair seat so body weight is on center of seat or stool.
2. *Knees* bent at slightly greater than right angles. DO NOT CROSS KNEES because this prevents adequate circulation in lower limbs.
3. *Lower Legs* vertically positioned from knee to ankle with backs of knees free from contact with chair seat.
4. *Feet* flat on floor, slightly apart with weight evenly distributed.

D. **Position of Operating Stool for Application of Principles of Body Mechanics**

1. Adjust operating stool to correct height.
    a. Position stool seat to level opposite lower border of knee cap.

5

    b. Sit on stool with feet flat on floor, lower legs and thighs
     aligned at right angles, and upper thighs centered on stool
     seat. (Figure 17*A*).
  2. Position operating stool so field of operation is in correct align-
    ment for operator's normal erect sitting position. (Figure 18*A*)
    a. Align center of stool seat opposite patient's upper arm.
    b. Sit close to, but avoid resting against patient.

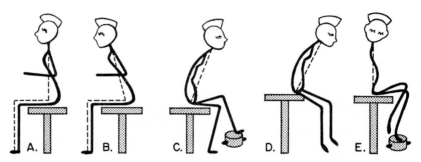

FIGURE 17.—Working position, sitting. *A*. Correct: back straight, head balanced over vertebral column in vertical position, thighs firmly on chair seat, operating stool at knee height from floor, knees positioned at angle slightly greater than 90°, feet flat on floor. *B*. Correct: back straight, head balanced over vertebral column in forward position. *C*. Incorrect: stool too low, head forward, shoulders slumped, one foot resting on rheostat. *D*. Incorrect: stool too high, head forward, shoulders slumped, operator sitting on edge of stool. *E*. Incorrect: stool too high, head tipped to one side, vertebral column curved, torso weight balanced on one thigh, legs crossed, weight of lower limbs supported by foot resting on rheostat.

VI. **POSITION OF CHAIR IN RELATION TO UNIT EQUIPMENT**
  (Figure 18)

  With the patient positioned comfortably in the chair, the operator needs ready access to unit equipment. If the operator must lean or stretch across the patient, he can be asked to rise while the chair is repositioned.

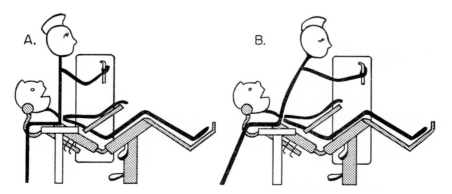

FIGURE 18.—Dental chair and operating stool positions. *A*. Correct: patient positioned in dental chair so operator can reach unit equipment; operating stool approximately opposite patient's upper arm to allow accessibility to field of operation. *B*. Incorrect: dental chair too far from unit equipment, so operator must stretch across or lean against patient.

VII. **POSITION OF FIELD OF OPERATION**
(Figure 19)

A. **Mandibular Field:** occlusal plane at about 15° angle to floor when mouth is open (incisal edges of anterior teeth slightly higher than occlusal surfaces of posteriors).

B. **Maxillary Field:** occlusal plane at 40° angle to floor.

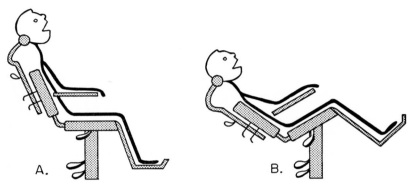

FIGURE 19.—Field of operation position. The field of operation should be approximately at the level of the operator's elbow. *A.* Shows position when operator is standing. *B.* Shows position when operator is sitting.

VIII. **LIGHT ADJUSTMENT**

A. **Position Dental Light:** as close as possible to the field of operation but not in the pathway of bracket table or motor arm.

B. **Adjust Focal Area**

The focal area is rectangular, with the long axis of the rectangle parallel with the patient's lips.

1. Adjust light so top of focal area is just below the patient's nostrils.
2. Avoid directing the primary beam into the patient's eyes.

IX. **ADJUSTMENT OF EQUIPMENT FOR DISMISSAL OF PATIENT**

A. Raise chair and backrest to erect position, then lower chair until platform is at lowest level.
B. Remove bracket table, motor arm, rheostat and operating stool from patient's pathway.
C. Remove patient's bib or towel, then assist him from the chair, since vertigo may result from reclined position.

X. **TECHNICAL HINTS**

A. Avoid postural habits which produce fatigue and reduce efficiency; change position frequently to increase circulation.

B. Exercise lower limbs whenever possible; avoid undue pressure on backs of legs which will decrease circulation.

    1. Place foot flat on floor, then curl toes under several times to relieve muscle tension, increase circulation.

    2. In sitting position, cross one leg over other, point toes and rotate foot downward and around in circular motion several times to relieve muscle tension, increase circulation.

C. Position instruments so they can be reached conveniently during operating procedures: use mobile Mayo stand behind patient or adjustable-height bracket table; place water and air syringes in holders attached to bracket table rim.

D. Engage in controlled activities to maintain physical fitness, to strengthen muscles not used during working procedures, and to enhance mental and emotional outlook.

E. Wear clothing that promotes good body mechanics: uniform that permits comfortable arm movement; shoes that support arches firmly and allow sufficient toe movement.

XI. FACTORS TO TEACH THE PATIENT

A. Patient cooperation assists the operator to achieve adequate visibility and accessibility, which permit thorough, safe and efficient instrumentation with minimum patient discomfort.

B. Operator works from seated position to reduce fatigue and maintain alertness.

SUGGESTED READINGS

Reception of the Patient

BRAUER, J. C. and RICHARDSON, R. E.: *The Dental Assistant*, 3rd ed. New York, Blakiston Division, McGraw-Hill, 1964, pp. 34–57.

Chair Positioning

GLICKMAN, IRVING: *Clinical Periodontology*, 2nd ed. Philadelphia, Saunders, 1958, pp. 573–576.

MCGEHEE, W. H. O., TRUE, H. A., and INSKIPP, E. F.: *A Textbook of Operative Dentistry*, 4th ed. New York, McGraw-Hill, 1956, pp. 83–90.

MORRIS, H. B.: An Operating Stool Can Conserve the Dentist's Health, N. Y. S. Dent. J., *26*, 69, February, 1960.

Body Mechanics

GOLDEN, S. S.: Human Factors Applied to Study of Dentist and Patient in Dental Environment: A Static Appraisal, Am. Dent. A. J., *59*, 17, July, 1959.

GREEN, E. J. and BROWN, M. E.: Body Mechanics Applied to the Practice of Dentistry, Am. Dent. A. J., *67*, 679, November, 1963.

HIATT, W. H. *et al.*: Health and Physical Fitness of Dentists (with Implications), J. Dent. Med., *16*, 211, October, 1961.

HOWORTH, M. B.: Posture in Adolescents and Adults, Am. J. Nursing, *56*, 34, January, 1956.

KILPATRICK, H. C.: *Work Simplification in Dental Practice*. Philadelphia, Saunders, 1964, pp. 484–502.

STOLL, F. A. and McCORMICK, HARRIET: Body Mechanics for Dental Hygienists and Other Means for Preventing Fatigue from Standing, Am. Dent. Hygienists' A. J., *24*, 60, July, 1950.

WEINER, E. M.: The Feet of the Dentist, New York J. Dent., *25*, 65, February, 1955.

WINTERS, M. C.: *Protective Body Mechanics in Daily Life and in Nursing: A Manual for Nurses and Their Co-workers*. Philadelphia, Saunders, 1952, pages 19, 22–24.

Chapter 7

PERSONAL AND MEDICAL HISTORY

FOR safe, scientific dental and dental hygiene care, a meaningful, complete patient history is necessary. Study of the history prior to each appointment guides and directs the services to be performed. Taking the history must be a carefully thought out procedure. Skill is required since tact, ingenuity, and judgment are taxed to the fullest in the attempt to obtain both accurate and complete information from the patient.

The significance of the history cannot be overestimated. Oral conditions reflect the general health of the patient. Dental procedures may complicate existing pathological conditions elsewhere in the body. General health and nutritional status influence tissue healing, a factor of importance to outcomes which may be expected from the care given.

When there is any question about the history as described by the patient or an abnormal condition observed by the dentist or dental hygienist, consultation with the patient's physician is mandatory to gain complete understanding of the case.

Frequently it is necessary to supplement the general patient history with special studies such as a dietary survey. Detailed information about the diet would be shown in a record of foods eaten over a period of a week. This information is particularly useful in the analysis of periodontal conditions and in dental caries control (see pages 345–366).

I. OBJECTIVES FOR OBTAINING THE HISTORY

Each item of a patient history has its own specific uses as suggested in Tables 2 and 3 (pages 73–76). A carefully prepared history guides the appointment planning and procedures and aids the dentist and patient as suggested in the items below.

A. Identifies those patients who require antibiotic or other premedication.

B. Provides information about systemic conditions which may have oral manifestations, and therefore supplements the findings of the oral inspection.

C. Contributes to an awareness of conditions which necessitate precautions, modifications, or adaptations during appointments, including the possible need for emergency care.

D. Permits appraisal of the general health and nutritional status which in turn contribute to the probability of success in patient care and instruction.

E. Gives insight into emotional and psychological factors, attitudes, and prejudices which may affect present appointments as well as the required continuing care.

F. Suggests the time interval needed for recall appointments.

(69)

G. Aids the dentist in making the diagnosis and in obtaining data for treatment planning.

H. Assists the dentist in making necessary referrals to physicians or specialists.

I. Leads to better understanding of the factors which motivate the patient and the patient's appraisal of his own oral health problems.

II. USE OF HISTORY FORMS

The wide variety of forms in current use is an indication of the many applications made during history taking. Although forms are available commercially, many dentists prefer to prepare their own for printing.

Two general methods for obtaining the history are by interview and by questionnaire to be completed by the patient. The form is designed in accord with the method used.

A. Characteristics of an Adequate History Form

The length or the number of items included are not necessarily indications of the value of the form. The extensive and involved form may be equally as practical or impractical as the brief check-list which permits no detailed description. Success in use depends on function and the clear common understanding of the meaning of the recorded information by all who will refer to it.

1. Provides ample space for conveniently noting details of importance which pertain to the particular problems of the individual patient.
2. Provides for ready identification of special needs of the patient when the history is reviewed prior to each appointment in a series or at a recall appointment.
3. Provides ample space to record the patient's own words whenever possible in the interview method or for the patient to write freely on a questionnaire.
4. Provides space for notes concerning patient attitudes and prejudices as stated or displayed during the history taking or other phases of the appointment.
5. Size consistent with the complete patient record forms for filing and ready availability.

B. Types of Forms

The personal contact of the interview method develops rapport between the patient and the operator and more detail can be obtained. However, when a patient completes a questionnaire he may provide information which he might hesitate to say directly to the interviewer.

1. Interview form: list of specific items with adjacent spaces for writing.
   a. Item transposed into question for patient.
   b. Information recorded in the patient's own words when feasible.
2. Interview form: list of general topics only with spaces for recording details.

        a. Master list of specific items to be transposed into questions for the patient.

        b. Information recorded in form of notes to be transferred to permanent record; patient's own words used when feasible.

    3. Questionnaire to be completed by the patient.

        a. Series of questions phrased in terminology readily understandable by all patients; spaces provided for checking or for answers to be written.

        b. Patient is given form, writing board and pen.

        c. Completed history reviewed at the dental chair and discussed with the patient for clarification of answers as necessary.

C. Routines for Taking the History

Two general methods are commonly used. In one, the complete history is taken during the initial appointment. In the second method only a brief history to obtain the most pertinent data is taken at first, which is followed at a succeeding appointment with a complete history. In the second method it is expected that rapport will be greater and the patient more at ease. The history is reviewed at the time of each recall appointment and the information corrected and supplemented.

Notation of date and recording or review of the history should be entered in the patient's record of operations. This is not only important to the completion and review of records, but may be a necessary reference in the event a legal complication arises.

III. GENERAL PROCEDURES FOR THE INTERVIEW

In long-range planning for the patient's health, much more is involved than asking questions and receiving answers. The rapport gained at the time of the interview contributes to the continued cooperation of the patient.

A. Participants: dental hygienist alone with the patient or parent of child patient. The history should never be taken in the waiting room when other patients are present.

B. Setting

    1. Consultation room or office preferred: away from the atmosphere of the operatory where the patient's thoughts would be on the techniques to be performed.

    2. Operatory: may be the only available place where privacy is afforded.

        a. Seat patient comfortably in upright position.

        b. Turn off running water, dental light, and close the door.

        c. Sit on operating stool to be at eye level with the patient.

C. Pointers for the Interview

Interviewing involves communication between individuals. Communication implies the transmission or interchange of facts, attitudes, opinions or thoughts by words, gestures or other means.

Through tactful but direct questioning, communication can be successful and the patient will give such information as he knows. Frequently the patient is unaware of a health problem.

The attitude of the dental hygienist should be of friendly understanding, reassurance and acceptance. Genuine interest and willingness to listen when a patient wishes to describe symptoms or complaints not only aids in establishing the rapport needed, but frequently provides insight into the patient's real attitudes and prejudices. Self-confidence, gentle efficiency and skill promote a feeling of confidence on the part of the patient and help to put him at ease. Familiarity with the items on the history form will permit directing questions informally rather than item for item as a fixed routine.

IV. ITEMS INCLUDED IN THE PATIENT HISTORY

Detail obtained through the history depends on the objectives for patient care. Items included should be directed to obtain information pertinent to dental diagnosis and treatment and dental hygiene care. In addition, recognition of symptoms of systemic conditions not previously diagnosed provides opportunities for timely referral to a physician.

In specialized practices emphasis concerning particular phases of care is required. The age group most frequently served would influence the nature of the items included. The important consideration in any practice or clinic is to select items that provide practical useful data which can be readily applied during patient care.

Tables 2 and 3 include items most frequently used. The listed suggestions and hints for effects on appointment procedures are as the items apply in particular to dental hygiene care.

V. TECHNICAL HINTS

A. For patients with special health problems which require premedication or other adaptation of procedure, print in red ink with a fine pen in $\frac{1}{2}$ to $\frac{3}{4}$ inch letters diagonally across all permanent record pages the identifying word such as DIABETIC, HEPATITIS, CARDIAC, or RHEUMATIC.

B. Analyze the usefulness of items on the patient history form periodically and plan for revision as scientific research reveals new information which must be applied.

VI. FACTORS TO TEACH THE PATIENT

A. The importance of having the personal and medical history prior to performance of dental and dental hygiene techniques.

B. The interrelationship of the medical and dental professions.

C. The relationship between oral health and general physical health.

D. Advantages of cooperation in furnishing information which will help dental personnel to interpret observations accurately and assure the dentist that the correct diagnosis and treatment plan has been made.

TABLE 2.—ITEMS FOR THE PERSONAL HISTORY

Items to be Recorded in Patient History	Considerations	Suggested Effects on Appointment Procedures
1. NAME ADDRESS: residence and business TELEPHONE NUMBERS: residence and business NAME OF PARENT or guardian MARITAL STATUS	Accurate recording necessary for business aspects of dental practice.	Aids in establishment of rapport.
2. SEX	Certain diseases are more common to one sex than the other.	Referral to physician upon observations of disease symptoms.
3. BIRTHDATE	Whether patient is of age or a minor. Certain diseases and oral conditions are more common to specific age groups. Characteristics affecting appearance and healing capacity of oral tissues varies with age.	If a minor, approval of plan for care must be secured from parent or guardian. Instruction emphasis varies with age group.
4. BIRTHPLACE	Presence of fluoride in water supply. Food habits. Certain diseases are more common to certain areas.	Recognition of dental fluorosis if excess fluoride. Instruction on diet adapted to cultural patterns.
5. RACE	Certain diseases are more common to one race than another. Cultural influences on food selection and dietary.	Instruction on diet adapted to cultural patterns.
6. OCCUPATION: Present and former	May be a factor in the etiology of certain diseases and dental stains. May affect diet or oral habits (biting objects).	Adapt techniques for removal of extrinsic stains. Patient instruction applied.
7. PREVIOUS DENTAL CARE AND NAME OF DENTIST	Extent and frequency of required dental needs. Determine patient's interest in oral health.	Patient instruction applied to needs.
8. REFERRED BY AND ADDRESS	Identification of person to whom to send referral thank you letter.	
9. REQUEST OR CHIEF COMPLAINT	If patient has pain.	The chief complaint should be relieved first.
10. LAST PHYSICAL EXAMINATION	Validity of medical history.	When reason to question validity, verify with physician before proceeding with dental hygiene care.
11. NAME, ADDRESS AND TELEPHONE NUMBER OF PHYSICIAN	For consultation.	Consultation with physician required (1) For condition requiring premedication. (2) When disease symptoms are suspected but patient does not state. (3) In an emergency.

TABLE 3.—ITEMS FOR THE MEDICAL HISTORY

Items to be Recorded in Patient History	Considerations	Suggested Effects on Appointment Procedures
1. GENERAL HEALTH AND APPEARANCE	Patient's appraisal of his own health.	Response, cooperation and attitude expected.
2. RECENT ILLNESSES	Nature of disease. Length of convalescence.	
3. PRESENTLY UNDER TREATMENT OF PHYSICIAN	Nature of illness. Type and duration of treatment.	Relate to other items in history.
4. PRESCRIBED MEDICATION: past and present	Nature and purpose. Possible effect on oral tissues.	Instruction such as dietary recommendations may be limited.
5. X-RAY TREATMENT: past and present	Frequency.	Limitation of exposures to dental x-ray.
6. SELF-MEDICATION HABITS	Type. Frequency. Attitude toward professional care.	Response to instruction.
7. MOUTH HABITS	Bruxism. Clenching teeth. Biting foreign objects or lips, cheeks, tongue.	Possible need for periodontal care. Instruction concerning habits.
8. SMOKING HABITS	Frequency. Effects on teeth and oral mucosa.	Stain removal from teeth; instruction in personal care.
9. DAILY DIETARY	Special recommendations of physician: past and present. Vitamin supplements. Appetite. Regularity of meals. Food likes and dislikes. Use of alcohol.	Instruction in diet for oral health. Prognosis for success of dental hygiene techniques.
10. HEIGHT AND WEIGHT	Obesity or possible malnutrition.	Instruction emphasis placed on diet.
11. EYES	Purpose for correction by eyeglasses. Abnormal appearance may be symptomatic of some diseases.	Remove glasses and place in a safe place during appointment. Necessary adaptations in techniques and instruction for blind or partially blind.
12. EARS	Deafness or degree of deafness.	Necessary adaptation in methods of instruction.
13. NASAL SINUSES, TONSILS AND ADENOIDS	Mouth breathing as possible cause of gingivitis and malocclusion.	Patient instruction emphasis placed on personal oral care. Breathing difficulties or initiation of gagging may hinder techniques.
14. CARDIAC	Determine the extent of heart damage through consultation with physician.	May require premedication to prevent infection. Shorten length of appointment to prevent fatigue. Be prepared to administer emergency care (see Table 15, page 471).

TABLE 3. (Continued)

Items to be Recorded in Patient History	Considerations	Suggested Effects on Appointment Procedures
15. RHEUMATIC FEVER	Determine heart damage through consultation with physician.	See "Cardiac" above.
16. HYPERTENSION	High, normal, or low.	When high, shorten length of appointment.
17. BLOOD DISEASES	Determine severity through consultation with physician. Possible oral manifestations.	Frequent recall appointments to prevent heavy deposit accumulation thus lessening trauma to the gingival tissue (see pages 433–435).
18. BLEEDING TENDENCY	Determine severity through consultation with physician.	If prolonged bleeding, premedication may be necessary. Short appointments required. Involve only quadrant or half of teeth and gingiva at a time. Refer hemophiliac to dentist before proceeding.
19. DIABETES	Determine severity through consultation with physician.	Avoid trauma to tissues. Expect prolonged healing time. Need frequent recall. Be prepared to administer emergency care for diabetic coma or insulin shock (see pages 442–443).
20. RESPIRATORY	Rate and ease of respiration. Persistent cough.	Short appointment required. Wear face mask if condition may be communicable.
21. GASTROINTESTINAL	Determine if patient is restricted to a specific diet prescribed by physician.	Patient instruction in accord with prescribed diet and medication.
22. COMMUNICABLE DISEASES	Stage of disease; expected communicability.	If epidemic as in common cold or virus infections, patient may be asked to reappoint at termination of disease. Wear face mask.
22A. INFECTIOUS OR SERUM HEPATITIS	Date of termination of disease. Possibility of patient being a carrier.	Personal attention to all minor breaks in skin of hands of operator. Exceptional care in sterilization of instruments.
22B. TUBERCULOSIS	Determine whether case is active or passive through consultation with physician.	Passive: use supplementary sterilization measures. Active: techniques performed only under hospital procedures.
23. EPILEPSY	Determine frequency of epileptic seizures. Determine medications being prescribed through consultation with physician.	If gingival hyperplasia is present, adapt oral prophylactic techniques (see page 401). Dentist may wish to refer patient to periodontist. Administer first aid procedures if seizure occurs.
24. ALLERGIES	Determine substances to which patient is allergic.	Avoid using drugs to which patient is allergic.

TABLE 3. (Continued)

Items to be Recorded in Patient History	Considerations	Suggested Effects on Appointment Procedures
25. PHYSICAL DISABILITIES	Extent of disability. Record nature of condition: Cerebral palsy. Multiple sclerosis. Arthritis. Poliomyelitis. Other.	Adjust physical arrangements for convenience of patient. Adapt techniques and instruction (see pages 407–419)
26. ENDOCRINE INVOLVEMENTS	Possible oral manifestations. Record nature: Puberty. Menopause. Thyroid or other.	Adapt techniques and instruction (see pages 449–456).
27. PREGNANCY	Month, parturition date. Possible oral manifestations. Patient discomfort.	Adjust physical arrangements for convenience of patient. Adapt instruction and techniques (see pages 458–465). Need for change in recall plan.
28. OTHER	Record: Mental retardation. Psychiatric conditions. Psychological aspects. Emotional problems expressed by patient. Factors of importance not previously covered.	For mental retardation see pages 388–397.

SUGGESTED READINGS

Patient History

American Dental Association, Council on Dental Therapeutics: *Accepted Dental Remedies*, 29th ed. Chicago, American Dental Association, 1964, pp. 1–8.

ASH, M. M., HARD, DOROTHY, and TONDROWSKI, VICTORIA: Role of the Hygienist in the Detection of Disease, Am. Dent. A. J., *59*, 546, September, 1959.

BRAUER, J. C. and RICHARDSON, R. E.: *The Dental Assistant*, 3rd. ed. New York, Blakiston Division, McGraw-Hill, 1964, pp. 312–215.

BURKET, L. W.: *Oral Medicine*, 4th ed. Philadelphia, Lippincott, 1961, pp. 8–13.

CHERASKIN, E.: The Oral Diagnostic Procedure, in Finn, S. B.: *Clinical Pedodontics*, 2nd ed. Philadelphia, Saunders, 1962, pp. 87–89.

GORDON, S. G. and HALPERN, I. L.: Medical Aspects of Dental Patient History, Oral Surg., Oral Med. & Oral Path., *15*, 1270, October, 1962.

GRANT, DANIEL, STERN, I. B., and EVERETT, F. G.: *Orban's Periodontics*, 2nd ed. St. Louis, Mosby, 1963, pp. 224–231.

KERR, D. A., ASH, M. M., and MILLARD, H. D.: *Oral Diagnosis*. St. Louis, Mosby, 1959, pp. 64–102.

Management of Dental Problems in Patients with Cardiovascular Disease, Report of a Working Conference Jointly Sponsored by the American Dental Association and American Heart Association, Am. Dent. A. J., *68*, 333, March, 1964.

MILLER, S. C.: *Oral Diagnosis and Treatment*, 3rd ed. New York, Blakiston Division, McGraw-Hill, 1957, pp. 10–16.

THOMA, KURT and ROBINSON, H. B. G.: *Oral and Dental Diagnosis*, 5th ed. Philadelphia, Saunders, 1960, pp. 9–20.

Interviewing

FENLASON, A. F.: *Essentials in Interviewing*. New York, Harper, 1952.

GARRETT, ANNETTE: *Interviewing, Its Principles and Methods*. New York, Family Service Association of America, 1942. 123 pp.

KAHN, R. L. and CANNELL, C. F.: *Dynamics of Interviewing*. New York, John Wiley, 1963. 368 pp.

Chapter 8

THE ORAL INSPECTION

INSPECTION of the oral cavity follows the recording of the patient history. Procedures for the appointment and succeeding care depend on the needs of the patient as evidenced by the history and the oral conditions observed.

Information is obtained by three general methods of inspection: visual, tactile through the use of instruments, and radiographic. Inspection lends itself to a visual means of instruction which contributes to the patient's understanding and to the success of the services performed. When the patient is acquainted with the general objectives and reasons behind the plan of procedure, he is more cooperative and appreciative.

The oral tissues are sensitive indicators of the general health of the individual. Changes in these structures are frequently the first indication of subclinical disease process in other parts of the body. The dental hygienist is not qualified to diagnose, but it is her responsibility to observe, record and call to the attention of the dentist deviations from the normal appearance of the oral cavity. The prerequisites in accomplishing this are knowledge and understanding of the normal morphology and function (anatomy and physiology) of the body which can be applied to the intelligent recognition of oral conditions.

A thorough oral inspection has application in the total care program for the patient as suggested below.

1. Gives understanding of the oral health problems of the patient in order to define the techniques to be performed and the instruction needed.

2. Serves as a visual instructional device when showing the patient the clinical findings in order to promote greater interest and cooperation.

3. Provides a means of comparison of individual oral inspections over a series of routine recall appointments and thus to determine the effects of dental hygiene care and the success of patient instruction.

4. Contributes to the prevention of oral disease by early recognition of deviations from normal tissues and calling such deviations to the attention of the dentist.

5. Provides information for continuing records of the patient's oral diagnosis and treatment planning by the dentist.

INSTRUMENTS

The mouth mirror, explorers, and periodontal probe are used with the assistance of a source of air under pressure for the tactile and visual inspection. These instruments are used continuously throughout the oral prophylaxis to guide procedures and evaluate the completion of the case. The dexterous and efficient use of inspection instruments markedly influences the accuracy of operation and minimization of time spent for the total appointment.

I. THE MOUTH MIRROR

A. Purposes and Uses

1. To provide indirect vision.
2. To provide indirect illumination.
3. To retract cheek, lip, tongue.

B. Description

1. Surfaces
    a. Plane (flat).
    b. Magnifying (concave).
    c. Front Surface (reflecting surface is on front of the lens rather than back as with the plane or magnifying mirror. The front surface eliminates "ghost" images.)
2. Diameters: vary from $\frac{5}{8}$ to $1\frac{1}{4}$ inches.
3. Attachments: threaded plain stem or cone socket to be joined to handle of chosen length and diameter.

C. Technique for Use

1. Use pen grasp with fulcrum on tooth surfaces (see page 141).
2. Retraction
    a. Use petroleum jelly or other lubricant on dry or cracked lips and corners of mouth.
    b. Adjust fingers holding the mirror so that the angles of the mouth are protected from undue pressure of shank of mirror handle.
    c. Insert mirror and remove carefully to avoid hitting the teeth since this can be very disturbing to the patient.
3. Maintain clear vision
    a. Warm mirror with water, rub along buccal mucosa to coat mirror with thin transparent film of saliva, and request patient to breathe through his nose, to prevent condensation of moisture on mirror.
    b. Discard scratched mirrors.

D. Care of Mirrors

1. Dismantle mirror and handle for sterilization.
2. Examine carefully after scrubbing with brush prior to sterilization to assure removal of debris around back, shank and rim of reflecting surface.
3. Handle carefully during sterilization procedures to prevent other instruments from scratching reflecting surface.
4. Consult manufacturer's specifications for sterilizing or disinfecting procedures which may cloud mirror, particularly the front surface type.

II. EXPLORERS

A. Uses

1. To detect, by tactile sense, irregularities of the tooth surfaces.

2. To direct scaling procedures through identification of calculus, cemento-enamel junction, and other irregularities of tooth surface which may complicate or delay efficient techniques.
3. To distinguish carious lesions for charting of the teeth.

B. Description

1. Shapes: a wide variety of shapes are available including sickle, right angle, pigtail, tapered, and contra-angled wire end.
2. Single or paired
    a. Single: adaptable to all tooth surfaces; universal.
    b. Paired: working ends or shanks curved to facilitate accessibility to all tooth surfaces; one is mirror image of the other.

C. Technique for Use

1. Use pen grasp with fulcrum on nonmobile tooth (see page 141).
2. Maintain sharp tip of explorer on tooth surface to protect gingival tissue.
3. Vary angle of working end to tooth structure.
    a. Use right angle when exploring occlusal pits for dental caries.
    b. Use acute angle (5° to 20°) when exploring near or under gingival margin.
4. Apply light grasp to permit tactile sense to be a guide.

D. Care of Explorers

1. Sharpen and retaper dull explorer tip (see page 33).
2. With explorer tip sharp and tapered, the following may be expected:
    a. Increased tactile sensitivity with less pressure required.
    b. Prevention of unnecessary trauma to the gingival tissues.
    c. Decreased operating time.
    d. Increased patient comfort.
3. Handle explorers carefully: avoid accidental dropping or pressure against tip when sterilizing or storing instruments.

III. PERIODONTAL PROBE[1,2]

A. Purposes and Uses

The dentist, particularly the periodontist, uses the probe as an aid to diagnosis and treatment planning. The dental hygienist may assist the dentist in the specific measurement and charting of periodontal pockets (see pages 260–262).

In the dental hygiene appointment, the probe is an indispensable aid to planning and carrying out the procedures for patient care and instruction. Effective use of the probe aids in the following:

1. Distinguishing dental hygiene cases from those requiring periodontal treatment.
2. Identification of the location, shape and depth of the gingival sulci for definition of scaling procedures.
3. Selection of appropriate scalers.
4. Planning length and number of appointments required to perform the complete oral prophylaxis.

5. Outlining and presenting instruction in personal care procedures.
6. With observations noted in the patient's permanent record, opportunity for continuing study of the patient's gingival health is provided.

B. Description

1. Shape: tapered, rod-like blade with a blunt and rounded tip.
2. Blade: marked in millimeters; projects from shank at an obtuse angle to permit access to all tooth surfaces.

C. Technique for Use

1. Use pen grasp with fulcrum on nonmobile tooth (see page 141).
2. Insert blade along tooth surface and into pocket with a firm but gentle pressure until tissue resistance indicates depth of sulcus (Figure 20).
3. Apply blade in line with long axis of tooth for accuracy.
4. Identify depth of pocket by millimeter marks on the blade.
5. Proceed in uniform manner around each tooth and from tooth to tooth.
6. Record findings on appropriate chart designed to show areas being inspected.

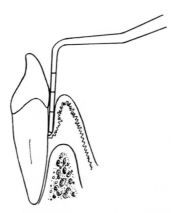

FIGURE 20.—Periodontal probe in position for measuring depth of gingival sulcus or periodontal pocket. The probe is inserted until tissue resistance is felt at the bottom of the sulcus or pocket. The blade must be held parallel to the long axis of the tooth for accurate measurement. (Modified from Miller, *Textbook of Periodontia*, Blakiston Division, McGraw-Hill Book Co.)

IV. INSTRUMENTS FOR APPLICATION OF AIR

A. Purposes

With appropriate, timely application of air to clear saliva and debris and/or dry the tooth surfaces, the following can be accomplished:

1. A thorough, more accurate inspection of the teeth and gingival tissues.
2. Visibility of the field of operation which facilitates positive scaling techniques and minimizes the time required for scaling.

3. Dry dental calculus can be observed more readily on the tooth surface.
4. Tooth surfaces are dried for the application of solutions: disclosing solution page 192; topical fluoride solution page 204.

B. **Compressed Air Syringe**

1. Description
    a. Air source: tank of compressed air with tubing attachment to syringe.
    b. Air tip: with contra-angled working end adjustable for maxillary and mandibular fields of operation.
2. Technique for use
    a. Use palm grasp around handle of syringe; thumb depresses release button on handle.
    b. Make controlled, short, gentle applications of air.
        (1) Teeth, particularly cervical areas, may be sensitive to air.
        (2) Forceful application may direct saliva and debris out of the oral cavity or into the throat region which may cause the patient to cough.
        (3) Avoid startling the patient by forewarning him that air is to be applied.
3. Care
    a. Clean inside of air tip with pipe cleaner prior to sterilization.
    b. Sanitize syringe by careful wiping with gauze wipe moistened in disinfecting solution.

C. **Manual Chip Blower**

This instrument is not commonly used because of the greater efficiency of the compressed air syringe. Consideration is given here because of the precautions required for sterilization.

1. Description: rubber bulb attached to air tip with contra-angled working end.
2. Technique for use
    a. Hold rubber bulb firmly in palm; index finger and thumb steady shank of blower to prevent action against the tissues; remaining fingers depress bulb.
    b. Remove from proximity to oral tissues when pressure on bulb is released to prevent suction of debris and saliva into the air tip and bulb.
3. Care: separate air tip and bulb and clean inside of air tip with pipe cleaner prior to sterilization.

PROCEDURE FOR THE ORAL INSPECTION

I. **ADVANTAGES OF FOLLOWING A ROUTINE ORDER**

A. The possibility of overlooking details of importance is minimized.
B. Efficiency is increased and time conserved.
C. A professional atmosphere is maintained which will inspire the patient's confidence.

6

II. ORDER OF INSPECTION

Inspection begins as the patient is received and ushered to the dental chair. The recommended order of inspection (Table 4) provides for a systematic observation from the external features of the body and face to the vestibule, oral cavity proper, throat region, and finally to the gingiva and teeth which are in the specific field of operation for dental hygiene appointment techniques.

III. EVALUATION OF OBSERVATIONS

A. Compare appearance of tissues with normal.
B. Outline appointment procedures in accord with the needs of the patient.

IV. PREPARATION OF RECORDS

A. Reasons for preparing complete, accurate, clear, neat records.
1. For ready use by the dentist in preparation of the diagnosis and treatment plan.
2. For reference at future appointments during the continuing dental and dental hygiene care of the patient.
3. For reference in the event a legal complication arises.
B. Use a record form with adequate space for recording details.
C. Prepare permanent records in ink.
D. Use abbreviations and symbols only when their meaning will be clear to all who read them.

V. TECHNICAL HINTS

A. Employ adequate light for visibility to all parts of the oral cavity.
B. Provide the patient with a hand mirror to observe proceedings. The instructional value of the inspection is increased.
C. Establish rapport before tactfully discussing dental hygiene care.
D. Reserve comment at all times on questions involving diagnosis. Record questions for reference to the dentist.

THE IMMEDIATE FIELD OF OPERATION; THE TEETH AND GINGIVA

The techniques of the dental hygiene appointment are applied principally to the teeth, the gingiva and the gingival sulcus. Detailed knowledge and understanding of the anatomy and normal clinical appearance of this field of operation are prerequisite to making the oral inspection and performing techniques intelligently.

It is not within the scope of this book to describe the entire oral cavity or the anatomy of individual teeth. A brief outline of the anatomy and clinical appearance of the gingiva and gingival sulcus is included, however, to serve as a quick reference during the study of the oral inspection, the deposits on the teeth, and the techniques of the oral prophylaxis.

(Text continued on page 85)

TABLE 4.—THE ORAL INSPECTION

Order of Inspection	To Observe	Suggested Relation to Appointment Procedures
1. OVER-ALL APPRAISAL OF PATIENT	Posture, gait. Respiration. State of fatigue. Facial expression. Facial profile. General health status: eyes, hair, weight-height proportions.	Response, cooperation and attitude to be expected. Length of appointment. Use of face mask when patient shows evidence of upper respiratory infection. Classification of occlusion.
2. SKIN	Color, texture. Traumatic lesions. Eruptions. Growths.	Possible need for postponement of appointment when extensive lesions exist. Instruction: general dietary and nutritional factors.
3. LIPS	Cracks, angular cheilosis. Blisters, ulcers. Traumatic lesions; irritation from biting habits. Abrasions.	Care during retraction. Need for applying cream or petroleum jelly. Possible need for postponement of appointment if lesions can interfere with procedures or patient can be uncomfortable.
4. BREATH ODOR	When patient opens mouth.	May indicate need for emphasis on personal oral care procedures.
5. EASE OF OPENING MOUTH	Muscle tone and elasticity. Freedom of movement of temperomandibular joint.	Ease or difficulty of accessibility or visibility during instrumentation. Instruction: adaptation of toothbrush size and technique.
6. LABIAL AND BUCCAL MUCOSA MUCOBUCCAL FOLDS RETROMOLAR AREAS FRENUMS OPENING OF STENSON'S DUCT	Color, size, texture, contour. Abrasions; traumatic lesions; cheekbite. Ulcers, growths. Moistness of membranes.	Avoidance of sensitive areas during retraction, radiographic film placement, or oral physical therapy instruction.
7. HARD PALATE	Height, color, contour. Appearance of rugæ. Tori, growths, ulcers.	Placement of radiographic films. Instruction in toothbrushing on palatal surfaces.
8. TONGUE	Color, size, texture, consistency. Appearance of papillæ. Muscle tone; mobility. Fissures.	Large muscular tongue affects convenience of retraction and gag reflex during instrumentation or radiographic film placement. Instruction: tongue brushing; dietary factors.
9. SUBLINGUAL AREA UNDERSURFACE OF TONGUE SUBMAXILLARY AND SUBLINGUAL GLAND DUCTS OPENINGS	Color, size, texture, consistency of tissue. Ulcers, growths. Traumatic lesions. Abrasions.	Care of sensitive areas during instrumentation, placement of cotton roll holders, saliva ejector, or radiographic films.

TABLE 4. (Continued)

Order of Inspection	To Observe	Suggested Relation to Appointment Procedures
10. SOFT PALATE AND UVULA	Color, size, shape. Ulcers, growths.	Effect of large or enlarged uvula on gag reflex; relation to techniques applied to posterior lingual regions.
11. TONSILAR REGION	Size of tonsils. Color and appearance of membranes.	Effect of enlarged tonsils on gag reflex: adjustment of techniques. Need for face mask when patient shows evidence of throat infection. Instruction: adapt procedures for toothbrushing lingual surfaces of posterior teeth to prevent gagging.
12. GINGIVA Free Attached Interdental papillæ	Color, size, contour, consistency, surface texture, position. Abrasions; toothbrush trauma. Fistulous openings. Ulcers, growths.	Scaler selection. Care of sensitive areas during techniques. Instruction: personal care procedures; dietary and nutritional factors.
13. GINGIVAL SULCI	Depth.	Scaler selection. In conjunction with extent of calculus: planning length and number of appointments. Aid to identification of cases requiring periodontal care.
14. TEETH	Morphology, location.	Scaler selection. Adaptation of instruments.
	Edentulous areas.	Fulcrum selection. Instruction: personal care procedures for adjacent teeth.
	Eruption.	Instrumentation adaptation to tissue flaps. Instruction: need for preservation of primary teeth.
	Mobility.	Fulcrum selection (see page 141)
	Proximal contact relation; areas of food impaction.	Instruction: use of dental floss; need for restoration of contact areas.
	Biting and chewing habits.	Instruction: discuss problems such as unilateral chewing, biting hard objects.
	Attrition. Abrasion. Erosion.	Care during techniques to avoid sensitive areas. Instruction: correction of habit contributing to the condition.
	Hypersensitive areas (exposed cementum).	Care during techniques to avoid sensitive areas. Indication for application of desensitizing agent (see page 209).

TABLE 4. (Continued)

Order of Inspection	To Observe	Suggested Relation to Appointment Procedures
14. TEETH (*Continued*)	Decalcified areas and carious lesions.	Adapt techniques to avoid altering the lesions. Instruction: dental caries preventive procedures. Instrument selection.
	Calculus, soft deposits and stains.	Length and number of appointments; plan for recall frequency. Instruction: preventive procedures. Instrument selection.
	Restorations.	Adaptation of scalers to margins. Selection of polishing agents.
15. DENTURES Complete. Removable partial. Fixed partial. Tissue adjacent to denture.	Calculus, soft deposits and stains. Areas of food retention. For tissues: see items 6, 7, 8, 9, 10, 12 of this Table.	Selection of cleansing procedures. Instruction: Personal care procedures for dentures and supporting teeth; use of dental floss under fixed partial denture; need for digital massage of adjacent oral mucosa.
16. APPRAISAL OF STATE OF ORAL CLEANLINESS	Extent of accumulated food debris, materia alba, plaques, stains. Color, size, contour, consistency and surface texture of gingiva.	Instruction: personal care procedures; diet selection; need for routine recall appointments.
17. OCCLUSION	Major classification. Malaligned teeth or groups of teeth. Effects of oral habits.	Adapt instrumentation and radiographic film placement. Instruction: for personal care for malaligned teeth.

I. THE TEETH: DEFINITIONS RELATED TO CLINICAL TECHNIQUES

A. **Anatomical Crown:** that part of the tooth covered by enamel.

B. **Anatomical Root:** that part of the tooth covered by cementum.

C. **Clinical Crown:** that part of the tooth which has been denuded of epithelium and projects into the oral cavity.

D. **Clinical Root:** that part of the tooth covered by attached periodontal tissues.

II. THE NORMAL GINGIVA

A. **Definition:** the part of the oral mucous membrane which is firmly attached to the alveolar process and the surfaces of the teeth, and surrounds the necks of the teeth.

B. **Histology of Outer Surface Layer:** stratified squamous epithelium.

C. **Description of the Parts of the Gingiva** (Figure 21)
1. *Free gingiva*
   a. Unattached.
   b. Surrounds tooth in collar-like fashion.
   c. Forms the wall of the gingival sulcus.
   d. Extends from gingival crest to epithelial attachment.
   e. Demarcated from adjacent attached gingiva by shallow linear groove, the *free gingival groove*, which is 0.5 to 1.5 mm. from the crest.[3]
2. *Gingival crest* (margin of the free gingiva)
   a. Edge of gingiva closest to incisal or occlusal of tooth.
   b. Marks opening to gingival sulcus.
3. *Attached gingiva*
   a. Attached to cementum and alveolar bone.
   b. Extends from free gingival groove to alveolar mucosa.
   c. Lines of demarcation.
      (1) From alveolar mucosa by definite line, the *mucogingival junction*, created by light pink of attached gingiva uniting with red of alveolar mucosa.
      (2) From mucosa on floor of mouth by line similar to mucogingival junction.
      (3) No line in palate because of dense structure and firm attachment of entire palatal mucosa.
4. *Interdental papilla*
   a. Extends into and fills the interproximal area (depending on relationship of adjacent teeth).
      (1) Tapered when teeth are closely spaced or overlapped.
      (2) Flat when teeth are widely spaced.
   b. Bound by proximal surfaces of teeth, the contact areas, and the crest of the alveolar bone.
   c. Tip and lateral borders are the continuation of the free gingiva; other parts are attached gingiva.

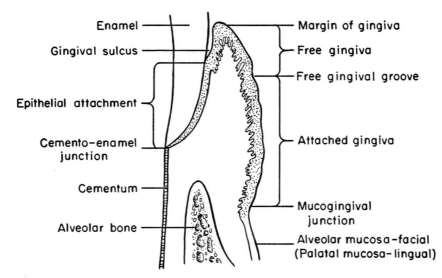

FIGURE 21.—Diagram illustrating the parts of the gingiva and adjacent tissues.

D. **Clinical Appearance of the Gingiva** (Figure 22)

  1. Color
      a. Coral pink.
      b. Wide range of normal: varies with complexion.
      c. Pigmentations associated with race.
  2. Size: closely related to contour and position.
  3. Contour
      a. Festooned appearance with intermittent prominences corresponding to contour of roots.
      b. Interdental depressions which taper toward free gingiva and blend with conical interdental papilla.
      c. Gingival crest tapered, with knife-like edge adapted closely to tooth.

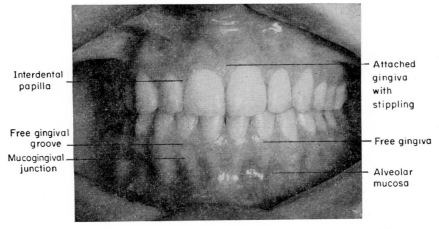

FIGURE 22.—Normal clinical appearance of the gingiva of a young adult.

  4. Consistency
      a. Firm, resilient.
      b. Tightly bound to underlying bone (except free gingiva).
  5. Surface texture
      a. Free gingiva: smooth.
      b. Attached gingiva: stippled (minutely "pebbled").
      c. Interdental papilla: free gingiva smooth, central portion stippled.
  6. Position (varies with age)
      a. Childhood: gingiva covers varying portion of anatomical crown depending on eruption stage of tooth.
      b. Adolescence and young adulthood (teeth fully erupted)
          (1) Clinical crown may be equivalent to the anatomical crown.
          (2) Gingival crest at level of enamel contour.
      c. Advancing age: gingival crest will be below the enamel contour with continuing eruption of the teeth due to attrition.

III. **THE GINGIVAL SULCUS (CREVICE)**

 A. Between the free gingiva and the tooth.

 B. Bounded by tooth surface and the epithelial covering of the free gingiva which clings closely to the tooth surface.

 C. Extends from gingival crest to the epithelial attachment (approximately 1.8 mm.[4]).

IV. **THE EPITHELIAL ATTACHMENT**

 A. Attached to tooth surface in vicinity of cemento-enamel junction, at a level varying with degree of eruption.

 B. Consists of epithelium which is the continuation of the lining of the gingival sulcus.

 C. Forms the base of the gingival sulcus.

FACTORS TO TEACH THE PATIENT

 I. Reasons for the careful oral inspection.

 II. Purposes of the instruments of inspection.

 III. Clinical characteristics of the normal gingiva.

 IV. Relationship of conditions observed in the oral inspection to personal daily oral care procedures.

 V. General dietary and nutritional influences on the health of the oral tissues.

 VI. How the oral cavity tends to reflect the general health.

REFERENCES

1. BEUBE, F. E.: *Periodontology*, New York, Macmillan, 1953, pp. 376–377.
2. GLICKMAN, IRVING: *Clinical Periodontology*, 2nd ed. Philadelphia, Saunders, 1958, pp. 548–549.
3. SICHER, HARRY: *Orban's Oral Histology and Embryology*, 5th ed. St. Louis, Mosby, 1962, p. 231.
4. *Ibid.*, p. 253.

SUGGESTED READINGS

BURKET, L. W.: *Oral Medicine*, 4th ed. Philadelphia, Lippincott, 1961, pp. 13–19.

COLBY, R. A., KERR, D. A., and ROBINSON, H. B. G.: *Color Atlas of Oral Pathology*, 2nd ed. Philadelphia, Lippincott, 1961. xiv & 201 pp.

CHERASKIN, E.: Oral Diagnostic Procedure, in Finn, S.B.: *Clinical Pedodontics*, 2nd ed. Philadelphia, Saunders, 1962, pp. 82–103.

GLICKMAN, IRVING: *Clinical Periodontology*, 2nd ed. Philadelphia, Saunders, 1958, pp. 468–479.

GREENE, J. C. and VERMILLION, J. R.: Oral Hygiene Index: A Method for Classifying Oral Hygiene Status, Am. Dent. A. J., *61*, 172, August, 1960.

GREENE, J. C. and VERMILLION, J. R.: Simplified Oral Hygiene Index, Am. Dent. A. J., *68*, 7, January, 1964.

MASSLER, MAURY, KOPEL, HUGH, KELNER, MORRIS, and WERTHER, RAY: Oral Habits, J. Dent. Child., *22*, 132, Third Quarter, 1955. (Labial Frenum, p. 141.)

MASSLER, MAURY and SCHOUR, ISAAC: *Atlas of the Mouth*, 2nd ed. Chicago, American Dental Association, 1958, Plates 20, 34, 42–49.

MILLER, S. C.: *Oral Diagnosis and Treatment*, 3rd ed. New York, Blakiston Division, McGraw-Hill, 1957, pp. 4–9, 17–32.

ORBAN, B. J. and WENTZ, F. M.: *Atlas of Clinical Pathology of the Oral Mucous Membrane*, 2nd ed. St. Louis, Mosby, 1960, 148 pp.

SIMON, L. G.: The Role of the Dental Hygienist in the Detection of Cancer, Am. Dent. Hygienists' A. J., *27*, 310, October, 1953.

THOMA, K. H. and ROBINSON, H. B. G.: *Oral and Dental Diagnosis*, 5th ed. Philadelphia, Saunders, 1960, pp. 1–8, 21–77.

Field of Operation

BEUBE, F. E.: *Periodontology.* New York, Macmillan, 1953, pp. 3–14.

GLICKMAN: op. cit., pp. 9–22.

GOLDMAN, H. M., SCHLUGER, SAUL, COHEN, D. W., CHAIKEN, B. S., and FOX, LEWIS: *Introduction to Periodontia,* 2nd ed. St. Louis, Mosby, 1962, pp. 15–32.

GOLDMAN, H. M., SCHLUGER, SAUL, and FOX, LEWIS: *Periodontal Therapy.* 2nd ed. St. Louis, Mosby, 1960, pp. 25–36.

PERMAR, DOROTHY: *A Manual of Oral Embryology and Microscopic Anatomy,* 3rd ed. Philadelphia, Lea & Febiger, 1963, pp. 113–121.

SICHER, HARRY: *Orban's Oral Histology and Embryology,* 5th ed. St. Louis, Mosby, 1962, pp. 220–271.

Chapter 9

INSPECTION OF THE OCCLUSION

THE dental hygienist, by studying the occlusion of each patient, can contribute significantly to the complete dental care and instruction. Recognition of malocclusion assists the dentist in his referral of patients to the orthodontist, gives many valuable points of reference for patient instruction, and determines necessary adaptations in radiographic and oral prophylaxis techniques.

As in other phases of oral inspection, it cannot be overemphasized that the dental hygienist does not diagnose. It is her role to interpret to the patient* the dentist's recommendations at his request.

I. OBJECTIVES FOR OBSERVING OCCLUSION

Recognition of the patient's occlusion and understanding the oral health problems of malocclusion can aid in accomplishing the following:

A. Relate the influence of the patient's malocclusion, appearance and/or speech, to other evidences of his psychological problems or needs.

B. Adapt techniques of instrumentation during the oral prophylaxis and radiography to malpositioned teeth or groups of teeth.

C. Plan personalized instruction in relation to such factors as oral habits, masticatory efficiency, personal oral care procedures and predisposing factors to dental and periodontal disease.

D. Plan the frequency of recall appointments for professional care on the basis of deposit retention areas, particularly those which are difficult to reach in routine personal care.

E. Assist the dentist by recording the general features of malocclusion for special consideration by the dentist who may wish to refer the patient to an orthodontist.

II. DEFINITIONS

A. **Occlusion:** the contact of the teeth in the mandibular arch with those in the maxillary arch in functional relation during any and all mandibular movements.

1. *Normal (Ideal) Occlusion:* the ideal mechanical relation between the teeth of the maxillary arch and the teeth of the mandibular arch.

   a. All teeth in maxillary arch in maximum contact with all teeth in mandibular arch in a definite pattern.

   b. Maxillary teeth slightly overlapping the mandibular teeth on the facial surfaces.

---

* The word "patient" is used to mean patient *and* parent when patient is a child.

2. *Malocclusion:* any deviation from the ideal relation of the maxillary arch and/or teeth to the mandibular arch and/or teeth.

3. *Centric Occlusion*
   a. The maximum occlusal contact relationship of the teeth when mandible is in its centric relation.
   b. Centric relation: the most unstrained, retruded anatomic and functional position of the heads of the condyles in the glenoid fossæ of the temperomandibular joints.

B. **Types of Facial Profile** (Figure 23)

   1. *Mesognathic:* having slightly protruded jaws which give the facial outline a relatively flat appearance (straight profile).

   2. *Retrognathic:* having prominent maxilla and a deficient, retruded mandible (convex profile).

   3. *Prognathic:* having prominent, protruded mandible and normal (usually) maxilla (concave profile).

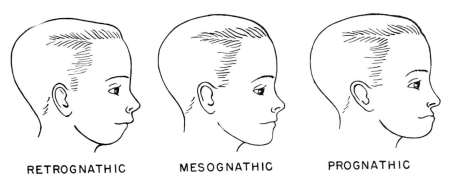

RETROGNATHIC   MESOGNATHIC   PROGNATHIC

FIGURE 23.—Types of facial profiles.

C. **Malrelations of Groups of Teeth**

   1. *Crossbites*
      a. Anterior: maxillary incisors are lingual to the mandibular incisors.
      b. Posterior: maxillary or mandibular posterior teeth are either buccal or lingual to their normal position; this may occur bilaterally or unilaterally (Figure 24).

   2. *Edge-to-Edge Bite:* incisal surfaces of maxillary teeth occlude with incisal surfaces of mandibular teeth instead of overlapping as in ideal occlusion (Figure 25).

   3. *End-to-End Bite:* molars and bicuspids occlude cusp-to-cusp as viewed mesiodistally (Figure 26).

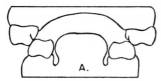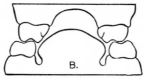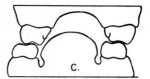

FIGURE 24.—Posterior crossbite. *A.* Mandibular teeth lingual to normal position. *B.* Mandibular teeth buccal to normal position. *C.* Unilateral crossbite: right side normal; left side, mandibular teeth buccal to normal position.

FIGURE 25

FIGURE 26

FIGURE 25.—Edge-to-edge bite. Incisal surfaces occlude.

FIGURE 26.—End-to-end bite. Molars in cusp-to-cusp occlusion as viewed from the buccal.

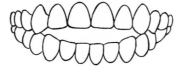

FIGURE 27.—Openbite. Lack of incisal contact. Posterior teeth in their normal occlusion.

FIGURE 28

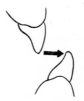

FIGURE 29

FIGURE 28.—Normal overbite of anterior teeth.

FIGURE 29.—Excessive overbites. *A.* Deep Overbite. *B.* Anterior Crossbite with Deep Overbite.

FIGURE 30

FIGURE 31

FIGURE 30.—Overjet. Maxillary incisors are labial to mandibular incisors and there is a horizontal distance between labioincisal surfaces of the mandibular incisors and the linguoincisal surfaces of the maxillary incisors.

FIGURE 31.—Underjet. Maxillary incisors are lingual to mandibular incisors and there is a horizontal distance between the labioincisal surfaces of the maxillary teeth and the linguoincisal surfaces of the mandibular teeth.

4. *Openbite:* lack of occlusal or incisal contact between maxillary and mandibular teeth because either or both have failed to reach the line of occlusion. The teeth cannot be brought together and a space remains due to the arching of the line of occlusion (Figure 27).

5. *Overbite:* the vertical distance by which the maxillary incisors overlap the mandibular incisors (Figure 28).
   a. *Deep Overbite:* mandibular incisors contact palate or lingual gingiva of maxillary anterior teeth when teeth are in centric occlusion (Figure 29*A*).
   b. *Anterior Crossbite with Deep Overbite:* maxillary incisors contact mandibular lingual gingival tissue when teeth are in occlusion (Figure 29*B*).

6. *Overjet:* The horizontal distance between the labioincisal surfaces of the mandibular incisors and the linguoincisal surfaces of the maxillary incisors (Figure 30).

7. *Underjet* (maxillary teeth are lingual to mandibular teeth): the horizontal distance between the labioincisal surfaces of the maxillary incisors and the linguoincisal surfaces of the mandibular incisors (Figure 31).

D. **Malpositions of Individual Teeth**

1. *Labioversion:* a tooth which has assumed a position labial to normal.

2. *Linguoversion:* position lingual to normal.

3. *Buccoversion:* position buccal to normal.

4. *Supraversion:* elongated above the line of occlusion.

5. *Torsoversion:* turned or rotated.

6. *Infraversion:* depressed below the line of occlusion. (Example: primary tooth that is submerged or ankylosed).

DETERMINATION OF THE CLASSIFICATION OF OCCLUSION

The determination of the classification of occlusion is based upon the principles of Edward H. Angle, which he presented in the early 1900's. He defined normal occlusion as "the normal relations of the occlusal inclined planes of the teeth when the jaws are closed,"[1] and based his system of classification upon the relationship of the maxillary first permanent molars.

Although authorities have since agreed that the maxillary first permanent molars do not occupy a fixed position in the dental arch, Angle's system serves to provide an acceptable basis for a general classification useful to the dental hygienist. A more comprehensive picture of malocclusion is made by the orthodontist who studies the relationships of the position of the teeth to the jaws, the face and the skull.

Four general classes of malocclusion are described below. These are designated by Roman numerals. Since the mandible is movable and the maxilla is stationary, the classes describe the relationship of the mandible to the maxilla. For example, in Distoclusion (Class II) the mandible is distal, whereas in Mesioclusion (Class III) the mandible is mesial to the maxilla, as compared to the normal position.

Normal or ideal occlusions are found in only 2 per cent of the population. Another 27 per cent have slight malrelationships which do not require orthodontic care. The remaining 71 per cent with malocclusions sufficiently severe to require orthodontic treatment have been studied[2,3] and the following percentages by classification are typical:

	Per Cent
Class I. (Neutroclusion)	76
Class II. (Distoclusion) Div. 1	18
Class II. (Distoclusion) Div. 2	5
Class III. (Mesioclusion)	1

I. **NORMAL (IDEAL) OCCLUSION** (Figures 22 and 32)

A. *Facial Profile:* mesognathic; relatively flat.

B. *Molar Relation:* the mesiobuccal cusp of the maxillary first permanent molar occludes with the buccal groove of the mandibular first permanent molar.

C. *Cuspid Relation:* the maxillary permanent cuspid occludes with the distal half of the mandibular cuspid and the mesial half of the mandibular first bicuspid.

II. **MALOCCLUSION**

A. **Class I or Neutroclusion** (Figure 32)

1. Description
   a. *Facial Profile:* same as Normal Occlusion (I, A, above).
   b. *Molar Relation:* same as Normal Occlusion (I, B, above).
   c. *Cuspid Relation:* same as Normal Occlusion (I, C, above).
   d. Malposition of individual teeth or groups of teeth.
2. General Types of Conditions which Frequently Occur in Class I.
   a. Crowded maxillary or mandibular anterior teeth.
   b. Protruded or retruded maxillary incisors.
   c. Anterior crossbite.
   d. Posterior crossbite.
   e. Mesial drift of molars resulting from premature loss of teeth.

B. **Class II or Distoclusion** (Figure 32)

1. Description: mandibular teeth posterior to normal position in their relation to the maxillary teeth.
   a. *Facial Profile:* retrognathic; maxilla protrudes; lower lip is full and often rests between the maxillary and mandibular incisors; the mandible appears retruded or weak.
   b. *Molar Relation*
      (1) The buccal groove of the mandibular first permanent molar is distal to the mesiobuccal cusp of the maxillary first permanent molar by at least the width of a bicuspid.
      (2) If the distance is less than the width of a bicuspid the relation should be classified as "tendency toward Class II."

   c. *Cuspid Relation*
      (1) The distal surface of the mandibular cuspid is distal to the
          mesial surface of the maxillary cuspid by at least the
          width of a bicuspid.
      (2) If the distance is less than the width of a bicuspid the re-
          lation should be classified as "tendency toward Class
          II."
2. Divisions of Class II Malocclusions.
   a. *Division 1*
      (1) Description: the mandible is retruded and all maxillary
          incisors are protruded.

Normal (Ideal) Occlusion.

Molar relationship: mesiobuccal cusp of maxillary first permanent molar occludes with
   the buccal groove of the mandibular first
   permanent molar.

Class I: Neutroclusion. Molar relationship
   same as Normal, with malposition of individual teeth or groups of teeth.

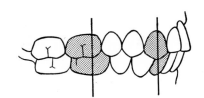

Class II: Distoclusion.

Molar relationship: buccal groove of the mandibular first permanent molar is distal to the
   mesiobuccal cusp of the maxillary first permanent molar by at least the width of a
   bicuspid.

Division 1: mandible is retruded and all maxillary incisors are protruded.

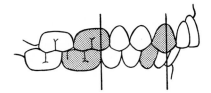

Division 2: mandible is retruded and one or
   more maxillary incisors are retruded.

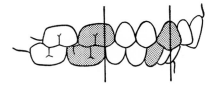

Class III: Mesioclusion.

Molar relationship: buccal groove of the mandibular first permanent molar is mesial to
   the mesiobuccal cusp of the maxillary first
   permanent molar by at least the width of a
   bicuspid.

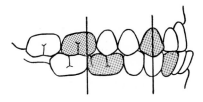

FIGURE 32.—Normal occlusion and classification of malocclusions.

(2) General types of conditions which frequently occur in Class II, Division 1 malocclusion.
    (a) Deep overbite.
    (b) Excessive overjet.
    (c) Abnormal muscle function (lips).
    (d) Short mandible.
    (e) Short upper lip.
b. *Division 2*
    (1) Description: the mandible is retruded, and one or more maxillary incisors are retruded.
    (2) General types of conditions which frequently occur in Class II, Division 2 malocclusion.
        (a) Maxillary lateral incisors protrude while both central incisors retrude.
        (b) Crowded maxillary anterior teeth.
        (c) Deep overbite.
        (d) Pleasing facial appearance (usually).
c. *Subdivision:* One side is Class I, the other side is Class II (may be Division 1 or 2).

C. **Class III or Mesioclusion** (Figure 32)

1. Description: mandibular teeth are anterior to normal position in relation to maxillary teeth.
a. *Facial Profile:* prognathic; lower lip and mandible are prominent.
b. *Molar Relation*
    (1) The buccal groove of the mandibular first permanent molar is mesial to the mesiobuccal cusp of the maxillary first permanent molar by at least the width of a bicuspid.
    (2) If the distance is less than the width of a bicuspid the relation should be classified as "tendency toward Class III."
c. *Cuspid Relation*
    (1) The distal surface of the mandibular cuspid is mesial to the mesial surface of the maxillary cuspid by at least the width of a bicuspid.
    (2) If the distance is less than the width of a bicuspid the relation should be classified as "tendency toward Class III."
2. General Types of Conditions which Frequently Occur in Class III Malocclusion.
a. True Class III: maxillary incisors are lingual to mandibular incisors and do not occlude with them.
b. Maxillary and mandibular incisors are in edge-to-edge occlusion.
c. Mandibular incisors very crowded, but lingual to maxillary incisors.

OCCLUSION OF THE PRIMARY TEETH[4]

I. **NORMAL** (Ideal)

A. **Cuspid Relation:** Same as permanent dentition.

    1. With primate spaces (see page 488 for definition).
        a. Mandibular: between mandibular cuspid and first molar (Figure 33).
        b. Maxillary: between maxillary lateral incisor and cuspid.
    2. Without primate spaces: closed arches.

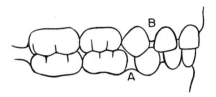

FIGURE 33.—Primary teeth showing primate spaces. *A*. Mandibular primate space between cuspid and first molar. *B*. Maxillary primate space between lateral incisor and cuspid.

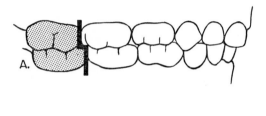

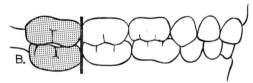

FIGURE 34.—Eruption patterns of first permanent molars. *A*. Terminal Step. Distal surface of mandibular second primary molar is mesial to the distal surface of the maxillary primary molar. Permanent molars erupt in normal occlusion. *B*. Terminal Plane. Distal surfaces of mandibular and maxillary second primary molars are on the same vertical plane. Permanent molars erupt in end-to-end occlusion.

B. **Second Molar Relation**

    1. The mesiobuccal cusp of the maxillary second primary molar occludes with the buccal groove of the mandibular second primary molar.
    2. Variations in distal surfaces relationships
        a. Terminal Step
            (1) The distal surface of the mandibular molar is mesial to that of the maxillary, thereby forming a mesial step (Figure 34*A*).
            (2) Morphological variation in molar size: maxillary and mandibular molars have approximately the same mesiodistal width.

7

    b. Terminal Plane
     (1) The distal surfaces of the maxillary and mandibular molars are on same vertical plane (Figure 34*B*).
     (2) The maxillary molar is narrower mesiodistally than the mandibular molar (occurs in high percentage of cases).
   3. Effects on occlusion of first permanent molars
    a. Terminal Step: first permanent molar erupts directly into proper occlusion (Figure 34*A*).
    b. Terminal Plane: first permanent molars erupt end-to-end.
     (1) With mandibular primate space: early mesial shift of primary molars into primate space; permanent mandibular molar shifts into proper occlusion.
     (2) Without primate spaces: late mesial shift of permanent mandibular molar into proper occlusion following exfoliation of second primary molar (Figure 34*B*).

II. **MALOCCLUSION OF THE PRIMARY TEETH: Same as permanent dentition.**

TECHNICAL HINTS

 I. Observe the patient's facial profile as he enters the room and is seated in the dental chair.
 II. Avoid mention of a dentofacial deformity which would make the patient feel self-conscious.
 III. Avoid suggesting to the patient or his parent the possible procedures which the orthodontist may use in the treatment of the case, as complications of the case become known only after the complete diagnosis.
 IV. To aid patient in closing to centric relation:
  A. Instruct him to curl his tongue and try to hold tip of tongue as far back as possible while closing.
  B. Ask him to "swallow and bite."
 V. When a small child has difficulty in occluding in centric relation the operator may firmly but gently press the cushions of the thumbs on the mucous membrane over the pterygomandibular raphe, holding the thumbs between the cheek and buccal surfaces of the teeth, as the patient is requested to close.
 VI. Study the occlusion of the patient with removable dentures with the dentures in place in the mouth.

FACTORS TO TEACH THE PATIENT

 I. Interpretation of the *general* purposes of orthodontic care (function and esthetics) to patients whom the dentist has referred to the orthodontist.
  A. Dependency of masticatory efficiency on the occlusion of the teeth.
  B. Influence of masticatory efficiency on food selection in the diet.
  C. Influence of masticatory efficiency and diet on the nutritional status of the body.
 II. Interpretation of the dentist's suggestions for the correction of oral habits which may contribute to malocclusion.

III. The space maintaining function of the primary teeth in prevention of malocclusion of permanent teeth.

IV. The role of malocclusion as a predisposing factor in the formation of dental caries and periodontal diseases.

V. Methods of reducing dental calculus and soft deposit retention in areas where teeth are crowded, displaced or otherwise not in normal occlusion.

VI. The relation of the occlusion and the position of the teeth to the patient's personal oral care procedures.
   A. Selection of the proper type of toothbrush.
   B. Application of thorough toothbrushing method or methods.
   C. Use of dental floss.

VII. Reasons for frequency of recall for the oral prophylaxis as they relate to malocclusion and position of individual teeth.

REFERENCES

1. ANGLE, E. H.: *Malocclusion of the Teeth*, 7th ed. Philadelphia, S. S. White, 1907.
2. BLAKE, S. R.: *A Study of the Incidence of Malocclusion and Facial Characteristics in Seattle High School Students, Aged 15 to 20 Years.* University of Washington, Master of Science in Dentistry Thesis, 1954, pp. 15, 41.
3. MOORE, ALTON: Seattle, School of Dentistry, University of Washington, personal communication.
4. BAUME, L. J.: Physiological Tooth Migration and Its Significance for the Development of the Occlusion.
   I. The Biogenetic Course of the Deciduous Dentition, J. Dent. Res., *29*, 123, April, 1950.
   II. The Biogenesis of Accessional Dentition, J. Dent. Res., *29*, 331, June, 1950.
   III. The Biogenesis of the Successional Dentition, J. Dent. Res., *29*, 338, June, 1950.
   IV. The Biogenesis of Overbite, J. Dent. Res., *29*, 440, August, 1950.

SUGGESTED READINGS

Occlusion

BEUBE, F. E.: *Periodontology.* New York, Macmillan, 1953, pp. 25–34, 319–321.
COHEN, M. I.: Recognition of Developing Malocclusion, *Dental Clinics of North America,* July, 1959, p. 299.
GRABER, T. M.: *Orthodontics.* Philadelphia, Saunders, 1961, pp. 127–189.
JACKSON, G. E.: Functional Consideration of the Problems of Occlusion, *Dental Clinics of North America,* July, 1959, p. 355.
MASSLER, MAURY, and FRANKEL, J. M.: Prevalence of Malocclusion in Children Aged 14 to 18 Years, A. J. Orthodont., *37*, 751, October, 1951.
MASSLER, MAURY and SCHOUR, ISAAC: *Atlas of the Mouth,* 2nd ed. Chicago, American Dental Association, 1958, Plates 26–33.
MILLER, S. C.: *Oral Diagnosis and Treatment,* 3rd ed. New York, Blakiston Division, McGraw-Hill, 1957, pp. 602–626.
MOSMANN, W. H.: Diagnosis and Prevention of Some Malocclusions, *Dental Clinics of North America,* March, 1962, p. 99.
OLSEN, N. H.: Space Maintenance, *Dental Clinics of North America,* July, 1959, p. 339.
THOMA, K. H.: *Oral Pathology,* 5th ed. St. Louis, Mosby, 1960, pp. 73–79.

Oral Habits

FINN, S. B.: Oral Habits in Children, in Finn, S. B.: *Clinical Pedodontics,* 2nd ed. Philadelphia, Saunders, 1962, pp. 314–329.
GRABER: op. cit., pp. 235–262.
HEMLEY, SAMUEL and KRONFELD, S. M.: Habits, *Dental Clinics of North America,* November, 1961, p. 687.

JARABAK, J. R.:   Controlling Malocclusions Due to Sucking Habits, *Dental Clinics of North America*, July, 1959, p. 369.
MASSLER, MAURY and WOOD, A. W. S.:   Thumbsucking, J. Dent. Child, *16*, 1, 1st Quarter, 1949.
SCHILLER, M. B.:   Dental Aspects in Speech Handicaps, Am. Dent. Hygienists' A. J., *35*, 171, October, 1961.
SHORT, M. J.:   Role of Dental Hygienist in Tongue Thrust Swallowing, Am. Dent. Hygienists' A. J., *37*, 86, 2nd Quarter, 1963.
SUBTELNY, J. D. and SUBTELNY, J. D.:   Malocclusion, Speech, and Deglutition, A. J. Orthodont., *48*, 685, September, 1962.

PART III

The Oral Prophylaxis

Chapter 10

INTRODUCTION TO THE ORAL PROPHYLAXIS

As used in this book and defined in this chapter, the term "oral prophylaxis" is limited in scope to the preventive services involved in the removal of deposits and stains from the teeth. Since "prophylaxis" actually means *prevention of disease*, then "oral prophylaxis" as *prevention of oral disease* is a term which includes much more than scaling and polishing of the teeth.[1] For example, restoring individual teeth, replacing missing teeth, adjusting the occlusion, and applying a topical fluoride solution for dental caries prevention are all disease preventing services. Since in practice many dental hygienists refer to the term "oral prophylaxis" as defined in this book, it is hoped that no confusion of terms will be created.

The fundamental aims of the oral prophylaxis lie in the prevention of periodontal diseases due to local irritants and the maintenance of the health of the supporting tissues of the teeth. These and other related contributory objectives suggested in this chapter should be foremost in the dental hygienist's mind as techniques and instruction are planned and carried out for the patient.

The dental hygienist defines techniques and their possible effects with a clear understanding of the specific field of operation, the teeth and their supporting structures. Within this area of operation occur deposits and stains which provide irritation to the soft tissues. The factors which contribute to the formation and retention of deposits and stains are significant to the application of methods for their removal and prevention. A scientific rather than a mechanical approach to clinical operations is important when working toward the goal of assisting the patient in obtaining and maintaining optimum oral health.

I. DEFINITIONS

A. **Oral Hygiene:** The science of mouth health and its preservation.*

B. **Prophylaxis:** Prevention of disease; preventive procedure.

C. **Oral Prophylaxis:** A series of scaling and polishing procedures whereby calculus, soft deposits and stains are removed from the clinical crowns of the teeth for *preventive* purposes.

*The term "oral hygiene" is used with a variety of meanings. It sometimes refers to the procedures used in the personal care of the mouth by the patient. It is used also to denote the cleanliness of the teeth and mouth and referred to as the "patient's oral hygiene."

D. **Odontexesis** (Periodontal Treatment): A series of scaling and polishing procedures whereby calculus, soft deposits and stains are removed from the clinical crowns of the teeth for *therapeutic* purposes.

II. OBJECTIVES FOR THE PATIENT

Objectives are primarily related to the health of the supporting structures of the teeth. The oral prophylaxis in itself cannot be expected to prevent dental caries (see pages 113–114).

A. Direct Objectives

1. Prevents periodontal diseases which may be caused by local irritants to the gingiva.
2. Assists in the maintenance phase of care for the patient who has undergone periodontal therapy.
3. Prepares the teeth for the topical application of fluoride solution.
4. Aids the patient in obtaining, so that he may maintain, oral cleanliness.
5. Assists in instructing the patient in the appearance and feeling of a thoroughly clean mouth as an aid in motivating him to develop adequate habits of personal oral care.
6. Improves oral esthetics.
7. Introduces the child to dental office procedures.

B. Indirect Objectives Related to the Effects of Removal of Deposits and Stains

1. Increases the resistance of the gingival tissues and therefore decreases their susceptibility to infection.
2. Aids in maintaining the normal color, size, contour, consistency, surface texture and position of the gingival tissues, and so promotes their normal function.
3. Aids in eliminating areas which can retain debris.
4. Aids in the prevention of halitosis due to retention of food debris and the stagnation of saliva.
5. Prepares the teeth and gingiva for dental operations including those performed by the operative dentist, prosthodontist, orthodontist, periodontist, pedodontist and the oral surgeon.

INTRODUCTION TO THE STUDY OF THE DEPOSITS AND STAINS ON THE TEETH

Deposits on the teeth are etiological factors in the production of poor oral health; poor oral health is a predisposing factor in the development of periodontal diseases which may be caused by local irritants to the gingiva. The degree of oral cleanliness, measured in part by the extent of deposits and stains on the teeth,* is one clinical feature of the state of oral health. Since the dental hygienist is a specialist in the preventive aspects of oral hygiene which are related to oral cleanliness, the importance of a clear understanding of the deposits and stains and their significance cannot be overestimated.

*For criteria for evaluating oral cleanliness, see Table 4, page 85.

Some deposit occurs in every mouth, even within 24 to 48 hours following an oral prophylaxis.[2]   To the average patient with limited knowledge of oral hygiene, the primary significance of the deposits and stains is their unsightliness.   Since all deposits are not evident at such cursory inspection, the patient needs to learn where and how the deposits occur and the measures which may be taken to reduce their harmful effects.

The specific techniques used in the oral prophylaxis have been developed on the basis of the properties and characteristics of the various deposits and stains and the relationship of these to the tooth surface and gingival tissue.

General objectives for possessing a detailed knowledge of deposits and stains are:

1. To give direction and meaning to the performance of the specific oral prophylaxis techniques.
2. To understand the role of deposits and stains in the initiation and progress of poor oral health and so plan for individualized patient instruction in personal care procedures and routine recall appointments.

I. LOCATION OF DEPOSITS AND STAINS IN THE ORAL CAVITY

A. **Primary Site:** tooth surfaces.

B. **Other Sites**

   1. *Mucous Membranes:* temporary surface retention of food and debris may occur, particularly in the depths of the mucobuccal and mucolabial folds.
   2. *Free Gingiva:* occasionally heavy deposits on the teeth may extend over the gingival crest.
   3. *Tongue:* surface papillæ provide retentive areas for food particles and desquamated epithelial cells.
   4. *Prosthetic appliances.*

II. GENERAL CLASSIFICATION OF DEPOSITS AND STAINS

A. **Soft Deposits**
   1. Food debris
   2. Dental plaque
   3. Materia alba

B. **Hard Deposit:** Dental calculus

C. **Stains**
   1. Extrinsic
   2. Intrinsic

FACTORS WHICH INFLUENCE THE ACCUMULATION AND RETENTION OF DEPOSITS AND STAINS

A lack of oral cleanliness can well be expected.   Many foreign substances enter the mouth and become involved with the normal processes.   The biochemistry and microbiology of the oral cavity are complex.   The anatomical structures and their physiological functioning are highly specialized.

While applying knowledge of these many factors to instructional and clinical services, an understanding of the entire gamut of basic, basic medical, dental hygiene, clinical and social sciences is utilized.

The etiology or theories of causative factors for each deposit and stain will be outlined with the description of each in the chapters following. This introductory section includes an overview of the features of the oral cavity and the characteristics and habits of the patient which influence the general accumulation and retention of deposits and stains.

I. **NATURE'S ATTEMPT TO PREVENT DEPOSITS: THE SELF-CLEANSING MECHANISMS**

The teeth by their anatomy, alignment and occlusion, the gingiva, the tongue, the cheeks, and the saliva, function in a relationship called the self-cleansing mechanism of the oral cavity.

A review of the self-cleansing mechanisms during and following mastication is included for relating the natural processes to the deviating influences. The steps below are described for food particles, but the same processes apply to many materials which enter into or influence the formation of the deposits. These materials include mineral and organic components of the saliva, microorganisms and foreign substances introduced into the oral cavity.

A. **Food Enters the Mouth** and is carried by the tongue, assisted by the lips and cheeks, to the occlusal surfaces for grinding.

1. Salivary flow: increases due to sensory reflex stimulation.
2. Saliva begins lubrication of food and oral tissues.

B. **The Teeth are Brought Together for Chewing** and the food moves over the occlusal surfaces.

1. Marginal ridges: tend to force particles toward occlusal, away from proximal region.
2. Contact areas: prevent entrance to interproximal area.

C. **Food is Forced Out by Pressure of Bite** and passes over the smooth facial and lingual surfaces.

1. Embrasures: provide spillways for the escape of particles.
2. Cervical enamel ridges: deflect particles away from free gingiva onto attached gingiva.
3. Gingival crest: prevents retention of particles by being positioned at a point below the height of contour of the cervical enamel ridge and by its close adherence to the tooth surface.
4. Interdental papilla: fills the interproximal area and prevents particles from entering.

D. **Food Particles are Brought Back by the Tongue to Occlusal Surfaces** for additional chewing; process is repeated until food is ready for swallowing.

1. Salivary flow: continues to be stimulated with repeated masticatory movements.
2. Saliva: moistens food and thus reduces its adhering capacity.

E. **Food Particles Remaining on the Teeth are Removed**

1. Tip of tongue: explores and attempts to dislodge remaining particles.
2. Lips and cheeks in conjunction with tongue: aid in natural rinsing process by forcing saliva over and between the teeth.
3. Saliva: continues to flow in increased amounts during rinsing and swallowing of particles, then gradually returns to its normal flow.

II. **FACTORS WHICH CONTRIBUTE TO DEPOSIT RETENTION**

In reality, absolute cleanliness never results from the natural self-cleansing mechanisms. If maximum possible benefits are to be obtained, it is necessary to visualize these processes in the "perfect" mouth. The tooth surfaces are smooth; the tooth form and occlusion are ideal; the gingiva is the correct size and contour and in normal relationship to the teeth; the tongue, lips, cheeks and masticatory muscles function in complete harmony; and the saliva is of adequate consistency and quantity for complete lubrication and rinsing of the tooth and gingival surfaces. In addition, the bacterial flora and biochemical constituents and processes must be consistent with normal.

The normal rarely exists. Suggested in this section are many of the common deviations. No attempt will be made to review their causes, as some are obvious and many are related to other areas of study.

A. **Tooth Surface**

1. Any irregularity in the normal smoothness provides a retentive area for deposits.
   a. Pits, grooves.
   b. Lines of fracture.
   c. Rough exposed cementum.
   d. Eroded areas.
   e. Carious lesions.
   f. Inadequately polished dental restorations.
2. Primary cuticle (Nasmyth's Membrane): the tenacious, transparent, colorless membrane which frequently covers the cervical third of the tooth for a few years after eruption until worn off.
   a. Permits incorporation of stains.
   b. Protects accumulations of microorganisms.

B. **Tooth Contour:** Altered shape interferes with self-cleansing mechanisms.

1. Congenital abnormalities
   a. Extra or missing cusps.
   b. Bell-shaped crown with prominent buccal and lingual contours tends to provide deeper retentive area in cervical third.
2. Anterior teeth with flattened proximal surfaces have faulty contact with adjacent teeth, permitting deposits to wedge between.

    3. Occlusal and incisal surfaces altered by attrition interrupt normal excursion of food during chewing.

    4. Dental restorations inadequately contoured allow food to enter interproximal area.

      a. Marginal ridge missing.

      b. Contact area: missing, improperly located, or of unnatural width.

    5. Dental appliances

      a. Orthodontic appliances.

      b. Fixed partial denture with deficient gingival margin or unusually shaped pontic.

      c. Removable partial denture: inadequately adapted clasps.

C. **Position of Teeth: Malocclusion**

    1. Irregular alignment of single tooth or groups of teeth make surfaces inaccessible or ineffective for self-cleansing.

      a. Crowded or overlapped.

      b. Rotated.

      c. Inclined or migrated; contact area usually missing.

      d. Extrusion beyond line of occlusion when tooth in opposing arch is missing or ineffective.

      e. Incomplete eruption.

        (1) Below line of occlusion.

        (2) Partially erupted impacted third molar.

    2. Lack of use of teeth eliminates or decreases function of self-cleansing process.

      a. Lack of opposing teeth.

      b. Openbite.

      c. Severe maxillary anterior protrusion.

      d. Severe crossbite with limited lateral excursion of mandible.

    3. Deep anterior overbite

      a. Mandibular teeth force food particles against maxillary lingual gingiva.

      b. Lingual inclination of mandibular teeth allows maxillary teeth to force food particles against mandibular labial gingiva.

D. **Gingiva**

    1. Deviations from normal position provide retentive areas.

      a. Receded, leaving normal depressed area of tooth at cemento-enamel junction uncovered.

      b. Extended to height of contour of teeth provides access to gingival sulcus.

      c. Reduced height of interdental papilla provides access to interdental space.

      d. Tissue flap over occlusal of erupting tooth.

      e. Periodontal pocket prevents free gingiva from adhering closely to tooth surface which increases retentive capacity of gingival sulcus.

    2. Deviation in size and contour: enlarged gingiva creates retentive area at gingival crest.

    3. Deviation in surface texture: poor tone and inadequate keratinization make gingiva susceptible to laceration and subsequent bleeding which releases blood elements for deposition on tooth surface.

E. **Tongue, Lips, Cheeks:** Limitations of normal activity prevent cleansing and rinsing functions.

    1. Congenital malformations
      a. Tongue
        (1) Tonguetie.
        (2) Macroglossia.
      b. Lips
        (1) Short upper lip.
        (2) Unusually small mouth opening.
    2. Muscle tone and elasticity diminished.
    3. Muscular coordination.
      a. Undeveloped in young child.
      b. Impaired in patients with a neuromuscular disease.

F. **Saliva**

    1. Decreased quantity limits lubricating and rinsing effects.
    2. Thick, viscid consistency (associated with less secretion) acts as agglutinating agent in attaching deposits to the teeth.
    3. Stagnation of saliva permitted.
      a. Decreased activity of tongue, lips and cheeks.
      b. Properties and quantity of saliva: thick, viscid saliva in smaller amounts stagnates more readily.

G. **The Act of Mastication**

    1. Decreased amount of chewing promotes swallowing before food, teeth and mucous membranes are adequately lubricated.
    2. Excessive pressure when teeth are occluded may force food into interproximal areas.

H. **Mouth Breathing**

    1. Dehydration of oral tissues results in insufficient lubrication of the tissue.
    2. Repeated access of air to saliva aids in the ready release of carbon dioxide which in turn contributes to calculus formation (see pages 123–124).

III. **THE INFLUENCE OF MICROORGANISMS IN ACCUMULATION AND RETENTION OF DEPOSITS**

A. Chromogenic bacteria and fungi produce pigments.
B. Filamentous organisms provide organic framework for attaching components of deposits to the teeth.
C. Massive growths may be adhesive and aid in retaining foreign materials.

IV. **THE EFFECTS OF DIETARY AND EATING HABITS**

A. **Physical Character of Foods Used in the Diet**

    1. Soft, moist, nondetergent foods.
      a. Adhere to tooth surface.
      b. Not returned readily to occlusal surface for continued chewing during mastication.

   c. Most effective in deposit formation if eaten at end of meal.
   d. Particles left on teeth provide food for bacterial proliferation.
  2. Firm, crispy, fibrous, detergent foods.
   a. Require more chewing, hence stimulate increased flow of saliva.
   b. Are effective in mechanical cleansing of teeth.
  3. Fluid in diet (especially water).
   a. Insufficient, especially following food ingestion, limits aid given to the natural cleansing process.
   b. Excessive, during meals.
    (1) Softens food which detracts from cleansing effects.
    (2) Promotes early swallowing of food before excess salivary flow is stimulated. Excess saliva is required for cleansing of teeth.

B. **Diet Selection**
 1. Masticatory deficiencies limit selection of firm abrasive foods.
 2. Tasteless, bland foods fail to stimulate as much salivary flow.
 3. Repeated use of foods containing natural pigments provides coloring matter for certain stains.

C. **Eating Habits**
 1. Insufficient mastication: "bolting" food.
  a. Mechanical cleansing effects of food not utilized.
  b. Salivary secretion insufficiently stimulated because of less time.
 2. Unbalanced chewing
  a. Unilateral chewing to avoid sensitive gingiva or teeth, edentulous areas.
  b. Decreased bite pressure to avoid pain from sensitive teeth.

V. **THE EFFECTS OF DRUGS, TOBACCO AND OTHER FOREIGN SUBSTANCES**

A. **Drugs**
 1. Internal effect of certain drugs alters quantity of saliva.
 2. External effect of coloring agents from certain drugs may provide material for staining.

B. **Tobacco**
 1. Increases salivary flow.
 2. Contains tar products which stain teeth.

C. **Dentifrices:** may contain staining agent.

D. **Metal-Containing Dust Inhaled by Industrial Workers:** Certain metals contain coloring agents effective in staining the teeth (see page 133).

VI. **PERSONAL ORAL CARE HABITS**

A. **Neglect**
 1. The natural self-cleansing mechanisms are inadequate, and must be supplemented by meticulous personal care.
 2. Incomplete or inadequate brushing of less accessible areas encourages deposit retention in those areas.

B. **Effects of Faulty Techniques in Creating Retentive Areas**
   1. Alteration of position or contour of gingiva (see page 106).
      a. Receded from vigorous brushing against free gingiva.
      b. Chronic horizontal or circular brushing may change shape of gingival crest.
   2. Vigorous repeated horizontal brushing may abrade the enamel and cementum and create a groove.
   3. Incorrect use of toothbrush, interdental stimulator, dental floss or tape may result in reduction in height of interdental papillae.

VII. **INDIVIDUAL CHARACTERISTICS RELATED TO ACCUMULATION AND RETENTION OF DEPOSITS**
   A. **Age**
      1. Greatest incidence of certain deposits and stains tends to be related to age groups.
      2. Effects on retentive areas of teeth and gingiva.
         a. Gingiva around erupting teeth.
         b. Natural physiological processes alter position, contour and surface texture of gingiva with aging.
         c. Physiological gingival recession and continued eruption due to attrition exposes cemento-enamel junction area.
      3. Indirect effect: lack of muscular coordination required for effective toothbrushing and rinsing.
         a. Undeveloped in young.
         b. Diminished in aged.
   B. **Awareness of Oral Cleanliness**[3]
      1. Self-cleansing efficiency depends in part on the individual's perception of debris by oral sensation (taste and touch).
      2. Tongue activity in cleansing decreased with lack of awareness.
   C. **Emotional Disturbances**
      1. Changes in salivary flow: fear and anxiety decrease flow.
      2. Neglected oral care habits frequently accompany poor mental hygiene.
      3. Poor diet selection, including excessive carbohydrates and other soft foods, is characteristic of the emotionally disturbed.[4]

FACTORS TO TEACH THE PATIENT

   I. The interrelationship of the natural self-cleansing mechanisms, personal oral care habits, and the professionally administered oral prophylaxis in preventing deposit retention.
  II. The application of the objectives of the oral prophylaxis to the individual patient's oral health.
 III. Types of foods which aid in cleaning the teeth as compared to foods which do not.
  IV. Information and techniques which will help to develop an awareness of oral cleanliness.
   V. Specific oral care procedures related to the individual's problem of deposit and stain retention.

REFERENCES

1. Bunting, R. W.: *Oral Hygiene*, 3rd ed. Philadelphia, Lea & Febiger, 1957, p. 233.
2. Hanke, M. T.: Studies on the Local Factors in Dental Caries, Am. Dent. A. J., *27*, 1379, September, 1940.
3. Goose, D. H. and Jones, H. P. A.: Introductory Study of the Self-Cleansing Action of the Mouth, Brit. Dent. J., *100*, 272, May 15, 1956.
4. Grant, D., Stern, I. B., and Everett, F. G.: *Orban's Periodontics*, 2nd ed. St. Louis, Mosby, 1963, pp. 549–552.

SUGGESTED READINGS

Baer, P. N.: Relation of the Physical Character of the Diet to the Periodontium and Periodontal Disease, Oral Surg., Oral Med., & Oral Path., *9*, 839, August, 1956.
Bunting, R. W.: *Oral Hygiene*, 3rd ed. Philadelphia, Lea & Febiger, 1957, pp. 94–120, 121–122, 233–234.
Kerr, D. A. and Ash, M. M.: *Oral Pathology*. Philadelphia, Lea & Febiger, 1960, pp. 94–95.
Miller, J.: Relationship of Occlusion and Toothbrushing with Caries Rate, J. Dent. Res., *40*, 1282, November-December, 1961. (Abstr.)
Miller, S. C.: *Textbook of Periodontia*, 3rd ed. New York, Blakiston Division, McGraw-Hill 1950, pp. 76–78.
O'Rourke, J. T. and Miner, L. M. S.: *Oral Physiology*. St. Louis, Mosby, 1951, pp. 38–103.
Swartz, M. L. and Phillips, R. W.: Comparison of Bacterial Accumulations on Rough and Smooth Enamel Surfaces, J. Periodont., *28*, 304, October, 1957.

Chapter 11

SOFT DEPOSITS

DENTAL PLAQUE

DENTAL plaque is a thin, tenacious, film-like deposit made up principally of microorganisms and mucinous substances from the saliva. It is removed by polishing procedures. Plaque is the most commonly found of all tooth deposits and occurs on the clinical crowns of the teeth particularly on surfaces not directly exposed to cleansing mechanisms. It often provides the basis for attachment of other deposits including food debris, materia alba and calculus. Stains become impregnated in dental plaque.

I. TERMINOLOGY

There is a wide variance in terminology used in the literature to describe the soft, extraneous material which adheres to tooth surfaces. Stephan[1] lists no less than 27 names which have been used by various authors. The substances listed are not all identical, but have never been classified specifically.

Collections of food debris and creamy-white materia alba may be distinguished clinically from the relatively thin, transparent deposits grouped under the general term "dental plaque." Since dental plaques vary in thickness, degree of adherence to the tooth surface, and percentage composition, a distinction between "film" and "plaque" is sometimes convenient.

A. **Film**
1. Common names used: "mucinous film," "mucinous plaque."
2. Characteristics
   a. Thin, viscous.
   b. High content of salivary mucin, fewer microorganisms.
   c. Lightly attached to tooth surface.

B. **Plaque**
1. Common names used: "bacterial plaque," "true plaque," "acid plaque."
2. Characteristics
   a. Thick.
   b. High content of microorganisms, less of mucin.
   c. Firmly attached to tooth surface.
   d. May be discolored by stains.

C. **Notes Concerning Interrelation of Film and Plaque**
1. Film may be considered as freshly formed plaque.
2. Film frequently occurs on the outer surface of plaque.
3. Thickness and extent of either vary on different teeth at different times and in different individuals.[1]

II. **CLINICAL CHARACTERISTICS**

Dental plaque may be thin and transparent and therefore seen only after the application of a disclosing solution, or it may be thick and discolored which gives the tooth a dull surface. Knowledge of the characteristics and composition is important to identification and removal (Table 5).

TABLE 5.—CLINICAL CHARACTERISTICS OF DENTAL PLAQUE
AND MATERIA ALBA

Characteristic	Dental Plaque	Materia Alba

CLINICAL APPEARANCE	*Tooth:* dull, dingy.
	Thin or freshly deposited plaque:
	  Transparent (seen only after application of disclosing solution).
	  or
	  Stained by substances from foods, tobacco, or chromogenic bacteria.
	Heavy or old plaque:
	  Matted, fur-like surface, usually stained.
		Soft, cheese-like, mealy substance.
		White or cream colored.
		Opaque.
		May extend over crest of free gingiva.
		Gingiva: frequently shows marginal redness.

DISTRIBUTION ON TEETH	Protected areas not readily exposed to self-cleansing mechanisms.
	Most frequent surfaces:
	  Facial (cervical third)
	  Proximal
	  Lingual: mandibular molars
	  Buccal: maxillary molars
		Surfaces not exposed to cleansing mechanisms.
		May cover entire crown of tooth out of occlusion.
		Proximal surfaces exposed when interdental papilla is of reduced height.
		Most frequent at cervical third of:
		  Labial: anterior
		  Buccal: maxillary molars
		  Lingual: mandibular molars.

COMPOSITION	Primarily protein. Mucinous & colloidal materials from saliva, Desquamated epithelial cells. Leukocytes. Living & dead microorganisms (large numbers, wide variety). Bacterial products & enzyme systems.	Food debris (gross). Mucin. Desquamated epithelial cells. Masses of bacteria and fungi multiplying profusely. Bacterial products. Purulent matter.
OCCURRENCE	All teeth. Tends to deposit more rapidly on teeth of caries susceptible persons. Film or plaque-like substance occurs on removable dentures.	All teeth not subjected to cleansing mechanisms.

RELATION TO TECHNIQUES OF ORAL PROPHYLAXIS	Clinical appearance does not reveal tenacity to tooth.
	Tenacity varies with thickness and age of deposit:
	  Thin: May be mildly tenacious and readily removed with abrasive.
	  Heavy: May be very tenacious and require repeated polishing with abrasive.
		Masses are readily removed with slight abrasive action.

RECURRENCE	Within 24 to 48 hours after oral prophylaxis.	Readily when teeth are not cleaned routinely by toothbrushing, action of detergent foods, or self-cleansing mechanisms.

III. MANNER OF FORMATION

Dental plaque is protein in nature and a product of oral metabolism. Its etiology has not been definitely established but it is evident that its formation is dependent on the ability of microorganisms and salivary protein components to adhere to the tooth surface.

The sources of the protein materials of which the plaque is composed are believed to be microorganisms and saliva rather than food. It has been shown that when teeth are thoroughly cleaned (plaque completely removed), the mouth placed at rest, and no food ingested, the plaque reforms readily. This research shows that the materials are provided by sources in the mouth.[2]

A. Etiological Theories

1. Bacterial

   Filamentous organisms form a strongly adherent mesh-like colony which provides a network for the inclusion of other microorganisms and plaque components.[3]
2. Mucinous (theory less strongly supported)

   Bacteria, acting upon carbohydrate, liberate organic acids which cause the precipitation of mucin from the saliva. The mucin forms the mucinous plaque.[4]

B. Predisposing Factors

1. Natural tendencies of the individual.
2. Saliva
   a. Consistency: thick, high mucin content.
   b. Stagnation around teeth makes components available for deposition.
3. Oral flora and the sources of nutrients for proliferation.
4. Lack of oral cleanliness: may affect amount of plaque and provide ready source of nutrients for bacterial proliferation.

IV. SIGNIFICANCE

Heavy plaques have an esthetic significance as they give teeth a dull, dingy, discolored appearance. In addition to their unsightliness, some plaques produce harmful effects while others are harmless. This may be related to the variation in physical properties and composition.

A. Protective Action

1. Mechanical: plaque acts as a barrier to prevent direct contact of saliva and food with the teeth.[2,3]
2. Buffering: plaque possesses high capacity (when acidogenic microorganisms do not predominate) for buffering weak acids which occur in foods, and acids produced from weak sugar solutions.[5]

B. Role in Deposit Retention: Plaques form the basis for attachment of materia alba, calculus, stains and bacterial outgrowths.

C. Role in Gingival Irritation: Thick plaque may be mechanically irritating and may produce or promote gingival marginal redness.

D. Role in Dental Caries Initiation: Dental caries is a disease of the dental calcified structures (enamel, dentin, cementum) which is

8

characterized by decalcification of the mineral components and dissolution of the organic matrix. The three major factors which are related to dental caries development are the fermentable carbohydrate foodstuffs, the enzymes of the oral microorganisms, and the tooth surface with physical and chemical composition subject to decalcification. A tooth rich in fluoride content will resist the process of dental caries (see page 199).

The type of diet of an individual influences the type of microorganisms present in the dental plaque. A diet which includes many fermentable carbohydrates encourages the multiplication of acidogenic (acid-forming) microorganisms. When a carbohydrate reaches the plaque during eating, the acidogenic microorganisms ferment the carbohydrate to an acid which is capable of decalcifying the tooth surface to form the initial area of early dental caries. This process may be outlined as follows:

Fermentable Carbohydrate	+	Action of Microbial Enzymes	=	Organic Acid
Acid	+	Enamel Surface	=	Enamel Decalcification (Initial Dental Caries)

The acid formation begins *immediately* following the contact of the dissolved carbohydrate with the tooth surface plaque. The pH level of the plaque is lowered, and does not return to normal pH for 1 to 2 hours[6] if left undisturbed by toothbrush, noncarbohydrate foods, or water. The frequency of eating foods containing fermentable carbohydrate is significant, as the number of times a day in which acid is formed on the tooth surface contributes to the extent and number of carious lesions.

For further understanding, more detail is outlined in the steps below.

1. *The plaque prior to carbohydrate contact.*
   a. Acidogenic microorganisms collect and are held by the plaque on the tooth surface, particularly in protected areas.
   b. Plaque retains nutrients useful for proliferation of the microorganisms.
   c. Normal pH: ranges from 6.4 to 7.0, different in different individuals, lower in caries susceptible individuals.
2. *Fermentable carbohydrate taken into mouth:* sugar solution enters plaque.
   a. Weak sugar solution: plaque is relatively impermeable to weak acids and weak sugar solutions and those that do permeate are buffered.
   b. Strong sugar solution: creates drastic change in osmotic pressure; draws sugar into the plaque.
      (1) Occurs rapidly when glucose or sucrose are present.
      (2) Starch molecules do not penetrate unless they are broken down (digested) by salivary amylase.
3. *Rapid acid formation with drop in pH of plaque.*[6,7]
4. *Buffering capacity of plaque lowered:* proves insufficient because of quantity and rapid formation of acid.
5. *Decalcification of enamel.*

    a. Critical pH considered to average 5.0 (may be 5.5 in some individuals) below which the enamel will decalcify.[7]

    b. Amount of decalcification depends on length of time and frequency that acid at pH below 5.0 maintains contact with tooth enamel.

  6. *pH of plaque returns to normal level in 1 to 2 hours.*[6]

MATERIA ALBA

Materia alba is a thick, cream-white, loosely attached deposit observed on the teeth as a result of uncleanliness and a nondetergent diet. It can be removed by the patient with the toothbrush. When a patient with excessive deposits of materia alba presents for an oral prophylaxis, it is well to give brushing instruction and request the patient to demonstrate toothbrushing in his mouth. By this means gross deposits will be removed prior to instrumentation.

I. CLINICAL CHARACTERISTICS

Materia alba has sometimes been called a "white soft plaque," a term which is readily understood when the composition is compared with dental plaque. Food debris is present in greater quantity in materia alba than in plaque, and there is marked profusion of molds, fungi and many types of bacteria which add bulk to the deposit. Other clinical characteristics are listed in Table 5, page 112.

II. MANNER OF FORMATION

A. Etiology

    1. Accumulation of food debris is associated with massive growth of microorganisms.

    2. Dental plaque usually aids in retention by providing a roughened sticky surface.

    3. Microorganisms gain nutrients from the accumulated food debris which promotes further proliferation.

    4. Accumulations remain undisturbed as cleansing mechanisms are absent.

B. Predisposing Factors

Of all the deposits found on the teeth, materia alba provides the most direct application for practically all of the factors related to the accumulation and retention of deposits as described in Chapter 10. Physical factors in the care of the teeth play an important role in its formation as this deposit is directly related to oral uncleanliness.

    1. Inadequate or neglected personal oral care habits.

    2. Soft diet containing many carbohydrates.

III. SIGNIFICANCE

Materia alba is unsightly due to the heavy accumulation of debris which gives the appearance of unclean teeth. Generally when materia alba covers the cervical third of a tooth, heavy dental plaque covers at least the central third.   In contrast to dental plaque, materia alba has no protective action.

A. **Gingival Irritation:** May produce or promote gingival marginal redness.
  1. The bulk of the debris serves as a mechanical irritant.
  2. Metabolic products of proteolytic organisms found in materia alba have been associated with gingival inflammation.[8]
  3. Toxic products of microorganisms may be absorbed through the gingival epithelium causing local inflammation.

B. **Breath Odor:** Decomposing food debris and purulent matter within the materia alba contribute to halitosis.

C. **Role in Dental Caries Initiation** (when acidogenic microorganisms are present).

Materia alba localizes large numbers of acid-forming microorganisms on the tooth surface and provides a wealth of nutrients for their proliferation.   Aid is given the underlying plaque in acid formation when fermentable carbohydrates are taken into the mouth (see page 114).

FACTORS TO TEACH THE PATIENT

I. The effects of thorough personal oral care procedures in the prevention of soft deposits.
II. Specific foods which have cleansing effects on the teeth compared with foods which cling to the teeth.
III. Specific foods containing glucose and sucrose as compared to foods containing starch.
IV. The cause and prevention of dental caries.

REFERENCES

1. STEPHAN, R. M.:   The Dental Plaque in Relation to the Etiology of Caries, Internat. Dent. J. 4, 180, December, 1953.
2. FOSDICK, L. S.:   Some New Concepts Concerning the Role of Sugar in Dental Caries, Oral Surg., Oral Med., & Oral Path., 5, 615, June, 1952.
3. BIBBY, B. G.:   Neglected Factors in the Study of Dental Caries, Am. Dent. A. J., 22, 222, February, 1935.
4. KIRK, E. C.:   A Consideration of the Question of Susceptibility and Immunity to Dental Caries, D. Cosmos, 52, 729, July, 1910.
5. FOSDICK, L. S.:   Theoretical Considerations of Certain Phases of the Caries Problem, Northwestern Univ. Bul., p. 4, Autumn, 1949.
6. STEPHAN, R. M.:   Changes in Hydrogen-Ion Concentrations on Tooth Surfaces and in Carious Lesions, Am. Dent. A. J., 27, 718, May, 1940.
7. STEPHAN, R. M.:   Intra-oral Hydrogen-Ion Concentrations Associated with Dental Caries Activity, J. Dent. Res., 23, 257, August, 1944.
8. KIMBALL, G. C.:   The Relationship of Materia Alba and Dental Plaque to Periodontal Disease, J. Periodont., 23, 164, July, 1952.

SUGGESTED READINGS

ANDLAW, R. J., BIBBY, B. G., and BUONOCORE, M. G.:   Cariogenicity of Foods, Dent. Prog., 3, 36, October, 1962.

BUNTING, R. W.:   *Oral Hygiene,* 3rd ed. Philadelphia, Lea & Febiger, 1957, pp. 121–125.

FOSDICK, L. S.:   Biochemical Aspects of Dental Caries, Dental Clinics of North America, July, 1962, p. 369.

GLICKMAN, IRVING: *Clinical Periodontology,* 2nd ed. Philadelphia, Saunders, 1958, p. 319.

KERR, D. A. and ASH, M. M.:   *Oral Pathology.* Philadelphia, Lea & Febiger, 1960, pp. 100–102, 109–123.

LEUNG, S. W.:   Saliva and Dental Caries, Dental Clinics of North America, July, 1962, p. 347.

VOLKER, J. F. and CALDWELL, R. C.:   The Etiology of Dental Caries, in Finn, S. B.:   *Clinical Pedodontics,* 2nd ed. Philadelphia, Saunders, 1962, pp. 613–634.

WILDMAN, J. D.:   A Cellular Study of Plaque, Dent. Prog., *2,* 211, April, 1962.

WILDMAN, J. D.:   Living Matrix of Plaque, Dent. Prog., *3,* 183, April, 1963.

Chapter 12

DENTAL CALCULUS

Dental calculus is a hard, calcified, tenacious mass which may occur on the clinical crowns of the natural teeth and on dentures and other dental appliances. It is removed from the teeth by scaling procedures. Complete removal followed by polishing to provide a smooth tooth surface is important in delaying attachment of new deposits.

A major purpose for performing the oral prophylaxis is to prevent periodontal disease initiated by local irritants. Of the factors considered causes for such periodontal disease, calculus plays an extremely important part.

Patients ask questions about calculus. If they do not ask, it behooves the dental hygienist to motivate their interest in understanding this oral problem. The patient should appreciate the need for frequent appointments for the removal of calculus, the length of the individual appointment, and the painstaking manner in which scaling procedures are carried out.

The patient also needs to be instructed in personal oral care procedures which will reduce calculus formation. When the soft deposits of beginning calculus are carefully removed within a short time after they collect, calcification cannot take place and hard calculus does not form. Thorough toothbrushing assisted by the action of detergent foods during chewing is believed to be the most effective way to retard calculus formation, although this method does not completely prevent it.

Understanding about calculus is, then, very important in the prevention of periodontal disease of local origin. A large part of clinical practice hours are devoted to removing the deposit from the teeth and providing instruction for patients.

I. CLASSIFICATION AND TERMINOLOGY

Dental calculus occurs on the clinical crown of the tooth. It is classified by its location on the tooth surface as related to the adjacent gingival tissue (Figure 35).

A. Supramarginal Calculus
1. Characteristics
   a. Located above the margin of the free gingiva.
   b. Visible in the oral cavity.
2. Other names
   a. Supragingival*
   b. Extragingival
   c. Coronal
   d. Salivary: a term formerly used to indicate that the source of the calculus was the saliva.

* The terms supra- and subgingival are at present probably the most widely used. Supra- and submarginal are more specific in their definition since the margin of the free gingiva is the dividing line between the two categories. The gingiva includes free, papillary and attached. Hence supra- and subgingival are not as accurate.

B. **Submarginal Calculus**

1. Characteristics
   a. Located beneath the margin of the free gingiva.
   b. Not directly visible in the oral cavity.
   c. Located within the confines of the gingival sulcus or perio-
      dontal pocket.
   d. Always extends to the bottom of the gingival sulcus or perio-
      dontal pocket; deepest deposit less calcified.
   e. When the gingiva recedes, the exposed parts of the sub-
      marginal deposits are classified as supramarginal.
2. Other names
   a. Subgingival
   b. Serumal: a term formerly used when it was believed that
      the source of the calculus was the blood.

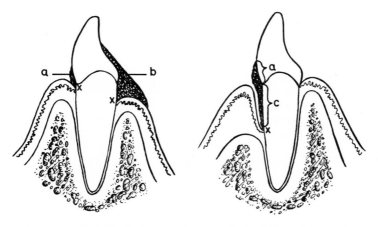

FIGURE 35.—Location of dental calculus. a. Supramarginal calculus. b. Extensive accumulation
of supramarginal calculus over crown, exposed root surface, and margin of the free gingiva.
c. Submarginal calculus along root surface to bottom of periodontal pocket. x. Bottom of pocket
or sulcus. Note level of crest of alveolar bone in relation to bottom of the sulcus. (Modified from
Miller, *Textbook of Periodontia*, Blakiston Division, McGraw-Hill Book Co.)

II. **COMPOSITION OF CALCULUS**

Calculus is made up of inorganic and organic constituents and water.
The chemical content of supramarginal and submarginal is similar.[1-3]
The organic matter and water content varies from as little as 10 per
cent to as high as 50 per cent depending on the age and hardness of the
deposit. The average fully calcified calculus has 75 to 80 per cent inorganic and 20 to 25 per cent organic matter and water.

Under the microscope it is apparent that calculus is deposited in
layers. On the surface of the deposit is a thick, matlike, soft layer of
microorganisms of many varieties mixed with epithelial cells, food
debris, and polymorphonuclear leukocytes.

A. **Inorganic**

The constituents are mainly salts of calcium, calcium phosphate
primarily, with small amounts of magnesium phosphate and calcium carbonate. Various trace elements have been identified.

At least two-thirds of the inorganic matter is crystalline, principally apatite. Hydroxyapatite predominates, which is the same crystal present in bone, enamel, dentin and cementum. (Dental enamel is the most highly calcified tissue in the body and contains 96 per cent inorganic salts as compared with dentin, 69 per cent, and cementum and bone with 46 per cent.[4]) Calculus also contains varying amounts of the crystalline salts brushite, whitlockite, and tetracalcium hydrogen triphosphate.[5] The inorganic elements are derived from the saliva.

B. Organic Matter and Water

The organic portion consists of microorganisms, salivary mucins, and desquamated cells. Substances identified in the organic matrix include fat, cholesterol, cholesterol esters, phospholipids, fatty acids, keratin, nucleoprotein, mucopolysaccharides, and a number of amino acids.[6]

The microorganisms are predominantly filamentous: Leptothrix, Leptotrichia, and Actinomyces. In early calculus, during the first five days, cocci are found in greater abundance than in older calculus. This was demonstrated in research studies using celluloid strips around teeth in the mouth when it was possible to examine the newly formed calculus at frequent intervals.[7-9]

III. CHARACTERISTICS OF CALCULUS WHICH INFLUENCE SCALING TECHNIQUES

A. Physical Character and Distribution

Identification of calculus prior to removal depends on knowledge of the appearance and extent of calculus as determined by clinical and radiographic examination. Selection of scalers and definition of techniques depend upon understanding of the texture, location, morphology and attachment of calculus. For complete dental hygiene care for the patient, calculus must be entirely removed and the tooth surface left smooth. Table 6 provides a summary of the clinical characteristics of calculus.

TABLE 6.—CLINICAL CHARACTERISTICS OF DENTAL CALCULUS

Characteristic	Supramarginal Calculus	Submarginal Calculus
COLOR	White, creamy-yellow, or gray. May be stained by tobacco, food or other pigments.	Light to dark brown, dark green or black. Stains derived from pigments of blood from irritated tissue lining the sulcus.
TEXTURE	Soft and sticky when first formed, prior to calcification. Moderately hard. Clay-like.	Soft and sticky when first formed prior to calcification. Dense and hard. Deposit deepest in sulcus not as hard as rest of deposit. Flint-like, brittle, depending on mode of attachment.

TABLE 6. (Continued)

Characteristic	Supramarginal Calculus	Submarginal Calculus
DISTRIBUTION ON TEETH	Uneven. May occur on a single tooth or group of teeth. Occurs with or without associated submarginal calculus. Deposits are related to openings of salivary ducts: 1. Buccal maxillary molar teeth. 2. Lingual mandibular anterior teeth. Collects more readily on: 1. Malpositioned teeth. 2. Nonfunctioning teeth.	Uneven. May occur on a single tooth or a group of teeth. Occurs with or without associated supramarginal calculus.
DISTRIBUTION ON INDIVIDUAL TOOTH	Above margin of free gingiva. May cover large portion of visible clinical crown.	Below margin of free gingiva. Within confines of gingival sulcus or periodontal pocket. Always extends to bottom of sulcus or pocket: lower border of soft deepest deposit is associated with line of epithelial attachment. As quantity of calculus increases, epithelial attachment moves accordingly toward apex of tooth. When gingiva recedes, submarginal becomes supramarginal: may become covered with deposits having color and texture of supramarginal.
FORM	Amorphous, bulky. Gross deposits may: 1. Form interproximal bridge between adjacent teeth. 2. Extend over margin of the gingiva. Shape of mass determined by anatomy of tooth, contour of gingival margin, and pressure of tongue, lips, cheeks.	Flattened to conform with pressure of free gingiva. Combinations of the following forms occur:[10-12] 1. Crusty, spiny or nodular formations. 2. Ledge or ring-like formations around the tooth. 3. Thin, smooth veneers. 4. Finger and fern-like formations. 5. Individual calculus islands.
RADIOGRAPHIC APPEARANCE	Radiopacity of enamel and dentin usually prevent calculus from producing radiographic image. Very dense deposits will be visible.	Gross deposits appear as irregularly shaped clumps or circular ledges on proximal surfaces. Tooth structure usually too radiopaque to permit lingual and facial calculus deposits to produce image. Calculus adjacent to epithelial attachment not calcified enough to be radiopaque (therefore calculus in radiograph does not indicate bottom of sulcus or pocket).
OCCURRENCE	Occurs in any age group. Occurs in almost all adults. Equally common to both sexes. Quantity has direct relationship to personal oral care procedures and physical character of diet.	Rarely occurs on primary teeth. Frequently occurs in adults. Equally common to both sexes. Quantity has direct relationship to personal oral care procedures and physical character of diet.

B. **Manner of Attachment to the Tooth Surface**

Calculus is more easily removed from some teeth or surfaces than others. The ease or difficulty may be related to the manner of attachment of the calculus.

1. Bacteria attach calculus to the tooth.

When calculus first begins to form, filamentous bacteria form a meshwork or matrix and attach themselves to the surface of enamel or cementum. The entire mechanism of the attachment of the bacteria has not been defined but four ways of attachment have been studied from sections under a microscope.[13-15] Two or more of these are generally involved in the attachment of any one piece of calculus. The four modes of attachment are listed below. The first two are most common.

2. Modes of attachment
   a. *Calculus is attached to the secondary cuticle.*
      (1) Secondary cuticle is a thin, homogenous, noncellular, keratinous structure covering the enamel and cementum.
      (2) Cuticle lies between the tooth and the calculus.
      (3) Attachment of calculus is superficial since there is no penetration into the tooth surface.
      (4) Calculus is most readily removed when attached by this means.
   b. *Cuticle is absent and bacterial matrix is attached to minute irregularities in the surface of the cementum or enamel.*
      (1) Irregularities of the cemental surface may be minute spaces previously occupied by fibers of the periodontal membrane before the recession of the epithelial attachment.
      (2) Irregularities of the enamel may be lamellæ or cracks.
      (3) Calculus attached by this mode can be removed readily.
   c. *Bacteria of matrix penetrate into the cementum to various depths.*
      (1) Complete calculus removal is difficult.
      (2) Impossible to remove calculus without removing some cementum.
   d. *Bacteria of matrix attach into areas of cemental resorption.*
      (1) Cemental resorption may occur when cementum is exposed following gingival recession.
      (2) Irregularities may be in the form of undercuts which would lock the calculus to the area.
      (3) Impossible to remove calculus without removing some cementum.

FORMATION OF CALCULUS

Two major steps referred to as the *Attachment Phase* and the *Precipitation and Crystallization Phase* make up the process of calculus deposition.[16] First, the organic material is laid down as a matrix, then, through a calcification process, the hard deposit results. Layers are added and calcification occurs irregularly so that microscopically the form appears in swirls, clumps or tiers. The two major phases described below should be visualized as a continuing process.

I. ATTACHMENT PHASE

A. **Location:** in protected area undisturbed by self-cleansing or tooth-brushing. Malposition of teeth, rough surfaces, previous deposits, and inadequate personal care favor deposition (see pages 105–109).

B. **Matrix Formation.** The organic matrix of calculus consists of microorganisms, primarily filamentous forms, and a fine fibrillar meshwork throughout the areas between the microorganisms as seen by electronmicroscopic examination.[17–19]

   The microorganisms collect together, multiply, and form the matrix which attaches itself to the tooth surface by the modes of attachment previously described.

C. **Soft calculus is formed:** composed of bacterial matrix, desquamated epithelial cells, leukocytes, food debris, mucin.

D. **Calcification Within the Matrix**

   There is general agreement that the elements that form calculus come primarily from the saliva, but serum and gingival exudate may also contribute particularly to the content of submarginal calculus which forms in close proximity to the soft tissues of the wall of the sulcus or pocket.

   A definite pattern of calcification occurs within the matrix: first, the crystals are laid down on the surface of and between the bacteria, then later inside them or in the spaces remaining after the organisms have degenerated.[17–19]

II. PRECIPITATION AND CRYSTALLIZATION PHASE

The mechanisms by which the inorganic elements are precipitated out of the saliva, collect in the bacterial matrix, and come to form the complex apatite structure in calculus are not fully known.

A. **Calcification Process**

   The exact mechanism of the calcification of dental calculus and other ectopic calcifications (such as urinary or renal calculi) has not been completely defined, nor has the normal calcification of bone, cartilage, enamel or dentin. Current research studies point to the probability that calcification of calculus may involve the same phenomena as for other calcifications in the body.

   In the oral cavity, a number of possible mechanisms are probably in operation simultaneously during calculus formation. Some of the contributing factors are described below. It is hoped that the reader will supplement the material presented here with the excellent reviews which have appeared in the literature.[2,5,10,20–22] There are many unanswered questions in this complex body process. Physical, biochemical, microbiological, physiological and pathological sciences are among those involved.

   1. *Physical-Chemical Factors*
      There are factors responsible for holding the inorganic salts in

solution and factors which allow the salts to precipitate out of the saliva.* In order for the salts to leave the saliva and be available to the calculus matrix, there must be an increased alkalinity of the saliva (pH increase).† When this happens, the inorganic salts become less soluble and precipitate out.

The amount of carbon dioxide in the saliva influences the alkalinity of the saliva as follows:

a. Carbon dioxide in solution in the saliva forms carbonic acid which makes the saliva acid. The carbonic acid keeps the inorganic salts in solution.

b. When the freshly secreted saliva enters the oral cavity, there is a loss of carbon dioxide as the saliva comes in contact with the air. The effects are as follows:

(1) Carbon dioxide tension of alveolar air (40 mm. mercury) is less than the carbon dioxide tension of saliva (60 mm. mercury).

(2) There is a tendency to equalize the tension between the air and the saliva which results in a decrease in carbon dioxide of the saliva.

(3) Equalization of tension occurs immediately upon contact with air at the openings of the salivary ducts (helps to explain the most common locations of supramarginal calculus).

(4) The decrease in carbon dioxide means that there is less carbonic acid in the saliva, therefore the inorganic salts cannot be held in solution and are precipitated out. The salts are then available for calculus formation.

2. *Bacteriological factors*

The exact role of bacteria in calculus formation is not clear. Some authorities have believed that bacteria, through their metabolic processes, produce environmental changes which lead to an alkaline pH of the saliva in which the inorganic salts cannot stay in solution.

Recent studies with germ-free animals suggest that bacteria are not essential to calcification. The germ-free mice were shown to be subject to calculus formation and a type of periodontal destruction.[25–27]

3. *Epitactic concept*[21,28]

This newer concept emphasizes the role of the calculus matrix in initiating calcification. It is suggested that a "primary seed" of the organic matrix provides the link for the crystallization of the inorganic salts to hydroxyapatite. A "local factor" must be present in any calcifying matrix as evidenced by the fact that calcification takes place only in specific sites in the body.[29] Mucopolysaccharides are believed to play a definite role as a local factor.[30]

---

*The approximate content of saliva: water 99 to 99.5 per cent and total solids 0.5 to 1.0. The solids include inorganic salts (chlorides, carbonates, and phosphates of sodium, calcium, potassium and magnesium); gases (carbon dioxide, oxygen, nitrogen); and organic substances (enzymes, serum albumin and globulin, urea, uric acid, creatine, amino acids and salivary mucin).[23]

†The normal pH of the resting saliva is within the range of 6.2 to 7.4. The average is considered to be 6.8.[23,24]

REACTION OF GINGIVA TO THE PRESENCE OF CALCULUS

Calculus serves as an irritant to the gingival tissue. The rough surface of the deposit accumulates bacteria and debris. The bacteria produce substances which are toxic to the gingiva. The inflammation which results is the response to the bacterial-chemical agents.[31]

I. CHARACTERISTIC CHANGES IN THE APPEARANCE OF THE GINGIVA

To understand the gingival changes a clear knowledge of the appearance of the normal gingiva is essential for comparison. See Figure 22 and pages 85–88 for a description of the normal. All of the changes which may be affected by calculus listed below do not occur in every patient (Figure 36).

A. **Color:** darkens toward red, magenta, or blue.

B. **Size:** enlarges or recedes.

C. **Contour**
  1. Margin of the free gingiva: becomes rounded.
  2. Interdental papilla: blunted or flat (varies with spacing of the teeth).

D. **Consistency:** spongy, nonresilient.

E. **Surface Texture:** stippling may be lost; may become glossy.

F. **Position.** (See also II. D., page 106.)
  1. Margin of the free gingiva: position changes because of enlargement or recession of tissue.
  2. Gingival sulcus: increased depth related to submarginal deposits.
    a. Calculus stimulates recession of epithelial attachment.
    b. Enlargement of tissue may place margin of free gingiva higher on the crown which makes the sulcus deeper.

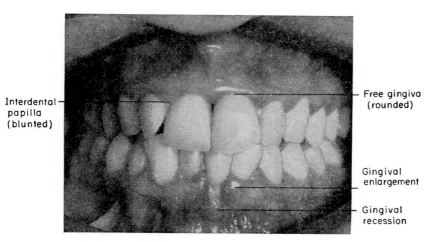

Interdental papilla (blunted)

Free gingiva (rounded)

Gingival enlargement

Gingival recession

FIGURE 36.—Gingival reactions to calculus on the teeth.

II. **TIME FACTOR IMPORTANT TO APPOINTMENT PLANNING**

The accumulation of calculus and the reaction of the surrounding tissue varies considerably in different individuals. The process should be understood as a long range one, requiring months and even years. The length of time before severe periodontal damage occurs also varies.

The presence of calculus is rarely painful or annoying to the individual because of the long range factor in its formation. The patient tends to become accustomed to its presence and is usually unaware of it until it accumulates in such quantity that it may be seen, or the gingiva bleed readily during toothbrushing.

PREVENTION OF CALCULUS FORMATION

To date there is no known therapeutic agent which successfully yet safely inhibits calculus formation or dissolves the calculus after it has calcified. It must be removed by prophylactic or periodontal instruments. Preventive measures are directed to the removal of the preliminary soft deposits of early calculus.

I. **METHODS OF CALCULUS CONTROL**

Chapter 10 lists in detail the many factors which contribute to the retention of the deposits on the teeth. All of these are directly or indirectly related to the retention of soft calculus. Mentioned below are a few of the important areas where the dental hygienist may assist the patient by means of oral prophylaxis procedures and patient instruction.

A. **Complete Removal of All Deposits During Scaling.**

When the calculus is completely removed and the tooth surface polished, the prompt reformation of calculus is delayed. The filamentous bacteria need a nucleus or rough spot for attachment. The conscientiously and thoroughly performed oral prophylaxis contributes to prevention.

Professional care for adequate supervision is arranged at appropriate intervals depending on the patient's rate of calculus formation. Some patients have light deposits and may require only two appointments each year, whereas others need a preventive scaling at two, three or four months' intervals.

B. **Oral Physical Therapy Measures.**

A daily regimen of personal care procedures to remove the soft preliminary deposits of calculus is the most effective preventive measure. Brushing must be thorough and exacting. Cleansing the teeth promptly after eating is more effective than at other times when food has been allowed to remain on the teeth. Toothbrushing can be supplemented by other oral physical therapy measures such as use of dental floss, rinsing, and interdental cleaning (see pages 302–315).

Removable dentures and other dental appliances must be cleaned promptly after eating to prevent deposit accumulation. Rinsing under running water is helpful when brushing is not possible immediately after eating.

C. **Diet.**

The dietary should include a sufficient amount of detergent foods to aid the self-cleansing mechanisms and oral physical therapy measures. A soft, sticky diet provides an important source of materials for deposits on the teeth.

II. CALCULUS INHIBITORS

An increasing amount of research is being conducted to find a practical, effective and safe method for calculus prevention. Any method will need to be based on facts concerning the nature of calculus and the mechanism of its formation. With recognition for the present incomplete knowledge about calculus, Leung[32] outlined four possible approaches: (1) prevent calcium precipitates from forming or, once formed, cause them to be dissolved, (2) prevent calculus from attaching to the tooth, (3) eliminate microorganisms for their role in attachment or in forming calcium precipitates, and (4) destroy the organic matrix or pre-calculus plaque. Although research has been directed along all four of these approaches, there have been hazards shown in the use of substances which will dissolve or otherwise harm, the tooth structure.

The most promising results have been obtained from experiments to destroy matrix material by enzymes and other potential inhibitors.[33,34] Investigation of the nature of the inhibitor used in commercial products is essential before practicing dentists and dental hygienists recommend these to patients.

FACTORS TO TEACH THE PATIENT

  I. The effect of calculus on the health of the periodontal tissues and therefore on the general health of the oral cavity.
 II. What calculus is and how it forms on the teeth.
III. Properties of calculus which will explain the need for detailed, meticulous scaling procedures.
 IV. The importance of routine appointments for removal of calculus.
  V. Measures which the patient may carry out to prevent calculus accumulation.

REFERENCES

1. GLOCK, G. E. and MURRAY, M. M.:   Chemical Investigation of Salivary Calculus, J. Dent. Res., *17*, 257, August, 1938.
2. HODGE, H. C. and LEUNG, S. W.:   Calculus Formation, J. Periodont., *21*, 211, October, 1950.
3. MANDEL, I. D. and LEVY, B. M.:   Studies on Salivary Calculus. I. Histochemical and Chemical Investigations of Supra and Subgingival Calculus, Oral Surg., Oral Med., & Oral Path., *10*, 874, August, 1957.
4. HODGE, H. C.:   Table 2, Chemical Contents of Enamel, Dentin, Cementum and Bone, in Sicher, Harry, ed.:   *Orban's Oral Histology and Embryology*, 5th ed. St. Louis, Mosby, 1962, p. 53.
5. LEUNG, S. W. and JENSEN, A. T.:   Factors Controlling the Deposition of Calculus, Internat. D. J., *8*, 613, December, 1958.
6. LEUNG, S. W.:   Salivary Calculus Deposition. Calcification in Biological Systems, American Association for the Advancement of Science, Washington, D. C., 1960.
7. MANDEL, I. D., LEVY, B., and WASSERMAN, B.:   Studies on Salivary Calculus. Histochemistry of Calculus Formation, J. Periodont., *28*, 132, April, 1957.
8. MANDEL, I. D.:   Experimental Calculus Formation, J. Dent. Res., *39*, 1092, November-December, 1960.

9. TURESKY, S., RENSTRUP, G., and GLICKMAN, I.:   Histologic and Histochemical Observations Regarding Early Calculus Formation in Children and Adults, J. Periodont., *32*, 7, January, 1961.
10. EVERETT, F. G.:   Calculus, Am. Dent. Hygienists' A. J., *30*, 121, July, 1956.
11. GREENE, J. H.:   Form, Location, and Classification of Subgingival Calculus, Am. J. Orthodont. & Oral Surg. (Section on Oral Surgery), *30*, 505, September, 1944.
12. EVERETT, F. G. and POTTER, G. R.:   Morphology of Submarginal Calculus, J. Periodont., *30*, 27, January, 1959.
13. ZANDER, H. A.:   Attachment of Calculus to Root Surfaces, J. Periodont., *24*, 16, January, 1953.
14. SHROFF, F. R.:   An Observation on the Attachment of Calculus, Oral Surg., Oral Med., & Oral Path., *8*, 154, February, 1955.
15. VOREADIS, E. G. and ZANDER, H. A.:   Cuticular Calculus Attachment, Oral Surg., Oral Med., & Oral Path., *11*, 1120, October, 1958.
16. GRANT, D., STERN, I. B., and EVERETT, F. G.:   *Orban's Periodontics*, 2nd ed. St. Louis, Mosby, 1963, pp. 101–102.
17. ZANDER, H. A., HAZEN, S. P., and SCOTT, D. B.:   Mineralization of Dental Calculus, Proc. Soc. Exp. Biol. and Med., *103*, 257, February, 1960.
18. GONZALES, F. and SOGNNAES, R. F.:   Electronmicroscopy of Dental Calculus, Science, *131*, 156, January 15, 1960.
19. McMILLAN, L., HUTCHINSON, A. C. W. and FOSDICK, L. S.:   Electron Microscopic Study of Dental Calculus, Dent. Prog., *1*, 188, April, 1961.
20. LEUNG, S. W.:   Calculus Formation. Salivary Factors. Dental Clinics of North America, November, 1960, p. 723.
21. MANDEL, I. D.:   Calculus Formation. The Role of Bacteria and Mucoprotein, Dental Clinics of North America, November, 1960, p. 731.
22. GRESSLY, F.:   Experimental Calculus Formation, Periodontics, *1*, 53, March-April, 1963.
23. BEST, C. H. and TAYLOR, N. B.:   *The Physiological Basis of Medical Practice*, 7th ed. Baltimore, Williams and Wilkins, 1961, pp. 594–595.
24. LANGLEY, L. L. and CHERASKIN, E.:   *The Physiological Foundation of Dental Practice*, 2nd ed. St. Louis, Mosby, 1956, p. 410.
25. BAER, P. N. and NEWTON, W. L.:   Occurrence of Periodontal Disease in Germ-free Rats, J. Dent. Res., *38*, 1238, November-December, 1959.
26. BAER, P. N. and NEWTON, W. L.:   Studies on Periodontal Disease in the Mouse. III. The Germ-free Mouse and Its Conventional Control, Oral Surg., Oral Med. & Oral Path., *13*, 1134, September, 1960.
27. FITZGERALD, R. J. and McDANIEL, E. G.:   Dental Calculus in the Germ-free Rat, Arch. Oral Biol., *2*, 239, August, 1960.
28. MANDEL, I. D.:   Histochemical and Biochemical Aspects of Calculus Formation, Periodontics, *1*, 43, March-April, 1963.
29. SOBEL, A. E.:   Local Factors in the Mechanism of Calcification, Ann. New York Acad. Sci., *60*, 713, April 27, 1955.
30. WEIDMANN, S. M.:   Review of Modern Concepts on Calcification, Arch. Oral Biol., *1*, 259, January, 1960.
31. ZANDER, H. A.:   Tissue Reaction to Dental Calculus and to Filling Materials, J. Dent. Med., *13*, 101, April, 1958.
32. LEUNG, S. W.:   Calculus—Its Formation and Possible Prevention, Pennsyl. D. J., *27*, 3, March, 1960.
33. DRAUS, F. J., LEUNG, S. W., and MIKLOS, F.:   Toward a Chemical Inhibitor of Calculus, Dent. Prog., *3*, 79, January, 1963.
34. JENSEN, A. L.:   Use of Dehydrated Pancreas in Oral Hygiene, Am. Dent. A. J., *59*, 923, November, 1959.

SUGGESTED READINGS

LEUNG, S. W.:   Calculus Research 1959: A Review, Am. Dent. A. J., *60*, 583, May, 1960.
LEUNG, S. W.:   Relation of Calculus, Plaque, and Food Impaction to Periodontal Disease, J. Dent. Res., *41*, 306, January-February, 1962.
LITTLE, M. F., WILEY, H. S., and DIRKSEN, T. R.:   Concomitant Calculus and Caries, J. Dent. Res., *39*, 1151, November-December, 1960.
SANDERS, W. E. and ROBINSON, H. B. G.:   Effect of Toothbrushing on Deposition of Calculus, J. Periodont., *33*, 386, October, 1962.
WILKINS, E. M.:   Review of Dental Calculus for Dental Hygiene Care and Instruction, Am. Dent. Hygienists' A. J., *38*, 9, 1st Quarter, 1964.

Chapter 13

STAINS OF THE TEETH

Discolorations of the teeth occur in three ways, (1) stain adhering directly to the surfaces of the teeth, (2) stain contained within calculus and soft deposits on the teeth, and (3) stain incorporated within the tooth structure. The dental hygienist is mainly concerned in her instructional and clinical techniques with the first two, since these may be removed by the techniques of the oral prophylaxis and in certain instances may be prevented by the patient's routine personal care.

The significance of stains is related primarily to their effect on the appearance of the teeth. In general, any detrimental effect on the teeth or gingival tissues is related to the soft deposit or calculus in which the stain occurs. Thick, bulky deposits of stain can conceivably be a source of irritation if they occur adjacent to the gingival crest. Certain stains provide an index for evaluating oral cleanliness and the patient's habits of personal care.

The reader is encouraged to refer directly to the articles listed in the references at the end of the chapter to gain appreciation for the limited amount of research which has been done in this area. The reports which have been made are inconsistent, particularly with reference to the occurrence and significance of the stains. For the most part, the etiology is not specific. A variety of terminology is the apparent result of the lack of definition of the causative factors.

I. DEFINITIONS FOR THE CLASSIFICATION OF STAINS

A. **Extrinsic:** stains which occur on the external surface of the tooth and which may be removed by techniques of the oral prophylaxis.

B. **Intrinsic:** stains which occur within the tooth substance and which cannot be removed by techniques of the oral prophylaxis.

C. **Exogenous:** stains which have developed or originated from sources outside the tooth. Exogenous stains may be extrinsic or intrinsic.

D. **Endogenous:** stains which develop or originate from within the tooth. Endogenous stains are always intrinsic and usually are discolorations of the dentin which are reflected through the enamel.

II. APPLICATION OF TECHNIQUES OF THE ORAL PROPHYLAXIS TO STAIN REMOVAL

A. Stains Occurring Directly on the Tooth Surface

1. Stains which are directly associated with the surface of the enamel or exposed cementum are removed by polishing techniques.

9

2. When stains are tenacious and require repeated polishing, precaution should be taken to avoid scratching the tooth surface with the abrasive agent.
3. If scalers are employed, techniques which may produce scratches on the tooth surface must be avoided.

B. **Stains Incorporated within Tooth Deposits:** when stain is included within the substance of the soft deposit or calculus, it is removed by the specific technique required for the deposit.

EXTRINSIC (EXOGENOUS) STAINS

Many stains are both described and classified by their colors, which is confusing for clinical designation. For example, there is a wide variety of green stains which occur on rather specifically different tooth surfaces. Green stains may result from chlorophyll preparations, from the metallic dust of certain minerals in industry, or from drugs. The most common green stain is not one of those listed above, but is a clinical entity with a specific occurrence pattern and no scientific name other than "Green Stain." The term Green Stain is applied to this particular stain, whereas green stains from other causes need to be clinically designated by their etiology.

The most frequently observed stains, Yellow, Green, Black Line, and Tobacco will be described first; the less common Orange, Red, and metallic stains will follow.

I. YELLOW STAIN

A. **Clinical Appearance:** dull, yellowish discoloration of the dental plaque.

B. **Distribution on Tooth Surfaces:** associated with presence of dental plaque.

C. **Occurrence**
1. Common to all ages.
2. More evident when personal oral care procedures are neglected.

D. **Etiology:** usually food pigments.

II. GREEN STAIN

A. **Clinical Appearance**
1. Light or yellowish-green to very dark green.
2. Embedded in dental plaque.
3. Shape: occurs in three general forms.
   a. Small curved line following contour of labial gingival crest.
   b. Smeared irregularly, may even cover entire facial surface.
   c. Streaked, following grooves or lines in enamel.
4. Lighter stain frequently superimposed by a soft, fuzzy yellow or gray debris.
5. Dark green more frequently associated with adequate personal toothbrushing habits; light green stain with inadequate (unclean teeth).[1,2]

6. Dark green occasionally becomes imbedded in surface enamel and may be observed as an intrinsic stain when superficial layers of deposit are removed.
7. Enamel under stain: sometimes decalcified.[3]

B. Distribution on Tooth Surfaces

1. Primarily labial and buccal; occasionally extends to proximal.
2. Most frequent: labial cervical third of maxillary anterior teeth.

C. Composition

1. Chromogenic bacteria and fungi.
2. Decomposed hemoglobin.
3. Inorganic elements: calcium, potassium, sodium, silicon, magnesium, phosphorous, and others in small amounts.[4]

D. Occurrence

1. May occur at any age; primarily found in childhood.
2. Sex: statistics vary.
   a. Males more frequently.[1,5]
   b. Females more frequently.[2]
3. Green stain tends to occur without other stains (except yellow) in the same mouth in nearly one-half the cases.[2,5]

E. Recurrence: tends to depend on fastidiousness of personal care procedures.

F. Etiology

The etiology of green stain has not been established. It is possible that causes may vary in different mouths. Differences of opinion exist as to the effects of oral uncleanliness, chromogenic bacteria, and gingival hemorrhage. The theories and predisposing factors have been reviewed in the literature.[1-4] A summary is given below.

1. Theories
   a. Chromogenic bacteria or fungi[6,7]
      (1) Retained and nourished in dental plaque.
      (2) Produce coloring substances.
   b. Blood pigments from hemoglobin are decomposed by bacteria.
2. Predisposing factors
   a. Means for retention and proliferation of chromogenic bacteria.
      (1) Dental plaque.
      (2) Materia alba and food debris.
      (3) Primary cuticle in young children before it has worn off during mastication.[8]
   b. Gingiva with hemorrhagic tendencies (as would occur, for example, when routine toothbrushing is neglected or a soft diet fails to provide gingival massage).

III. BLACK LINE STAIN

A. Other Names Used in the Literature

1. Black (most common).[9-11]

2. Mesenteric Line.[12,13]
3. Brown Plaque.[14]
4. Brown Stain.[5]

B. Clinical Appearance

1. Black or dark brown.
2. Continuous or interrupted fine line, 1 mm. wide (average), no appreciable thickness.
3. May be a wider band or even occupy entire gingival third in severe cases (rare).
4. Follows contour of gingival crest about 1 mm. above crest.
5. Usually demarcated from gingival crest by clear white line of unstained enamel.
6. Appears black at bases of pits and fissures.
7. Heavy deposits slightly elevated from the tooth surface, may be detected with an explorer.
8. Gingiva: firm, resilient, with little or no tendency to hemorrhage.
9. Teeth: tendency to lower incidence of dental caries.

C. Distribution on Tooth Surface

1. Labial, buccal and lingual; follows contour of gingival crest onto proximal surfaces.
2. Rarely on labial of maxillary anterior.
3. Most frequently: lingual and proximal surfaces of maxillary posterior teeth.

D. Composition[14]

1. Inorganic substances (possibly in form of calcium and magnesium phosphates or carbonates).
2. Mucin or its compounds precipitated from the saliva.
3. Filamentous and other bacteria.

E. Occurrence

1. All ages; more common in childhood.
2. More common in females.[10,11]
3. Frequently in clean mouths.
4. Line occurs more extensively and thicker when personal care is neglected.

F. Recurrence: tends to reform despite regular personal care, but quantity may be lessened if care is meticulous.

G. Manner of Formation

1. Etiology[14]
   a. Mucin is deposited on the teeth from the saliva.
   b. Bacteria (particularly filamentous forms) establish themselves in mucin.
   c. Inorganic salts become incorporated in mucin.
   d. Pigment is provided by mesenteric or chromogenic bacteria.
2. Predisposing factors: none apparent, except a natural tendency.

IV. TOBACCO STAIN

A. Clinical Appearance

1. Light brown to dark leathery brown or black.
2. Shape
   a. Diffuse staining of dental plaque.
   b. Narrow band which follows contour of gingival crest, slightly above the crest.
   c. Wide, firm, tar-like band may cover cervical third and extend to central third of crown.
3. May be incorporated in calculus deposit.
4. Heavy deposits (particularly from chewing tobacco) may penetrate the enamel and become intrinsic.

B. Distribution on Tooth Surfaces

1. Cervical third, primarily.
2. Any surface, as well as pits and fissures.
3. Most frequent: lingual surfaces.

C. Composition

1. Tar products of combustion.
2. Brown pigment from chewing tobacco.

D. Predisposing Factors

1. Natural tendencies: quantity of stain not proportional to amount of tobacco used, which indicates individual differences.
2. Personal oral care procedures: increased deposits with neglect.
3. Extent of dental plaque and calculus available for adherence.

V. ORANGE AND RED STAINS

A. Clinical Appearance: orange or red stain at the cervical third.

B. Distribution on Tooth Surfaces

1. More frequently on anterior than posterior teeth.
2. Both labial and lingual of anterior teeth.[15]

C. Occurrence: rare (red more rare than orange).

D. Etiology: chromogenic bacteria.[6,7]

VI. METALLIC STAINS[15-18]

A. Metals or Metallic Salts from Metal-Containing Dust of Industry

1. Clinical appearance: examples of colors on teeth.
   a. Copper or brass: green or bluish-green.
   b. Iron: brown to greenish-brown.
   c. Nickel: green.
   d. Cadmium: yellow or golden brown.

   2. Distribution on tooth surfaces.
      a. Primarily anterior; may occur on any teeth.
      b. Cervical third more commonly.
   3. Manner of formation.
      a. Industrial worker inhales dust through mouth, bringing metallic substance in contact with teeth.
      b. Metal imparts color to dental plaque.
      c. Occasionally stain may penetrate tooth substance and become exogenous intrinsic stain.

B. **Metallic Substances Contained in Drugs**

   1. Clinical appearance: examples of colors on teeth.
      a. Iron: black (iron sulphide).
      b. Manganese (from potassium permanganate): black.
   2. Distribution on tooth surfaces: general, may occur on all.
   3. Manner of formation.
      a. Drug enters plaque substance, imparts color to plaque.
      b. Pigment from drug may attach directly to tooth substance.

INTRINSIC STAINS

Knowledge of the stains occurring within the tooth structure provides information for patient instruction. The dental hygienist does not diagnose, and specification of a cause for an intrinsic stain is the responsibility of the dentist.

The techniques of the oral prophylaxis have no effect on intrinsic stains. The patient, desiring an improvement in the appearance of the anterior teeth, may request removal of the discoloration. The dentist generally employs one of two alternatives in the treatment of these teeth. Improvement in tooth color can be produced by bleaching in certain instances. In other cases it is necessary to prepare a jacket crown to cover the discoloration.

In this section, intrinsic stains are considered in five groups according to their etiology.

I. **BLOOD AND OTHER TISSUE BREAKDOWN PRODUCTS FROM DISEASED PULP**

It should be realized that all pulpless teeth do not discolor. Improved endodontic procedures have contributed to the prevention of many discolorations formerly associated with that cause.

A. **Clinical Appearance:** wide range of colors; may be light yellow-brown, slate gray, reddish-brown, dark brown, bluish-black, black. Others have an orange or greenish tinge.

B. **Manner of Formation**[3]

   1. Blood and other pulp tissue elements are made available for breakdown as a result of hemorrhages in the pulp chamber, root canal operations, or necrosis and decomposition of the pulp tissue.
   2. Pigments from the decomposed hemoglobin and pulp tissue penetrate into the dentinal tubules.

II. DRUGS AND METALS USED IN DENTAL OPERATIONS

A. Restorative Materials

1. Copper amalgam used for filling primary teeth may impart a bluish-green color.
2. Silver amalgam can impart a gray to black discoloration (generally associated with improperly mixed and prepared material).
3. Silver nitrate used in cavity base under restoration produces black discoloration.

B. Endodontic Therapy and Restorative Materials[19]

1. Silver nitrate: bluish-black.
2. Volatile oils: yellowish-brown.
3. Strong iodine: brown.
4. Aureomycin: yellow.
5. Silver-containing root canal sealer: black.

III. IMPERFECT TOOTH DEVELOPMENT

A. Enamel Hypoplasia[20,21]

1. Systemic Hypoplasia (chronologic hypoplasia resulting from ameloblastic disturbance of short duration): teeth erupt with white spots which over a long period of time may become discolored from food pigments or other substances taken into the mouth.
2. Local Hypoplasia (affects single tooth): white spots may become stained as in systemic hypoplasia.
3. Hereditary Amelogenesis Imperfecta (enamel is partially or completely missing due to a generalized disturbance of the ameloblasts): teeth are yellowish-brown.

B. Dental Fluorosis

1. Manner of formation
   a. Enamel hypocalcification resulting from ingestion of excessive fluoride ion content of the drinking water (more than one part per million) during the period of calcification.
   b. When the teeth erupt there are white spots or areas which later become discolored from oral pigments and appear light or dark brown.
   c. Severe effects produce cracks or pitting; the discoloration concentrates in these.
2. Classification[22,23]
   a. Very mild: enamel shows irregularly scattered, small, opaque, white areas; frequently only a few teeth are affected.
   b. Mild: enamel shows white opaque areas which involve up to one-half of the tooth surface.
   c. Moderate: entire enamel is affected and brown staining occurs in varying degrees.
   d. Severe: entire enamel is affected and discrete or confluent pitting is present.

C. Hereditary Dentinogenesis Imperfecta (dentin is abnormal as a result of disturbances in the odontoblastic layer during development): teeth are translucent, and vary in color from gray to brown.

IV. **BLOOD BORNE PIGMENTATION (rare):** Pigments circulating in the blood are transmitted to the dentin from the capillaries of the pulp. Example: prolonged jaundice early in life can impart yellow or greenish discoloration to the teeth.[24]

V. EXOGENOUS INTRINSIC STAINS

A. **Extrinsic Stains** which have become incorporated in the enamel: Examples: tobacco, traces of green stain.

B. **Drugs:** Example: ammoniacal silver nitrate used in treatment of sensitive areas such as exposed cementum, or for inhibition of decalcification for dental caries prevention.

C. **Stain in Dentin:** Example: discoloration resulting from a carious lesion.

TECHNICAL HINTS

I. Avoid making patient feel self-conscious by overemphasis of the appearance of stains which occur in spite of conscientious tooth-brushing habits.

II. Use tact when questioning patients with brown stain since nonsmokers do not appreciate having an assumption made concerning the etiology of the stain on their teeth.

III. Refer patient's questions concerning the removal of intrinsic stains to the dentist. Avoid expressing an opinion in terms of diagnosis or prognosis of treatment until the dentist has recommended a procedure.

FACTORS TO TEACH THE PATIENT

I. Factors which contribute to stain accumulation.

II. Personal care procedures which can aid in the prevention or reduction of stains.

III. Reasons for not using an abrasive dentifrice to lessen or remove stain accumulation.

IV. Reasons for the difficulty in removal of certain extrinsic stains during the oral prophylaxis.

REFERENCES

1. AYERS, POLLY: Green Stain, Am. Dent. A. J., *26*, 2, January, 1939.
2. SPRINGER, JAMES: A Clinical Study of Green Stain, Tufts Dental Outlook, *18*, 30, December, 1944.
3. BOYLE, P. E.: *Kronfeld's Histopathology of the Teeth*, 4th ed. Philadelphia, Lea & Febiger, 1955, p. 475.
4. SHAY, D. E., HADDOX, J. H., and RICHMOND, J. L.: An Inorganic Qualitative and Quantitative Analysis of Green Stain, Am. Dent. A. J., *50*, 156, February, 1955.
5. LEUNG, S. W.: Naturally Occurring Stains on the Teeth of Children, Am. Dent. A. J., *41*, 191, August, 1950.
6. GOADBY, K.: *Mycology of the Mouth.* London, Longmans, Green & Co., 1903, cited by Glickman, Irving: *Clinical Periodontology*, 2nd ed. Philadelphia, Saunders, 1958, p. 320.
7. BARTELS, H. A.: A Note on Chromogenic Microorganisms from an Organic Colored Deposit of the Teeth, Int. J. Orthodont., *25*, 795, August, 1939.
8. THOMA, K. H. and GOLDMAN, H. M.: *Oral Pathology*, 5th ed. St. Louis, Mosby, 1960, p. 205.
9. BEUBE, F. E.: *Periodontology.* New York, Macmillan, 1953, p. 54.

10. BUNTING, R. W.: *Oral Hygiene*, 3rd ed. Philadelphia, Lea & Febiger, 1957, pp. 126–127.
11. GLICKMAN, IRVING: *Clinical Periodontology*, 2nd ed. Philadelphia, Saunders, 1958, p. 320.
12. PICKERILL, H. P.: A Sign of Immunity, Brit. Dent. J., *44*, 967, September 1, 1923.
13. SHOURIE, K. L.: Mesenteric Line or Pigmented Plaque: A Sign of Comparative Freedom from Dental Caries, Am. Dent. A. J., *35*, 805, December, 1947.
14. BIBBY, B. G.: A Study of Pigmented Dental Plaque, J. Dent. Res., *11*, 855, December, 1931.
15. GLICKMAN: op. cit., p. 321.
16. BUNTING: op. cit., p. 129.
17. BOYLE: op. cit., p. 476.
18. MILLER, S. C.: *Oral Diagnosis and Treatment*, 3rd ed. New York, Blakiston Division, McGraw-Hill, 1957, p. 458.
19. INGLE, J. I.: Seattle, University of Washington, School of Dentistry, personal communication.
20. SICHER, HARRY: *Orban's Oral Histology and Embryology*, 5th ed. St. Louis, Mosby, 1962, pp. 100–101.
21. THOMA: op. cit., p. 98.
22. DEAN, H. T.: Investigation of Physiological Effects by Epidemiological Method, in *Fluorine and Dental Health*, F. R. Moulton, Ed. Washington, American Association for the Advancement of Science, No. 19, 1942.
23. ARNOLD, F. A.: Use of Fluoride Compounds for the Prevention of Dental Caries, Internat Dent. J., *7*, 54, March, 1957.
24. BUNTING: op. cit., p. 130.

SUGGESTED READINGS

American Dental Association, Council on Dental Therapeutics: Significance of Dental Changes Induced by Tetracyclines, Am. Dent. A. J., *68*, 277, February, 1964.
LARGENT, E. J.: *Fluorosis*. Columbus, Ohio State University Press, 1961, pp. 70–73.

Chapter 14

PRINCIPLES OF TECHNIQUE FOR THE ORAL PROPHYLAXIS

A STUDY of oral and dental anatomy and histology necessarily precedes the consideration of specific techniques since development of a thorough, efficient and safe technique depends on an understanding of the characteristics of the tissues being influenced. Knowledge of the specific anatomy of each tooth and its relationship to the other teeth in the permanent, mixed, or primary dentitions is essential to the understanding and use of the instruments designed to accomplish the oral prophylaxis. Familiarity with the appearance of the gingival tissues and their relationship to the teeth provides the basis for working in accord with the needs of the patient and the final objectives to be attained.

The clinical results obtained for the patient are dependent in part on the proficiency and thoroughness with which the oral prophylaxis is accomplished. Factors related to proficiency may be grouped under the following headings:

1. Appreciation of the extent of the patient's problem as revealed by the oral inspection and recommendations of the dentist. In other words: *knowing what is to be done before doing it.*
2. Visibility, accessibility and illumination of working area.
3. A planned sequence for procedure in the total appointment, and specifically, the order of instrumentation.
4. Use of correct and efficient instrumentation and related procedures.

The first factor has been described in previous chapters. The other three will be considered here as introduction to successive chapters devoted to specific instruments and techniques.

I. VISIBILITY AND ACCESSIBILITY OF WORKING AREA

A. Factors Influencing Adequate Vision and Accessibility

1. Patient and operator position (see pages 61–68).
2. Efficient use of direct or reflected (by mouth mirror) illumination for each tooth surface.
3. Adequate yet gentle retraction of lips, cheek, tongue with consideration for patient's comfort and operator's convenience.

B. Effects of Adequate Vision and Accessibility

1. Instrumentation will be more thorough with minimum trauma to the oral tissues.
2. Length of time required will be lessened, which contributes to less fatigue for the operator.
3. Patient cooperation will be increased because of shortened operating time and less discomfort.

II. ORDER FOR INSTRUMENTATION IN THE MOUTH

A variety of routines are in current use by practicing dental hygienists. The one selected depends on the method taught in the dental hygiene school attended or the method found most efficient by the practitioner. The important consideration is the use of an habitual routine.

A. Advantages of a Systematic Procedure

1. Insure thoroughness in removal of deposits and stains.
2. Demonstrate ease and smoothness of operation.
3. Increase efficiency through repeated routine.
4. Decrease operating time.
5. Increase patient's comfort.
6. Increase in patient's confidence in operator.

B. Suggested Procedure for Cases Requiring Multiple Appointments

1. Recommended order
   a. Dentition on right side.
      (1) Mandibular quadrant to midline.
      (2) Maxillary quadrant to midline.
   b. Dentition on left side.
      (1) Mandibular quadrant to midline.
      (2) Maxillary quadrant to midline.
2. Objectives for recommended order
   a. For efficient appointment planning for those cases having heavy calculus deposits.
      (1) When multiple appointments are required.
      (2) Provides logical division of the teeth for ease in scaling a specific segment (quadrant or two quadrants).
   b. For patient comfort.
      (1) Divides stress of instrumentation between mandible and maxilla at appropriate intervals.
      (2) Confines to one side of mouth any sensitivity resulting from tissue trauma after removal of heavy calculus.
   c. For patient instruction.
      (1) Comparison of appearance of teeth and tissue of completed and untouched side.
      (2) Observation of the comparative effects of toothbrushing between appointments.
      (3) Planning for future appointments through recall.
   d. For dental hygienist's appraisal of the anticipated final effects of the oral prophylaxis by comparing the two sides in terms of tissue response.

PRINCIPLES FOR THE USE OF INSTRUMENTS

I. INSTRUMENT PARTS

Instruments have three major parts: the *working end*, the *shank* and the *handle* or shaft. Examples of the working end are the blade of a scaler, the wood point of a porte polisher and the rubber polishing cup of a prophylaxis angle. The relationship of the parts of an instrument are illustrated by the scaler in Figure 37.

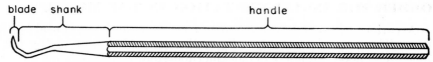

FIGURE 37.—Scaler to illustrate the parts of a typical instrument. The working end of the scaler is the blade.

II. INSTRUMENT SELECTION

A. Factors Influencing the Selection of Instruments

1. Nature, location and extent of deposit or stain to be removed.
2. Accessibility of the deposit or stain; area of mouth.
3. Topography of the tooth surface.
4. Size, contour, consistency and position of the free gingiva.
5. Design, size and function of the instrument.

B. Number of Instruments to Use

1. Number should be limited to a few well-selected instruments to increase efficiency in use and care of the instruments.
2. Familiarity with a variety of instruments.
    a. Provides opportunity to compare and select.
    b. Permits application of the general principles of use which pertain to all.

III. GRASP

A. Functions of the Instrument Grasp

The manner in which the instrument is held influences the entire procedure. A rigid grasp in which the instrument is gripped tightly, lessens the effectiveness of instrumentation. The appropriate grasp is firm, displays the confidence of the operator in the work being done, and provides the following effects:

1. Increased tactile sensitivity.
2. Positive control of the instrument with flexibility of motion.
3. Decreased hazard of trauma to the dental and periodontal tissues, which results in less postoperative discomfort for the patient.
4. Prevention of fatigue to operator's fingers, hand, and arm.

B. Types of Grasps

1. Pen
    a. Instrument held between thumb and index and middle fingers at the junction of the shank and the handle of the instrument.
    b. Shank rests against pad (side) of middle finger (not across the nail).
    c. Ring finger serves as fulcrum.
2. Palm
    a. Handle of instrument is held in palm by cupped index, middle, ring and little fingers.
    b. Thumb is free to serve as fulcrum.
    c. Limited applications
        (1) Porte polisher on maxillary facial surfaces.
        (2) Handpiece with mounted stone for instrument sharpening.

IV. FULCRUM

A fulcrum must always be used when instruments are applied to the teeth.

A. Definition

1. The support, or point of rest, on which a lever turns in moving a body.
2. The support, or point of finger rest on the tooth surface, on which the hand turns in moving an instrument.

B. Purposes

An effective, well-established fulcrum contributes to the following:

1. Stability for controlled action of the instrument.
2. Prevention of injury to the patient's oral tissues.
3. Comfort for the patient; confidence in operator's ability which results from the feeling of securely applied instruments.

C. Digits Used for Fulcrum

1. Pen grasp
   a. Ring finger.   Little finger is held close beside ring finger.
   b. Supplementary: pad of middle finger rests lightly on incisal or occlusal surface of tooth being scaled or polished.
      (1) Ring finger maintains regular fulcrum position.
      (2) Middle finger maintains its grasp on instrument.
   c. Fingers are slightly curved for support.
2. Palm grasp: thumb.

D. Location of Fulcrum Rest

The fulcrum must always be maintained on a *solid* tooth or teeth. The patient's chin, lips and cheeks are mobile and thus inadequate for providing stability.

1. Objectives
   a. For convenience to area of operation.
   b. For ready adaptation of instrument to the surface being explored, scaled or polished.
   c. For stability of instrument during stroke.
2. Adaptations for missing teeth
   a. Place cotton roll in the space to bridge the gap, but maintain fulcrum on firm tooth.
   b. Use patient's removable partial denture in place when it will not interfere with teeth being explored, scaled or polished.
   c. Place fingers of other hand as substitute in edentulous area.
3. Precautions in the selection of fulcrum tooth
   a. Mobile teeth should always be avoided.
   b. Consult radiographs for determination of adequacy of bony support for a tooth.
   c. Potential dangers in the use of inadequately supported teeth.
      (1) Fulcrum is unstable and inadequate for accomplishing purpose.
      (2) Unstable fulcrum leads to injury of tissue around tooth being explored, scaled or polished.
      (3) Trauma to tissues surrounding the fulcrum tooth.
         (a) Tearing of periodontal fibers.

(b) Tooth may become more mobile, or if lacking in bony attachment, may be removed.

    d. Incisor teeth are not recommended for fulcrum rests because of their frequent sensitivity to pressure.

E. Touch or Pressure Applied to Fulcrum

The fulcrum finger maintains a firm hold with moderate pressure to balance the action of the instrument being applied. Excessive pressure on the fulcrum rest can result in decreased stability for the controlled action of the instrument as well as fatigue in the operator's fingers and hand.

1. Mandibular fulcrums: heavy pressure on the movable mandible can cause fatigue and discomfort for the patient.
2. Maxillary fulcrums: since the maxilla is stationary, fulcrums on maxillary teeth should be used whenever possible for maxillary instrumentation to provide greater stability during instrumentation as well as comfort for the patient.

V. STROKE

A stroke is a single, unbroken movement made by an instrument. Strokes may be straight, in a horizontal or vertical direction, curved, to follow the contour of the tooth or gingival margin, or circular.

A. Factors Which Influence Selection of Stroke

1. Size, contour and position of gingiva.
2. Surface and section of surface being explored, scaled or polished.
3. Instrumentation zone: height of deposit on tooth (see page 156).
4. Size and shape of instrument used.

B. Nature of Stroke

1. Short, firm, controlled.
2. Directed to protect tissues.
3. Hand, wrist and arm act as a continuum to provide motion and pressure for instrumentation.
    a. Hand: to hold instrument and establish fulcrum.
    b. Wrist
       (1) Held so hand is straight from arm.
       (2) Relaxed to transmit energy from arm.
    c. Arm
       (1) To establish direction for stroke.
       (2) To limit size and length of stroke.
       (3) To provide energy for removing stains and deposits.
4. Effects from use of fingers only to activate instrument: finger muscles will tire readily, thus limiting tactile sensitivity required for control and efficiency.

C. Touch and Pressure Applied to Stroke

1. Explorer: light touch to provide for greatest degree of tactile sensitivity.
2. Scaler: light but secure touch until deposit is engaged, then controlled pressure for its removal.

3. Porte Polisher: firm, secure, even pressure during polishing stroke.
4. Prophylaxis angle: rubber cup is applied with light pressure in short but firm strokes.

VI. THOROUGHNESS OF PROCEDURE

Each particle of deposit and stain must be removed from the tooth surfaces. A firm technique with a painstaking approach will achieve both the complete removal of deposits and comfort for the patient. Since time is involved, a happy medium is possible with time minimized, yet the patient's tissues treated with maximum respect.

"Roughness, under the guise of increased diligence, should not be confused with thoroughness."[1] Roughness is generally associated with carelessness, and neither have any place in dental hygiene procedures. Possible effects of roughness are:

1. Infliction of unnecessary pain during operation.
2. Prolonged postoperative discomfort.
3. Production of excessive bleeding and debris which hinders the efficiency of the operator.
4. Production of tissue lacerations which retard healing.
5. Gouging of tooth surfaces which may produce postoperative sensitivity to touch and thermal changes.
6. Forcing of infected material into the deeper periodontal tissues which can lead to serious postoperative infection.

DEXTERITY DEVELOPMENT FOR THE USE OF INSTRUMENTS

This section is included particularly for the beginning dental hygiene student and the graduate dental hygienist who plans to return to practice after a period of retirement. A primary objective when learning or reviewing the techniques for the oral prophylaxis is to develop the ability to hold instruments correctly while employing them for use. However generally dexterous a person may be, the use of new or unusual instruments requires different procedures for coordination. Control is essential, and guided strength contributes to control.

Proficiency during techniques comes from repeated correct use of the instruments. Exercises for the fingers, hands and arms supplement experience. Directed exercises are needed for both hands, separately and together. To facilitate the development of dexterity, certain exercises have been selected to supplement other types of practice such as the use of instruments on a manikin. A regular period of time each day during the training period should be set aside for exercises.

I. SQUEEZING A BALL

A. Purposes

1. To develop general muscles of hand and arm.
2. To develop strength and control for use of palm grasp.

B. **Tennis Ball**
1. Hold ball in palm of hand, grip with thumb and all fingers.
2. Tighten and release grip at regular intervals.
3. One hand rests while other is holding the ball.

C. **Chip Blower**
1. Hold bulb in palm of hand, grip with middle, ring and little finger.
2. Use thumb and index finger to maintain nozzle in stationary position such as that required when directing air on the teeth.
3. Rest one hand while other is exercising the chip blower.

II. **STRETCHING A RUBBER BAND**

A. **Purposes**
1. To strengthen finger and hand muscles.
2. To develop control of finger movements.
3. To develop ability to separate ring and middle fingers, while keeping ring and little fingers together and index and middle fingers together.

B. **Rubber Band on Finger Joints without Use of Fulcrum**
1. Place rubber band at joint between first phalanx and second phalanx.
2. Stretch band by separating middle and ring fingers.
3. Place rubber band at joint between second phalanx and third phalanx and proceed as before.
4. Place rubber bands on both hands and do exercises together.
5. Use rubber bands of smaller size as strength and control increase.

C. **Rubber Band on Finger Joints with Use of Fulcrum**
1. Place rubber band on joint between first phalanx and second phalanx.
2. Establish fulcrum finger (ring finger) on table top with little finger closely adjacent to it; elbow and forearm free as they are during instrumentation. Stretch band by separating middle and ring fingers.
3. Touch thumb and index and middle fingers to simulate pen grasp for instrument. Stretch band by separating middle and ring fingers.
4. Variations.
   a. Hold instrument in pen grasp while doing the exercise.
   b. Do writing exercises with rubber band in place.
5. Rest one hand while other is being exercised.

III. **WRITING**

A. **Purposes**
1. To develop correct instrument pen grasp.
2. To propel instrument without moving fingers.
3. To practice use of instruments when mouth mirror is required.
4. To develop control and precision.

B. Circles and Vertical Lines

1. Hold long, well-sharpened, wooden lead pencil with pen grasp.
2. Establish fulcrum finger (ring finger) on table top; forearm and elbow free.
3. Inscribe counterclockwise circles and vertical lines on paper, rapidly and lightly at first, slowly and with more pressure later.
4. Accomplish writing by activation of the hand by the upper arm, without flexing or extending the thumb and fingers holding the pencil.
5. Practice each hand separately at first, then use pencil in each hand at the same time, alternating writing action to simulate adaptation of first the mirror and then the explorer, scaler or polisher.

C. Using Mouth Mirror

1. Hold mouth mirror with pen grasp in left hand close to pencil while practicing writing exercises (III B) through the mirror. Reverse hands.
2. Using engineer's graph paper and pen grasp with fulcrum as described earlier, follow the lines of the small squares while looking in mirror held with opposite hand.

D. Everyday Penmanship

1. Use pen grasp whenever possible for writing.
2. Practice word writing with the left hand to increase dexterity for handling mouth mirror.

IV. MOUTH MIRROR, COTTON PLIERS AND EXPLORER

A. Purposes

1. To develop ability to turn mouth mirror at various angles.
2. To develop dexterity in holding objects with cotton pliers while operating.
3. To establish desired grasp of explorer to assure maximum touch sensitivity.

B. Mouth Mirror

1. Hold mouth mirror with pen grasp, ring finger on table top as fulcrum finger with little finger closely adjacent to it, elbow and forearm free.
2. Practice turning mirror with fingers, adjusting as to the several surfaces of the tooth.
3. Hold a small object in opposite hand for viewing in mirror.
4. Practice crossing the mirror over fulcrum finger as in position for retracting lower lip with fulcrum finger while viewing lingual surfaces of mandibular anterior teeth in mouth mirror.

C. Cotton Pliers

1. Make small tight cotton pellets with thumb and index and middle fingers of each hand; then make one in each hand simultaneously.
2. Hold cotton pliers with pen grasp and establish fulcrum finger on table top; elbow and forearm free.

10

3. Practice picking up cotton pellets.
   a. Use in wiping motion on table top or other object.
   b. Move to different area to release pellet.

D. **Explorer**

1. Hold explorer with pen grasp and establish fulcrum finger on table top with upper arm and forearm free.
2. Use a rough-surfaced material such as sandpaper to feel with explorer tip until a light grasp permits maximum security of grasp and maximum sense of touch.

V. **TECHNICAL HINTS**

A. Time spent on exercises should be sufficient in any one period to cause moderate (but never severe) strain and fatigue of hand muscles, since to increase strength, muscles need to be over-worked.
B. To relax the muscles of the hands during a practice session, wash hands in warm water.

REFERENCE

1. GLICKMAN, IRVING: *Clinical Periodontology*, 2nd ed.   Philadelphia, Saunders, 1958, p. 585.

SUGGESTED READINGS

BUNTING, R. W.: *Oral Hygiene*, 3rd ed.   Philadelphia, Lea & Febiger, 1957, pp. 233–287.
GRANT, DANIEL, STERN, I. B., and EVERETT, F. G.: *Orban's Periodontics*, 2nd ed. St. Louis, Mosby, 1963, pp. 294–295.
HARD, D. G.:   A Method of Teaching Techniques in Oral Prophylaxis, J. Dent. Educ., *13*, 242, May, 1949.
TONDROWSKI, V. E.:   Preclinical Procedures for the Dental Hygiene Student, J. Dent. Educ., *20*, 321, November, 1956.

Chapter 15

SCALING PROCEDURES

SCALING is the process by which calculus is removed from the clinical crowns of the teeth. Each particle of calculus must be removed and the surfaces polished if dental hygiene care is to be effective and the objectives are to be accomplished (see page 102).

The reaction of the gingival tissue to the presence of calculus has been described on page 125. When deposits are completely removed and the tooth surfaces made smooth, the tissue will heal and assume normal characteristics. Areas once scaled need to be re-evaluated at a subsequent appointment. With even the most conscientious instrumentation, some fragments of calculus may remain and cause persistent irritation to the gingiva. The red or blue color of the inflamed area will be in distinct contrast to the normal pink of areas where no deposit remains.

To remove calculus completely, a high degree of scientific skill and understanding is required. Techniques must be exacting and thorough with consistent attention to fine detail.

THE SCALERS

Scalers, the dental prophylactic instruments used for calculus removal, have one or more cutting edges. Dental hygienists generally use three types, sickles, curets and hoes. Two other types of scaling instruments are used primarily by the dentist: chisels, for removal of gross supramarginal deposits, and files, for root planing after scaling.

Each scaler has its own design based on the specific purpose for which it is used. A scaler is selected for a particular operation depending on the location and extent of the calculus deposit to be removed, the topography of the tooth surface, and the characteristics of the adjacent gingival tissue.

When a scaler is to be used for the first time, the blade should be studied carefully and examined with a magnifying glass if necessary. A clear knowledge of the relationship of the cutting edges to the other parts of the instrument is important to the proper adaptation to the tooth surface as well as to the sharpening stone.

I. SICKLE SCALER

A. **Straight Sickle**

    1. Characteristics

       a. Two cutting edges on a straight blade (Figure 38*A*).

       b. Lateral surfaces of blade converge; tip of scaler is pointed.

       c. Cross section of blade is triangular.

       d. Shank is straight.

2. Adaptation
   a. To anterior teeth, or where accessibility permits using the blade in position with the long axis of the instrument handle parallel with the long axis of the tooth.
   b. With surface between cutting edges inclined at less than 90° angle toward tooth surface being scaled (Figures 39A and 39B).
3. Uses
   a. For removal of supramarginal deposits before applying curet to submarginal deposits.
   b. Fine, short-bladed sickle scaler: for submarginal calculus which is only a few millimeters below the gingival crest of anterior teeth.

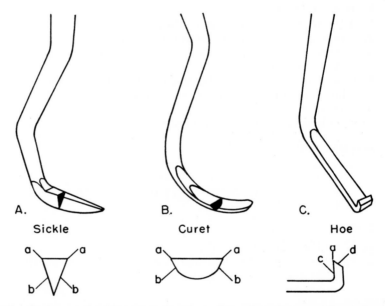

FIGURE 38.—Surfaces and cutting edges of scalers. The enlarged cross sections below the sickle and curet scalers show: *a.* cutting edges and *b.* lateral surfaces of blades. The side view of the hoe scaler shows: *a.* cutting edge, *c.* surface next to shank, and *d.* back surface of the blade.

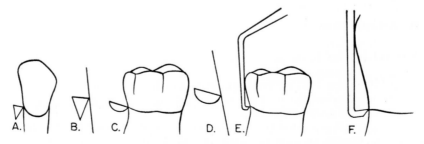

FIGURE 39.—Adaptation of scaler blade to tooth surface. *A.* and *B.* Sickle scaler, cross section to show adaptation to tooth at slightly less than 90° angle. *C.* and *D.* Curet scaler adapted at less than 90° angle. *E.* and *F.* Hoe scaler, showing contact of blade and shank with tooth.

(1) Straight blade cannot be adapted to curved root surface without traumatizing epithelial lining of gingival sulcus.

(2) Blade of large sickle is too wide, long, and bulky to gain access and provide tactile sensitivity required for removal of deep deposits.

B. Contra-angle or Modified Sickle Scaler

1. Characteristics: same as straight sickle with an angulated shank.
2. Adaptation: to proximal surfaces of posterior teeth (paired instruments to provide access to all proximal surfaces).
3. Use: same as straight sickle.

II. CURET SCALER

A. Characteristics

1. Two cutting edges (Figure 38B).
2. Slender, curved (spoon-shaped) blade.
3. Lateral surfaces of blade converge and terminate in a rounded, flattened end.
4. Cross section of blade is shaped like a half circle.
5. Blade has inner concave surface and outer convex, rounded surface.
6. Shank is curved or angulated.

B. Adaptation

1. To all surfaces of the teeth (paired instruments to provide access).
2. With instrument surface between cutting edges inclined at less than 90° angle toward tooth surface being scaled (Figures 39C and 39D).

C. Uses

1. For submarginal deposits.
2. For fine supramarginal calculus after gross deposits have been removed.

III. HOE SCALER

A. Characteristics

1. Single cutting edge (Figure 38C).
2. Blade turned at approximately a 100° angle to shank.
3. Edge of blade beveled at a 45° angle to terminal end of blade.
4. Shank is angulated.

B. Adaptation

1. Angular relationship between shank and handle of each hoe scaler in a set permits specific access to individual tooth surfaces.
2. With two point contact with tooth to stabilize the instrument and prevent nicking or scratching of the tooth surface (Figures 39E and 39F).
   a. Cutting edge in contact with tooth, apical to deposit depth.
   b. Shank in contact with crown.
3. With shank extending vertically, parallel with long axis of the tooth.

C. **Uses**
1. For readily accessible calculus deposits.
2. For submarginal calculus only when overlying gingival tissue is flabby and easily displaced; the hoe should never be forced to the bottom of the sulcus or pocket.

IV. **SPECIFICATIONS FOR THE SELECTION OF SCALERS**[1]

A. Effective in calculus removal with least possible trauma to gingival tissue and tooth structure.
B. Provide comfort to operator without causing fatigue or muscle cramp.
C. Includes minimum number in a set which permits maximum efficiency in calculus removal from each surface of each tooth.
D. Well balanced.
1. Blade should be centered in direct line with long axis of the handle.
2. Distance of cutting edges from junction of shank and handle (where instrument is held) should be optimum for permitting action of the scaler.
E. Handle of a diameter for grasp which prevents muscular fatigue and increases tactile sensitivity.
F. Light weight.
G. Blades of a shape which can be sharpened conveniently.
H. Material
1. Will maintain sharpness for an optimum length of time.
2. Can be sharpened readily.
3. Will not discolor or rust during use or sterilization.

PREPARATION AND PROCEDURE FOR SCALING

Prior to scaling, instruments and other equipment are prepared. The extent of the case must be appraised and the immediate field of operation inspected carefully. Inspection is a continuing process throughout the oral prophylaxis until complete removal of calculus is accomplished.

I. **PREPARATION OF SCALERS**

A. Scalers are sharpened and sterilized at the completion of an appointment to make ready for the next (see pages 28 and 34–43).
B. Alternate sharp scalers should be available for substitution during scaling procedures.
C. **Effects of Use of Sharp Scalers**
With scaler blade maintained with its original contour and cutting edges sharp, the following may be expected:
1. Prevention of unnecessary trauma to gingival tissues.
2. Increased tactile sensitivity.
3. Control of stroke with less pressure of instrument on tooth, lighter instrument grasp, and decreased pressure on fulcrum rest.
4. Reduced possibility of burnishing the calculus rather than removing it.

II. PATIENT INSPECTION FOR SCALING

A. Purposes

The preliminary observations made during the oral inspection (see pages 81–85) provide basic information for planning procedures and indicating the number of appointments required. A more specific inspection is required to define scaling techniques.

1. To determine exact location of calculus deposits.
2. To select scalers to be used.
3. To recognize irregularities of tooth surfaces or restorations which may interfere with scaling techniques.
4. During scaling procedures: to avoid unnecessary repetition and make each phase of the operation meaningful.
5. At expected completion of procedures: to assure complete removal of deposits.

B. Methods

Visual and tactile methods are used. Instruments have been described on pages 77–81. Access and visibility through adequate retraction and illumination are prerequisite to thoroughness. Inspection is accomplished through the integrated use of radiographs, periodontal probe, explorers, mouth mirror and compressed air. Disclosing solution application can contribute effectively during the final inspection after polishing.

1. Radiographic
   a. Bite-wing survey: provides a right-angle view of the crowns of the teeth and the relationship of the alveolar bone and the root which is most useful as a guide to scaling.
   b. Indications for use: helpful in all cases and should be mandatory before and after scaling of teeth with extensive calculus deposits and numerous dental restorations which involve the proximal surfaces.
   c. Suggestions for technique: slight underexposure of films aids in revealing less radiopaque deposits.
2. Visual
   a. Dry tooth surface with compressed air, maintaining retraction.
      (1) Observe area closely while applying air.
      (2) Use mouth mirror to reflect light through anterior teeth while the teeth are dry.
      (3) Note darkened opaque areas which may indicate presence of calculus. Confirm with exploration.
   b. Deflect gingival margin from tooth surface and inspect sulcus.
      (1) Direct warm air stream between tooth and gingival margin.
      (2) Use small cotton pellet in cotton pliers to dry a hypersensitive area.
   c. Use transillumination (see page 194).
3. Tactile
   a. Use periodontal probe to define sulcus depth.
   b. Use explorer to check tooth surface variations to the bottom of the sulcus.

C. **Characteristics to be Observed**
1. Depth of sulcus and height of alveolar bone: to define cases needing prompt consultation with dentist to outline needs for periodontal care following dental hygiene care.
2. Topography of the tooth surfaces.
3. Nature, location, extent and accessibility of deposits.
4. Color, size, contour, consistency and position of the free gingiva.
5. Abnormalities of the teeth which may interfere with instrumentation.
   a. Abrasion.
   b. Erosion.
   c. Developmental anomalies.
   d. Marked variations in the cemento-enamel junction.
   e. Deficient or overhanging dental restorations.
   f. Carious lesions.
   g. Areas of hypersensitivity.
   h. Malaligned teeth.

III. **PROCEDURE FOR SCALING**

The procedure for scaling varies with the severity of the case. Prerequisite to any procedure is the use of an efficient routine which will minimize time and assure little trauma to the patient.

One system, suggested below, is to scale a group of teeth as completely as possible before moving on to the next group. When there are gross deposits, yet it is expected that scaling will be completed in a single appointment, it may be helpful to remove gross supramarginal deposits systematically throughout the entire dentition, and then return to each area to complete the fine scaling.

For patients with excessive stains, it may be advisable to polish the gross stains before completing the scaling. By this method, better vision is provided for the finer aspects of scaling. A final repolishing is necessary after all calculus is removed.

With respect to the application of specific scalers, two methods are suggested. One is to complete a particular tooth or aspects of a group of teeth (for example, all buccal aspects of a quadrant), alternating scalers as needed. The second method is to apply a particular scaler to all applicable surfaces in a given quadrant followed by each successive scaler used in a similar manner.

A. **Suggested Procedure**
1. Inspect a group of teeth or quadrant. Follow a routine order for instrumentation.
2. Scale the group of teeth inspected.
3. Re-inspect for identification of remaining calculus and continue scaling as needed.
4. Move to n xt group of teeth or quadrant: follow same routine.

B. **Application for Case Requiring Multiple Appointments**
When the patient's tissues are enlarged, nonresilient, and have a tendency to hemorrhage readily upon application of instruments, it is usually impossible to be certain that the calculus is completely removed at the first appointment.

1. Scaling should be completed as nearly as possible to give the tissues the opportunity to return to normal before the next appointment.
   a. Postoperative instruction is given (see page 195).
      (1) Rinsing with a mild salt solution.
      (2) Personal oral care procedures.
   b. Next appointment scheduled: in several days to a week.
   c. Final inspection and complete scaling accomplished at succeeding appointment.
2. Scaling may be limited to a specific group of teeth (quadrant or maxillary and mandibular quadrants of one side of mouth as described on page 139) to provide for as near completion as possible in time allocated.
   a. Generalized removal of gross deposits inadvertently without directed effort to remove as much deposit as possible may do patient's gingival tissues more harm than good.
   b. Calculus roughened by partial removal is a source of greater irritation to the gingiva than the calculus prior to scaling. The tissues had been somewhat adjusted to the shape and surface texture of the deposit.
   c. Personal oral care procedures, particularly toothbrushing, force the gingival wall against the roughened calculus. Tissues are prevented from healing by the repeated source of irritation.

USE OF SCALERS: TECHNIQUES FOR THE REMOVAL OF CALCULUS

Development of ability, skill and efficiency for the successful removal of calculus through positive scaling techniques requires more than the development of dexterity for applying scalers to the tooth surfaces. A principle objective in technique is to accomplish a thorough removal of deposits with a minimum amount of trauma to the teeth and gingiva. In this delicate and exacting technique the dental hygienist must apply knowledge of the anatomical, histological and physiological characteristics of the tissues to the fullest advantage of the patient.

The purposes of scaling are not only to remove calculus from the clinical crowns of the teeth, but also to smooth the tooth surfaces to minimize the tendency for reaccumulation of soft deposits and calculus. The ultimate objective is to maintain the gingival tissue in a healthy state.

I. BASIC PRINCIPLES TO GUIDE TECHNIQUES

A. Positive procedures are guided by the appreciation of the need for the removal of each particle of calculus to assure maximum tissue response for oral health.

B. Technique is governed by knowledge of the nature and distribution of the calculus.

C. A thorough procedure is based on the realization of the importance of scaling in the over-all prevention of periodontal disease which may be due to local irritation of the gingival tissue.

D. Technique is directed by the knowledge of the function of each scaler and an awareness of the conditions under which instrumentation can be carried out most effectively. Each scaler should be used for the specific purpose and in the specific manner for which it was designed.

E. *The use of a scaler is governed by three major principles.*
   1. The grasp of the instrument.
   2. The control of the motion of the instrument.
   3. The tactile sense which the instrument affords.

II. STEPS IN THE REMOVAL OF CALCULUS

Calculus is removed by deliberate scaling in a routine order from tooth to tooth, and section by section of the calculus deposit itself on the individual surfaces. Each scaling stroke overlaps the previous one as the scaler is positioned progressively along the area of deposit.

Each stroke is planned so that a maximum amount of calculus is removed by a single stroke. The ultimate "positive scaling procedure" would be complete removal of the section of calculus by a single stroke. This is not usually possible except when the deposits are light and thin. Firm, adherent deposits require several strokes.

The five basic steps for the application of a scaler to remove an individual section of calculus are described here. These five steps are:

A. Grasp of instrument
B. Establish the fulcrum
C. Position the blade
D. Activate the scaler
E. Complete the stroke

A. Grasp of Instrument

1. Apply unstrained *pen* grasp (see page 140).
2. Use light grasp until deposit is engaged to permit tactile discrimination.
3. Tighten grasp only during scaling stroke for actual removal of deposit.
4. Return to light grasp immediately upon reaching height of deposit or length of stroke.

B. Establish the Fulcrum

1. Apply principles governing use of fulcrum (see page 141).
2. Use ring finger on solid tooth or teeth for major fulcrum rest.
3. Apply supplementary fulcrums whenever possible.
4. Use light but firm pressure of fulcrum finger on fulcrum rest during the preparatory steps to deposit removal.
5. Increase fulcrum pressure during activation of scaler to minimum required for balance of pressure of scaler on tooth being scaled and the grasp of the instrument.
6. Return to light but firm pressure immediately upon completion of stroke.

C. **Position the Blade for Deposit Removal**

1. *Preliminary or Exploratory Stroke:** the phase of scaling in which the instrument is held in a featherlike grasp in order to ascertain by tactile discrimination the amount and extent of calculus on the tooth surface below the gingival margin.
   a. Hold instrument with light grasp.
   b. Maintain light but firm pressure of fulcrum finger.
   c. Insert working end of scaler over deposit and continue carefully in direction of the apex of the tooth to the termination of the deposit. Tip of blade is in contact with the surface of the deposit or tooth at all times.
2. Adapt instrument for proper relationship of cutting edge of blade to tooth surface directly under deposit (Figure 39, page 148).
3. Hold cutting edge of blade firmly against the tooth surface just beneath the terminal border of the deposit for a moment before activating instrument.

D. **Activate Scaler**

1. *Working Stroke to Remove Deposit*
   a. Tighten grasp during working stroke (grasp is lightened immediately after).
   b. Move instrument firmly and deliberately.
   c. Make each stroke purposeful to avoid unnecessary repetition.
2. *Position of Scaler*
   a. *Keep cutting edge closely adapted to tooth surface during entire movement and at finish of stroke.*
   b. Utilize maximum length of blade: the use of the tip of the scaler is inefficient. It may scratch the tooth surface or the blade may break from undue pressure.
3. *Direction of Stroke*
   a. Vertical, in incisal or occlusal direction: for all scalers on all surfaces when scalers are used for submarginal calculus or calculus adjacent to gingival crest.
   b. Horizontal: for supramarginal calculus on central or incisal (occlusal) third of tooth when deposit is not related to gingival crest and cannot be removed as conveniently with a vertical stroke.
4. *Pressure of Scaler on Tooth Surface*
   a. Maintain minimum pressure for maximum efficiency in deposit removal.
   b. Balance pressure on fulcrum rest and grasp of instrument with pressure of scaler on the tooth surface.
5. *Control of Motion*
   a. Hand, wrist and arm act as a continuum to provide motion and pressure (see page 142).

---

* The preliminary or exploratory stroke is sometimes referred to as the "preparatory" stroke. If the term "exploratory" is used it should be distinguished from the meaning of the word as it applies to the use of an explorer. The scaler is not used as an explorer, and the calculus has been identified previously by using an explorer.

b. Position of hand holding instrument
    (1) Hold instrument firmly but comfortably in pen grasp.
    (2) Hold fingers grasping instrument immobile, close together and slightly curved.
    (3) Pivot hand around the fulcrum during stroke.
    (4) Rocking or rotary motion of arm propels the instrument.
6. *Length of Stroke*
    a. Short: deposit is removed in segments.
      (1) To permit accomodation of cutting edge of scaler to topography of tooth surface.
      (2) To maintain control and precision.
    b. Confine stroke to the *instrumentation zone*, which is the height of the deposit on the tooth surface. Most of the calculus is distributed in a zone which covers the area a short distance above and below the cemento-enamel junction.[2] There are variations depending on the position of the epithelial attachment, the use of the tooth in mastication, and other factors which were listed on pages 105 to 109.

E. Completion of Stroke

1. Hold instrument in place, just above instrumentation zone.
2. Lighten grasp as in preliminary stroke.

F. Continuation of Procedure

1. Move instrument laterally on tooth surface to adjacent undisturbed deposit, maintaining fulcrum.
2. Overlap strokes to insure complete removal of deposit.
3. Position scaler for next preliminary stroke; proceed with deposit removal.
4. Repeat until the tooth surface has been scaled completely.
5. Inspect scaled surface with explorer, using the aid of compressed air to ascertain complete removal of deposit.
6. Repeat scaling and recheck as indicated.

USE OF ULTRASONICS IN SCALING

Ultrasonic instrumentation is an adjunct to manual scaling but not a substitute. Because of the ease of removal of tooth deposits by ultrasonic techniques, the application is most effective with patients having gross stains, calculus and debris. The fine finish to provide smooth tooth surfaces and a high polish must be accomplished by conventional methods.

The mode of action and technique for use is considerably different from manual instruments. The efficiency in calculus removal by the two methods has been compared and very little difference has been observed except that the removal of fine submarginal calculus and root planing must be carried out by manual methods.[3,4] The effect on oral tissues compares favorably with manual, provided the instruments are used correctly and the principles of action are applied scientifically.[5] Histological studies have shown postoperative healing following ultrasonic scaling to be at least as satisfactory and in some instances, more satisfactory than hand scaling.[6,7]

In addition to the removal of gross deposits and stains, ultrasonics may be used in a variety of ways including the removal of overhanging restorations and in periodontal curettage and surgery. In orthodontics, ultrasonic instrumentation has been found effective for scaling prior to fitting and cementing appliances, and for the removal of excess cement after initial cementation and when appliances are removed.[8] Reference to the ultrasonic cleaning unit for instruments has been made on pages 26 and 28.

I. **MODE OF ACTION**[9–11]

The ultrasonic unit consists of an electric generator, a handpiece assembly, a set of interchangeable prophylaxis inserts and a foot control. The ultrasonic principle is based on the use of very high frequency sound waves.

A. The ultrasonic machine converts high frequency electrical energy into mechanical energy in the form of rapid vibrations.

B. The instrument tip vibrates at approximately 25,000 cycles per second with an amplitude of 1/1000 cm. The vibratory action fractures the deposit and causes it to be removed from the tooth.

C. Ultrasonic waves are dissipated in the form of heat. The heat is reduced by keeping the handpiece cooled internally and the working end cooled by a constant flow of water which is expelled through a metal tube or by means of an internal flow through the working end.

D. Effects of water: vibrating water forms minute vacuum bubbles which collapse with release of tremendous local pressure; the effect is cleansing to the area. Since it is necessary to have the instrument in contact with the deposit on the tooth surface if the deposit is to be removed, the bubbling cavitational action of the water has little if any actual influence on deposit removal.

II. **TECHNIQUE FOR USE**[5, 9, 12, 13]

A. **Preparation of Prophylaxis Inserts**

1. Tune according to manufacturer's specifications.
2. Instrument tips must be dull: if sharp they would nick and gouge the tooth surface.

B. **Preparation of Patient**

1. Use coverall and towel.
2. Topical anesthetic may be applied to allay gingival sensitivity.
3. Disclosing solution may be applied to aid in ready detection of deposits (see page 190).

C. **Aspiration of Water:** use an aspirator or effective saliva ejector.

D. **Instrumentation**

1. Use pen grasp for handpiece and apply fulcrum to appropriate, convenient tooth surfaces to stabilize the instrument and permit systematic coverage of tooth surfaces being scaled.
2. Application of working end: parallel to long axis of the tooth or at no more than a 15° angle to tooth surface.
3. Stroke
   a. Brush lightly over the deposit moving in a vertical direction from crown to submarginal area: 6 to 12 strokes usually suffice.

      b. Move instrument with smooth, light, quick, constant, and overlapping strokes.

      c. Increased number of strokes will not damage the tooth surface provided the instrument is blunt, the tip is not held perpendicular to the long axis of the tooth, and no positive pressure is used.

      d. Instrument tends to bind when inserted interproximally, and the excess pressure stops the vibration. Remove and reactivate the instrument.

4. Release foot pedal switch at regular intervals to aid in water control; stop to evaluate the tooth surfaces with an explorer periodically.

5. Complete procedure with manual instruments

      a. Remove remaining submarginal deposits and plane the surface smooth with curets.

      b. Polish with prophylaxis angle and polishing cup with mild abrasive.

E. Care of Prophylaxis Inserts

1. Autoclave; or wipe clean with disinfectant and place in cold disinfecting chemical.

2. Handle with care to avoid damage to working ends or internal mechanisms.

III. ADVANTAGES AND LIMITATIONS

A. Advantages

1. Calculus removal and tooth debridement may be accomplished with less effort than manual.

2. Less gingival hemorrhage which means less gingival injury and hence less postoperative discomfort can be expected.

3. Minimum tissue manipulation when tissues are hypersensitive (as in acute gingivitis, necrotizing ulcerative gingivitis).

4. Water jet cleanses the field of operation; aids visibility.

      a. Water flushes out the sulcus: no particles of calculus left to irritate the gingiva and delay postoperative healing.

      b. Spray of water may be beneficial to the gingival tissue.

5. Patient has a more comfortable appointment and less pain during instrumentation.

6. Operating time is reduced for removal of gross stains and calculus.

B. Limitations

1. Lack of tactile perception during instrumentation.

2. Some impeded visibility during operation; indirect vision with water-sprayed mouth mirror presents problems.

3. Will not complete the entire procedure: access to all areas is not possible, and fine submarginal calculus is not removed.

4. Polishing must be accomplished by conventional methods.

5. Patient and operator have discomfort and inconvenience of spraying or dripping of water.

USE OF A TOPICAL ANESTHETIC

Scaling can be an extremely uncomfortable procedure when teeth or gingiva are supersensitive. Injection of a local anesthetic by the dentist prior to scaling is the only answer to the problem for an isolated group of patients. When this procedure is followed, usually at least four appointments are required so that each quadrant may be anesthetized individually. The local anesthetic is used primarily for sensitivity of the teeth rather than the gingiva.

Topical anesthetics have been used with some degree of success for short duration desensitization of the gingiva. When the dental hygienist applies a topical anesthetic it is done under the direction of the dentist and in accord with the law of the state in which she practices.

In addition to the use during scaling, topical anesthetics may be helpful during radiographic technique (see page 230), for impression making, and by the dentist for such procedures as the incision of gingival abscesses, temporary relief from ulcers, wounds, or other injured areas, for replacement of periodontal dressings, and prior to the injection of a local anesthetic.

Topical anesthetics should be used with caution and care since toxic reactions are possible. It is essential to limit the concentration of the preparation, the area of application, and the total amount.

I. USES

    A. For patients who have a low pain threshold.
    B. For anxious patients.
    C. For psychological effect in gaining cooperation of apprehensive patients.
    D. For relief of gagging tendency.

II. ACTION OF THE TOPICAL ANESTHETIC

    The purpose is to desensitize the mucous membrane by anesthetizing the terminal nerve endings. A superficial anesthesia is produced which is related to the amount of absorption of the drug by the tissue. The absorption varies with the thickness of the stratified squamous epithelium covering and the degree of keratinization. The skin and lips are very resistant; the gingiva and cheek and palatal mucosa absorb drugs slowly; whereas the mucobuccal fold and sublingual tissue absorb more readily.

III. REQUIREMENTS OF AN ADEQUATE TOPICAL ANESTHETIC

    A. Produce effective lasting anesthesia.
    B. Miscible and stable in vehicle used.
    C. Anesthetizing agent readily released from the preparation when applied.
    D. Nonirritating to the tissues.
    E. Not induce hypersensitivity reactions or other toxic effect at the concentration required for anesthesia.
    F. Not delay healing.
    G. Be readily washed off with water.

IV. **PREPARATIONS USED: CHARACTERISTICS**

A number of preparations have been used in the form of ointments, solutions, troches, or powders. The American Dental Association, Council on Dental Therapeutics evaluates and classifies topical anesthetics.[14] Dobbs[15] indicates that the following anesthetics may be used topically in appropriate, safe percentages: Benzocaine, Pontocaine, Lidocaine (Xylocaine), Nupercaine, and Ravocaine. A few general properties and characteristics of the preparations made from these anesthetics are suggested below.

A. Oils, alcohols or glycols are used as the vehicle since most of the anesthetizing substances are only slightly soluble in water.

B. Most topical anesthetics are prepared in fairly concentrated form to allow for the resistance of the thick epithelial covering and viscid coating of saliva on the tissues.

C. The drugs are absorbed slowly due to their slight solubility and the resistance of the mucous membrane.

D. Alcohols or glycols in concentrated solutions may be irritating to the sensitive mucous membranes and therefore are inferior vehicles (per cent of alcohol or glycol should not be greater than 10 per cent).

E. Pastes or ointments are more effective than liquids but more difficult to apply.

F. Carbowaxes used as vehicles for topical anesthetics are somewhat hygroscopic, so that the jar in which the ointment is kept should be closed tightly.

G. Pressurized spray preparations need to be used with caution since it is difficult to control the amount of material expelled and to limit the area of application. Inhalation of the fine spray into the lungs can produce a toxic reaction. When the liquid flows into the throat (as may be possible with application of any type of preparation), coughing may be initiated.

V. **TECHNIQUE FOR APPLICATION OF A TOPICAL ANESTHETIC**

A. Explain purpose and anticipated effect to the patient.

B. Dry area with gauze wipe or cotton roll. Compressed air may be used with consideration for sensitive tissues.

C. Application
1. Liquid preparation: apply with cotton pellet saturated in the solution.
2. Paste or ointment: gently massage the ointment on the tissue surface with cotton pellet or apply into gingival sulcus with syringe.

D. Wait briefly for anesthetic to take effect before proceeding with scaling.

SUMMARY OF FACTORS WHICH MINIMIZE PATIENT DISCOMFORT AND PAIN

I. **FACTORS RELATED TO TISSUE SENSITIVITY**

A. Gingival Tissue: apply topical anesthetic.

B. Exposed Cementum and Dentin: apply desensitizing agent (see pages 210–211).

C. Protection of Lips and Corners of Mouth.
1. Apply petroleum jelly, cocoa butter, or other appropriate lubricant.
2. Dentist may prescribe appropriate medicated ointment for patient with tendency to develop herpes labialis.

D. Use warm water or mouth wash for patient's rinsing.

II. FACTORS RELATED TO THE USE OF SCALERS

A. Use the appropriate instrument for each tooth surface.
B. Scalers applied beneath the gingival margin must be as small as possible for efficient removal of deposits.
C. Scalers need to be sharp, yet the cementum can be damaged if sharp scalers are not applied correctly and carefully.
D. Control instrument by maintaining proper balance between grasp and fulcrum.
E. Apply a light grasp to assure tactile discrimination of calculus.
F. Establish fulcrum on a firm tooth or group of teeth.
G. Maintain correct relationship of cutting edge of blade to tooth surface during all steps of instrumentation.
H. Use short, effective strokes within the instrumentation zone to maintain control and precision.
I. Apply minimum effective pressure of scaler on tooth surface.
J. Minimize soft tissue manipulation.

III. FACTORS RELATED TO POSTOPERATIVE CARE (see pages 194–196)

A. Massage gingival tissue at completion of oral prophylaxis.
B. Apply an antiseptic solution.
C. Provide appropriate instruction in personal care.

TECHNICAL HINTS

I. BACTEREMIA FOLLOWING SCALING

Manipulation of the gingival tissues has been shown to produce a transient bacteremia in a significant percentage of cases.[5,16,17] Although transient and of no clinical significance in most instances, prophylactic antibiotic therapy is indicated for patients with a history of rheumatic fever or congenital heart defects (see pages 430–431). The frequency and severity of bacteremias are directly related to the degree of trauma.[18]

II. RETRACTION AND MAINTENANCE OF A CLEAR FIELD

A. Use of cotton rolls (this can be time consuming and should not be adopted as a routine procedure).
1. Aid in providing accessibility by placing a cotton roll in the mucobuccal or mucolabial fold adjacent to area being scaled.
   a. When patient is anxious and moves frequently.

　　　　b. When muscles of lips and cheeks are particularly taut.

　　　　c. When there is excess flow of saliva.

　　2. Aid in retraction of tongue and keeping field free from saliva by placing cotton roll under tongue.

　B. Maintenance of clear field and/or control of bleeding.

　　1. Application of pressure with cotton roll or pellet.

　　2. Application of 3 per cent hydrogen peroxide with cotton pellet, followed by patient rinsing and/or dry pellet applied with pressure.

　　3. Use of compressed air to deflect tissue and remove debris.

　　4. Frequent rinsing by patient.

III. ADAPTATION OF TECHNIQUES TO SPECIAL AREAS

　A. Adapt routine scaling procedures to malaligned teeth.

　　1. Adjust fulcrum finger for better access.

　　2. Redirect illumination by adequate adjustment of mouth mirror.

　B. Scale chalky, white, decalcified areas lightly, only for purpose of removing soft material. Do not allow blade to enter area of broken enamel or to fracture edge of lesion.

　C. Since decalcification frequently occurs beneath green stain, scaling should be attempted with caution and only to remove debris and materia alba.

　D. Ascertain by repeated use of explorer and radiographs that calculus and not some other irregularity of tooth structure or defective restoration is present.

　E. Scaling techniques are adapted for removal of calculus from removable dentures. Care must be taken not to scratch the denture surface.

IV. INSTRUMENTATION

　A. Facilitate scaling procedures by removing gross deposits of materia alba and food debris.

　　1. Request patient to demonstrate correct toothbrushing method in his mouth before instrumentation.

　　2. Apply 3 per cent hydrogen peroxide with cotton pellet and request patient to rinse thoroughly.

　B. Observe patient's reactions during instrumentation.

　　1. For anticipation of sudden movements which might result in accidental trauma to soft tissues.

　　2. For indication that patient is experiencing undue pain caused by operator.

　　3. For indication that excess saliva has collected.

　C. Round off sharp edges on back surface of sickle scalers or corners of hoes to prevent laceration of adjacent soft tissues.

　D. Unnecessary scaling after deposit is removed is injurious, particularly at the cemento-enamel junction where the cementum is thin. The cementum may be removed and a hypersensitive area left.

　E. Cultivation of a keen tactile sense permits the operator to recognize completion of scaling.

　F. Fulcrums on soft tissue give the patient a feeling of pressure being applied, and the impression that the operator is heavy handed.

　G. Repolish area when additional scaling has been necessary after routine polishing has been completed.

V. SUGGESTED PROCEDURE WHEN A SCALER BLADE IS BROKEN DURING OPERATION

The procedure used by a dental hygienist in a specific dental office should be in accord with the dentist's own philosophy. It is recommended that this be discussed with the dentist at an appropriate time along with other procedures and policies.

The principle objective in the location of a broken scaler tip is to know *positively* that the tip has been *removed*. With this in mind, excessive rinsing, application of compressed air or other procedures which could cause the removal of the scaler tip unknowingly would be out of order. A general procedure is suggested here.

A. Cease operation immediately. Do not alarm the patient by describing the accident.

B. Before the patient is permitted to swallow or rinse, examine the immediate field of operation, the floor of the mouth and the area of the mucobuccal fold. Do not apply compressed air if there is a possibility of forcing the scaler tip into the gingival sulcus. Area may be dried with cotton or gauze wipe.

C. If scaler tip is not removed in Step B, make periapical and bite-wing radiographs of the area.

D. Consult dentist for assistance in removal of tip in accord with previously discussed policy.

VI. PROTECTION OF THE OPERATOR: Wear rimmed glasses for protection from bits of calculus or debris which may accidentally get in the eyes. Wear plain glass lenses when correction is unnecessary.

FACTORS TO TEACH THE PATIENT

I. The nature, occurrence and etiology of calculus.

II. The importance of the complete removal of calculus to the health of the oral tissues in the prevention of periodontal diseases.

III. Relation of the accumulation of deposits to the patient's personal oral hygiene procedures.

IV. Basic reasons for need and advantages of more than one appointment to complete the oral prophylaxis.

V. Needed frequency of recall appointments for oral prophylaxis in relation to the individual tendency to accumulate deposits.

REFERENCES

1. GRANT, DANIEL, STERN, I. B., and EVERETT, F. G.: *Orban's Periodontics*, 2nd ed. St. Louis, Mosby, 1963, pp. 284, 287.

2. GLICKMAN, IRVING: Clinical Periodontology, 2nd ed. Philadelphia, Saunders, 1958, pp. 589–590.

3. STENDE, G. W. and SCHAFFER, E. M.: Comparison of Ultrasonic and Hand Scaling, J. Periodont., *32*, 312, October, 1961.

4. McCALL, C. M. and SZMYD, L.: Clinical Evaluation of Ultrasonic Scaling, Am. Dent. A. J., *61*, 559, November, 1960.

5. SCHAFFER, E. M.: Objective Evaluation of Ultrasonic Versus Hand Instrumentation in Periodontics, Dental Clinics of North America, March, 1964, p. 165.

6. GOLDMAN, H. M.: Histologic Assay of Healing Following Ultrasonic Curettage versus Hand-Instrument Curettage, Oral Surg., Oral Med., & Oral Path., *14*, 925, August, 1961.

7. SCHAFFER, E. M., STENDE, G., and KING, D.: Healing of Periodontal Pocket Tissues Following Ultrasonic Scaling and Hand Planing, J. Periodont., *35*, 140, March-April, 1964.

8. JARABEK, J. R.: The Cavitron—An Auxiliary in Clinical Orthodontics, Illinois D. J., *30*, 604, September, 1961.

9. EWEN, S. J. and SORRIN, S.: Ultrasonics and Periodontal Therapy, Dental Clinics of North America, March, 1964, p. 145.

10. EWEN, S. J.: General Ultrasonic Theory and Periodontal Therapy, New York J. Den., *32*, 278, October, 1962.

11. EWEN, S. J.: Ultrasound and Periodontics, J. Periodont., *31*, 101, April, 1960.

12. EWEN, S. J. and TASCHER, P. J.: Clinical Uses of Ultrasonic Root Scalers, J. Periodont., *29*, 45, January, 1958.

13. EWEN, S. J. and TASCHER, P. J.: Instrumentation in Ultrasonic Periodontal Therapy, J. Periodont., *30*, 67, January, 1959.

14. American Dental Association, Council on Dental Therapeutics: *Accepted Dental Remedies*, 29th ed. Chicago, American Dental Association, 1964, pp. 32–33, 39–40.

15. DOBBS, E. C.: *Pharmacology and Oral Therapeutics*, 12th ed. St. Louis, Mosby, 1961, pp. 378–385.

16. American Dental Association, Council on Dental Therapeutics: op. cit., pp. 3–4.

17. WINSLOW, M. B. and KOBERNICK, S. D.: Bacteremia After Prophylaxis, Am. Dent. A. J., *61*, 69, July, 1960.

18. BENDER, I. B., SELTZER, S., TASHMAN, Sylvia, and MELOFF, GERTRUDE: Dental Procedures in Patients with Rheumatic Heart Disease, Oral Surg., Oral Med., & Oral Path., *16*, 466, April, 1963.

SUGGESTED READINGS

Scalers and Scaling Procedures

BARNES, J. E. and SCHAFFER, E. M.: Subgingival Root Planing: A Comparison Using Files, Hoes, Curettes, J. Periodont., *31*, 300, September, 1960.

BEUBE, F. E.: *Periodontology*. New York, Macmillan, 1953, pp. 64–96.

BODECKER, C. F.: Difficulty of Completely Removing Subgingival Calculus, Am. Dent. A. J., *30*, 703, May, 1943.

BUNTING, R. W.: *Oral Hygiene*, 3rd ed. Philadelphia, Lea & Febiger, 1957, pp. 244–254.

GAGE, C. A.: Discomfort During Scaling Can Be Reduced, Am. Dent. Hygienists' A. J., *31*, 157, October, 1957.

GLICKMAN, IRVING: *Clinical Periodontology*, 2nd ed. Philadelphia, Saunders, 1958, pp. 547–618.

GOLDMAN, H. M., SCHLUGER, S., FOX, L. and COHEN, D. W.: *Periodontal Therapy*, 2nd ed. St. Louis, Mosby, 1960, pp. 106–133.

HARD, D. G.: The Conservative Treatment of Periodontal Disease, Am. Dent. A. J., *44*, 725, June, 1952.

HINE, M. K. and SWENSON, H. M.: Role of Prophylactic Procedures in the Treatment of Periodontal Disease, Am. Dent. A. J., *45*, 301, September, 1952.

HIRSCHFELD, LEONARD: Subgingival Curettage in Periodontal Treatment, Am. Dent. A. J., *44*, 301, March, 1952.

MILLER, S. C.: *Textbook of Periodontia*, 3rd ed. New York, Blakiston Division, McGraw-Hill, 1950, pp. 260–306.

MOSKOW, B. S.: Response of the Gingival Sulcus to Instrumentation: A Histological Investigation. I. The Scaling Procedure, J. Periodont., *33*, 282, July, 1962.

O'BANNON, J. Y.: Gingival Tissues Before and After Scaling the Teeth, J. Periodont, *35*, 69, January-February, 1964.

ORBAN, B. J. and MANELLA, V. B.: A Macroscopic and Microscopic Study of Instruments Designed for Root Planing, J. Periodont,. *27*, 120, April, 1956.

SCHWARTZ, M.: Magnetic Instrument for the Recovery of Broken Curette Fragments and Other Steel Bodies, J. Periodont., *29*, 195, July, 1958.

WAERHAUG, JENS, ARNO, ARNULF, and LOVDAL, ARNE: The Dimension of Instruments for Removal of Subgingival Calculus, J. Periodont., *25*, 281, October, 1954.

Topical Anesthesia

DOBBS, E. C.: Drugs Which Act on the Skin and Mucous Membranes, Dental Clinics of North America, July, 1963, p. 473.

GRUBER, L. W.: New Fields of Application for Xylocaine as Applied to Dentistry, I. Xylocaine Ointment as a Topical Anesthetic in Dentistry, Oral Surg., Oral Med., & Oral Path., *5*, 281, March, 1952.

PING, R. S., WHITE, J. G., and SPEAR, L. B.:   Dyclonine Hydrochloride as a Topical Anesthetic in Dentistry, Oral Surg., Oral Med., & Oral Path., *10*, 623, June, 1957.

RAPOPORT, LEONARD and DOBBS, E. C.:   A Quantitative Estimation of the Potency of Ten Topical Anesthetic Preparations, Am. Dent. A. J., *47*, 430, October, 1953.

TAINTER, M. L. and MOOSE, S. M.:   Studies in Topical Anesthetics.   I. Efficacy of Certain Common Anesthetics When Used on the Gums, Am. Dent. A. J., *23*, 309, February, 1936.

TAINTER, M. L., THRONDSON, A. H., and MOOSE, S. M.:   Studies in Topical Anesthesia.   II. Further Observations on the Efficacy of the More Common Local Anesthetics When Used on the Gums and Oral Mucosa, Am. Dent. A. J., *24*, 1480, September, 1937.

Ultrasonics

ALLEN, E. F. and RHOADS, R. H.:   Effects of High Speed Periodontal Instruments on Tooth Surface, J. Periodont., *34*, 352, July, 1963.

ASHBY, B. E.:   Role of an Ultrasonic Unit in a Public Health or School Health Program, Am. Dent. Hygienists' A. J., *36*, 159, 4th Quarter, 1962.

EWEN, S. J.:   Ultrasonic Wound—Some Microscopic Observations, J. Periodont., *32*, 315, October, 1961.

GOLDMAN, H. M.:   Curettage by Ultrasonic Instrument, Oral Surg., Oral Med., & Oral Path., *13*, 43, January, 1960.

JOHNSON, W. N. and WILSON, J. R.:   Application of the Ultrasonic Dental Unit to Scaling Procedures, J. Periodont., *28*, 264, October, 1957.

KOLL, LUCILLE: Ultrasonics in Dental Hygiene, Am. Dent. Hygienists' A. J., *34*, 60, April, 1960.

KORN, N. A.:   Instrumentation: Hand and Mechanical, Am. Dent. Hygienists' A. J., *38*, 21, 1st Quarter, 1964.

ZANDER, H. A., KOHL, J. T., and KELLER, H.:   New Tool for Dental Prophylaxis, Am. Dent. A. J., *63*, 636, November, 1961.

Chapter 16

INTRODUCTION TO POLISHING TECHNIQUES

THE natural and restored surfaces of the teeth are polished after calculus has been removed during scaling procedures. This is followed by polishing removable dentures. A combination of motor-driven and hand instruments is employed with a wet abrasive agent.

Polishing must be performed carefully to prevent damage to the dental and gingival tissues. The epithelium of the gingival crest can be denuded when there is excess movement of polishing instruments and abrasive against this tissue. Because of the possibility of removing tooth structure, it is advisable to polish the cementum and the region of the cemento-enamel junction by hand polishing methods, using the finest grade of abrasive. A combination of motor-driven and hand methods may be used on the enamel surfaces.

I. OBJECTIVES FOR POLISHING

The process of polishing removes stains, films, and dental plaque from the clinical crowns of the teeth and provides smooth, shiny tooth surfaces. Well-polished tooth surfaces offer the following advantages:

A. Smooth tooth surfaces, free from deposits and stains, resist the tendency for the attachment of new deposits.

B. The excursion of food during mastication is easier so that less accumulation of debris results.

C. The patient can recognize and appreciate the appearance and feeling of a clean mouth which will aid in motivating him to practice adequate routines of personal oral care.

D. The properly instructed patient will obtain more effective results from his personal care techniques.[1]

II. INSTRUMENTS FOR POLISHING

The description and techniques for use of each of the instruments listed here will be included in the chapters following.

A. **Motor-Driven:** prophylaxis angle and handpiece attachments for rubber cup and bristle brush (see pages 178 and 179).

B. **Manual**

1. Porte polisher with wood point (see pages 173–177).
2. Straight orangewood stick, 8 inches long and $\frac{3}{16}$ of an inch in diameter with wedge-shaped end is adaptable for use on facial surfaces and facial aspects of proximal surfaces.
3. Dental tape and floss (see page 186).
4. Linen polishing strips (see page 188).

(166)

III. RECOMMENDED POLISHING ROUTINE

A routine system of polishing should be followed. The advantages of a systematic procedure consistent to all oral prophylaxis procedures have been described (see page 139).

A. Remove gross stains and plaques from enamel surfaces above gingival crest with rubber cup on prophylaxis angle.

B. Polish exposed cementum, region of the cemento-enamel junction or enamel surfaces adjacent to gingival crest with wood point in porte polisher.

C. Polish proximal surfaces, particularly the contact areas, and gingival surfaces of fixed partial dentures, with dental tape.

D. Apply disclosing solution (see pages 190–192).

E. Repolish with wood point in porte polisher.
  1. To remove remaining plaques revealed by disclosing solution.
  2. To provide glossy smooth surfaces on all teeth.

F. Use dental floss for removal of remaining particles of polishing abrasive.

G. Rinse patient's mouth thoroughly to remove abrasive particles which could be a source of irritation in the gingival sulcus.

H. Polish removable dentures (see pages 181–183).

IV. APPOINTMENT PLAN FOR PATIENT WITH EXTENSIVE CALCULUS

It is frequently advantageous for the patient with heavy calculus to have the deposits removed at one or more appointments as required and to return for a final appointment for polishing. Such a procedure permits the gingival tissue to heal after the source of irritation has been removed.

Motivation and instruction in personal oral care procedures must be provided in order that the patient will supplement the effects of scaling with routine care between appointments. Irritation which could result from use of a polishing abrasive will be minimized if the gingival tissues have been given an opportunity to return to normal size and position.

ABRASIVES USED IN POLISHING PROCEDURES

Abrasive agents are applied with polishers to remove dental stains and plaque. Abrasives selected will produce smooth tooth surfaces, but will not remove tooth structure unnecessarily, abrade gingival epithelium, or produce excessive frictional heat.

I. DEFINITIONS

A. **Abrasive:** a material composed of particles of sufficient hardness and sharpness to cut or scratch a softer material when drawn across its surface.

B. **Abrasion:** the wearing away of surface material by friction.

C. **Polishing:** the production, especially by friction, of a smooth mirror-like surface that reflects light evenly in all directions.[2] Polishing involves little loss of structural material of the surface being abraded.

II. CHARACTERISTICS OF ABRASIVE PARTICLES[3]

During polishing, sharp edges of abrasive particles are moved along the surface of a material, abrading it by producing microscopic scratches or grooves. The rate of abrasion, or speed with which structural material is removed from the surface being polished, is governed by characteristics of the abrasive particles as well as by the manner in which they are applied.

A. **Shape:** irregular-shaped particles with sharp edges produce deeper grooves, thus abrade faster than rounded particles with dull edges.

B. **Hardness:** particles must be harder than the surface to be abraded; harder particles abrade faster.

C. **Body Strength:** particles fracture into smaller sharp-edged particles during use; particles of greater impact (body) strength abrade faster.

D. **Attrition Resistance:** effective abrasive particles do not dull or become impregnated in the surface being abraded; particles with greater attrition resistance abrade faster.

E. **Size**
1. Particles of larger size produce deeper cuts or grooves in the surface being abraded; larger particles abrade faster.
2. Grades of abrasive and polishing agents
   a. *Grit:* denotes size of abrasive particle in a range of 6, coarse to 220, fine.
   b. *Powders or Flours:* denote size of particles smaller than 220 grit; dry particles are graded in order of increasing fineness as F, FF, FFF; particles imbedded in papers are graded 0, 00, 000.

III. METHOD OF APPLICATION OF ABRASIVES

A. **Quantity Applied:** the more particles applied per unit time, the faster the rate of abrasion.

1. Particles suspended in water or other vehicles are present in quantities proportional to the thickness of the paste. These vehicles act as lubricants to reduce the amount of frictional heat produced.
2. Dry powders or flours represent the greatest quantity that can be applied per unit time. Frictional heat is proportional to the rate of abrasion, therefore the use of *dry agents* is *contraindicated* for polishing natural teeth because of the potential danger of thermal injury to dental pulp.

B. **Speed of Application:** the greater the speed of application, the faster the rate of abrasion.

1. Particles drawn over a surface rapidly will fracture rapidly, producing shallower grooves in the abraded surface.
2. *Rapid abrasion* increases frictional heat: *contraindicated*.

C. **Pressure of Application:** the heavier the pressure applied, the faster the rate of abrasion.

    1. Particles to which pressure is applied produce deep grooves at first, but fracture according to their impact strength; with sufficient pressure, particles may disintegrate.

    2. *Pressure* increases frictional heat: *contraindicated.*

IV. EFFECTS OF POLISHING ON TOOTH STRUCTURE

Abrasive agents are used to produce esthetic, smooth tooth surfaces which are resistant to reaccumulation of stains and deposits. The high degree of calcification of dental enamel makes it quite resistant to abrasion by polishing agents normally employed for the oral prophylaxis, while cementum and dentin, which contain a higher percentage of organic matter and water, are less resistant to abrasion (see page 120).

Dental calculus, which contains from 75–80 per cent inorganic salts (see page 119), must be removed with scalers. If an attempt were made to remove this deposit with abrasives, tooth structure could be damaged and the amount of frictional heat generated could injure the dental pulp.

Research under *in vitro* conditions has demonstrated that abrasive agents can remove tooth structure. Bailey and Phillips found that 4 microns (0.000016 inch) of enamel were removed with fine pumice applied with a rubber cup revolved at 5800 r.p.m. for 5 seconds.[4] Allen and Rhoads used the rubber cup and pumice on extracted teeth for 30 to 120 seconds with 1 to 16 ounces pressure, and reported average losses of 1.15 mm. of root structure and 0.05 mm. of enamel.[5] In another study, the authors found that flour of pumice and levigated alumina produced three times the amount of enamel abrasion produced by stannic oxide, while various calcium carbonates removed very little tooth structure.[6]

The rate and degree of abrasion depend on interrelated factors: abrasive particle characteristics, method of application, and characteristics of the surface being abraded. Awareness of the effects of these factors will assist the operator to conserve tooth structure and maintain tooth vitality while the desired results of polishing are accomplished.

V. ABRASIVE AGENTS[7]

Preliminary polishing of roughened or stained surfaces is accomplished with the use of coarser abrasives. Final polishing and polishing of less resistant surfaces, such as cementum and ductile metals, require the use of a finer grade of abrasive.

A. **Coarser Abrasives:** used as pastes to remove gross stains and to polish porcelain.

    1. *Silex:* composed of sand, silicon dioxide or other forms of crushed quartz.

        a. XXX Silex: fairly abrasive.

        b. Super-fine Silex: finer grade than XXX.

    2. *Flour of Pumice:* composed of porous volcanic stone, chiefly silica with aluminum, potassium and sodium; specifications for particle size are listed in *The National Formulary.*

> *a.* Coarse and medium grades: too abrasive for use on natural teeth.
> *b.* Fine pumice: mildly abrasive.
> *c.* Superfine pumice: less abrasive than F, above.
> 3. *Kieselguhr* (diatomite): composed of siliceous remains of minute aquatic plants (diatoms); mildly abrasive.
> 4. *Tripoli:* composed of fine silicious powder; mildly abrasive, similar to superfine flour of pumice.

B. **Coarser Abrasives:** used to polish amalgam alloy restorations.

> 1. *Emery:* composed of natural oxide of aluminum (corundum) and other metallic oxides present as impurities; finer grades contain greater quantities of alumina; glued to linen strips or to paper disks for dental use.
> 2. *Sand* (silicon dioxide, silica): quartz crushed to powder fineness; glued to paper disks or linen strips for dental use.
> 3. *Aluminum Oxide, Pure* (alumina): purified form of bauxite available in various grain sizes; used as paste or glued to linen strips or paper disks. Extremely fine particles of aluminum oxide are called levigated alumina.
> 4. *Flour of Pumice, Superfine:* described above; used as paste or impregnated in rubber wheels.

C. **Finer Abrasives:** used as pastes to polish cementum and external surfaces of removable dentures, and to obtain final, high gloss on enamel surfaces.

> 1. *Whiting* (chalk): composed of precipitated calcium carbonate; available in various grades.
> 2. *Tin Oxide* (putty powder): manufactured by treating at a high temperature, the product of reaction between tin and concentrated nitric acid.
> 3. *Recrystallized Kaolinite:* a special fraction of anhydrous aluminum silicate obtained by heating kaolinite.[8]

D. **Finer Abrasives:** used as pastes to polish gold, platinum, stainless steel and acrylics, and to obtain final smooth finish on amalgam restorations.

> 1. *Whiting* (chalk): described above.
> 2. *Rouge* (Jeweler's rouge): iron oxide, a fine red powder; also used in cake form or impregnated on paper or cloth (crocus cloth); dirty to handle.
> 3. *Chromium Oxide:* fine powder; used to polish stainless steel.

VI. **PREPARATION OF ABRASIVES FOR CLINICAL USE**

When used for polishing natural teeth, abrasive agents are mixed with water or another lubricant that will facilitate particle movement across the surface to be abraded and thus reduce frictional heat.

A. **Mix Ingredients**

> 1. Place small amount of water or flavored mouthwash in dappen dish.
> 2. Add dry agent to saturation.
> 3. Stir to mix.

B. **Obtain Correct Consistency**

1. For motor-driven polishing: consistency of commercial dentifrice; moist, yet transportable in rubber cup from dish to patient's mouth.
2. For hand polishing: particles moist but discrete; less moisture is required because less frictional heat is generated with slower technique and saliva dilutes consistency of mixture during use.

VII. COMMERCIAL PREPARATIONS FOR DENTAL PROPHYLAXIS

Commercial dental prophylaxis preparations are available as powders or pastes. Powders are mixed with a flavoring agent. Stable pastes are formed when abrasive particles are moistened and held together in vehicles such as glycerin, propylene glycol or sorbitol. Selection of a preparation is based on its qualities of abrasiveness, consistency, and taste. See pages 308 to 309 for a description of dentifrice ingredients.

VIII. TECHNICAL HINTS

A. Observe tooth surfaces frequently during polishing to avoid over-polishing and unnecessary reduction of tooth structure.
B. Polish external surface of acrylic removable denture with fine grade abrasive only; do not use abrasive on internal surface, to avoid alteration of surface contour.
C. Remove all coarse abrasive particles from surfaces being polished, then apply a finer agent with a fresh wood point or rubber cup.
D. Add 1 or 2 drops of water as the mixture dries during the polishing procedure. Wet surface of mouth mirror under faucet and add water from mirror surface.

IX. FACTORS TO TEACH THE PATIENT

A. Highly polished tooth surfaces and restorations provide less potential for reaccumulation of deposits and stains than rougher unpolished surfaces.
B. Polishing agents employed in the dental office are too abrasive for routine daily home use.
C. Polishing procedures performed in routine professional oral prophylaxes do not "wear away" tooth surfaces.

REFERENCES

1. GRANT, DANIEL, STERN, I. B., and EVERETT, F. G.: *Orban's Periodontics*, 2nd ed. St. Louis, Mosby, 1963, p. 299.
2. SKINNER, E. W. and PHILLIPS, R. W.: *The Science of Dental Materials*, 5th ed. Philadelphia, Saunders, 1960, p. 577.
3. Ibid., pp. 579–580.
4. BAILEY, L. R. and PHILLIPS, R. W.: Effect of Certain Abrasive Materials on Tooth Enamel, J. Dent. Res., *29*, 740, December, 1950.
5. ALLEN, E. F. and RHOADS, R. H.: Effects of High Speed Periodontal Instruments on Tooth Surface, J. Periodont., *34*, 352, July, 1963.
6. GERSHON, S. D., POKRAS, H. H., and RIDER, T. H.: Dentifrices, p. 323, in Sagarin, Edward: *Cosmetics Science and Technology*, New York, Interscience Pub., 1957.
7. SKINNER and PHILLIPS: op. cit., pp. 577–578.
8. STOLL, F. A. and WERNER, A. R.: Clinical Observations of a New Polishing Agent for Dental Prophylaxis, Am. Dent. Hygienists' A. J., *37*, 79, 2nd Quarter, 1963.

SUGGESTED READINGS

DOBBS, E. C.:   *Pharmacology and Oral Therapeutics*, 12th ed. St. Louis, Mosby, 1961, pp. 66, 71–76, 514–517.

GERSHON, S. D., POKRAS, H. H., and RIDER, T. H.:   Dentifrices, pp. 296–360, in Sagarin, Edward: *Cosmetics Science and Technology*. New York, Interscience Pub., 1957.

GLICKMAN, IRVING: *Clinical Periodontology*, 2nd ed. Philadelphia, Saunders, 1958, p. 569.

MERICLE, M. R. and MUHLER, J. C.:   Studies Concerning the Antisolubility Effectiveness of Different Stannous Fluoride Prophylaxis Paste Mixtures, J. Dent. Res., *42*, 21, January–February, 1963.

SKINNER, E. W. and PHILLIPS, R. W., *The Science of Dental Materials*, 5th ed. Philadelphia, Saunders, 1960, Ch. 35.

Chapter 17

THE PORTE POLISHER WITH WOOD POINT

THE porte polisher is a prophylactic hand instrument constructed to hold a wood polishing point at a contra-angle. As suggested in the previous chapter, polishing with the prophylaxis angle and rubber cup generally precedes porte polishing. Time is saved by the removal of gross stains before the finer polishing. A comparison of the porte polisher and the prophylaxis angle is made in Table 7.

Hand polishing is accomplished by pressure of the wood point on the tooth surfaces as a moist abrasive is applied. The firm, carefully directed, rhythmic strokes impart a vigorous massage to the periodontal tissues. This is particularly beneficial to the periodontal ligament since the periodontal fibers serve as a cushion for the slight movement of the tooth which occurs as the pressure of the instrument is applied. Fones described the beneficial effects to the gingival margin.[1] He suggested that the slight bumping of the wood point on the tissue causes a light pressure and release which has a massaging effect in producing a stimulation of the peripheral circulation.

I. PURPOSES AND USES

The entire polishing procedure may be accomplished with the porte polisher although this is unusual in routine practice because of the time factor. Patients can be very appreciative of smooth, quiet hand polishing. With certain patients, under particular circumstances, and for selected procedures, porte polishing is specifically indicated. Functions, purposes, and uses are suggested here.

A. Removes stains, films, and dental plaque from the natural and restored surfaces of the teeth.

B. Provides a high, smooth polish which helps the tooth surfaces to resist deposit accumulation.

C. Effectively polishes cervical areas of teeth which are hypersensitive to the heat produced by even a slowly revolving rubber polishing cup. A superfine, unflavored abrasive mixed with water only is appreciated by these patients.

D. Adapts to tooth surfaces which are inaccessible to the prophylaxis angle, such as the following:

   1. Exposed proximal surfaces of the teeth of patients who have undergone periodontal surgery.

   2. Lingual surfaces of lingually inclined mandibular molars, or distal surfaces of maxillary third permanent molars.

E. Method of choice for application of certain desensitizing agents for exposed cementum and dentin (see page 210).

F. Useful for the bedridden patient when portable motor-driven equipment is not available (see page 330).

G. Helpful for orientation of small children, handicapped, or other patients apprehensive of motor-driven equipment.

(173)

II. **CHARACTERISTICS OF A PORTE POLISHER**

Several types of porte polishers are available for use. Practical features which influence selection are suggested below.

A. Can be taken apart conveniently for cleaning and sterilization.
B. Will not rust or discolor when given ordinary care.
C. Has convenient adjustment for attachment of wood points of various widths.
D. Is light weight for comfort of operator during use.
E. Has handle of diameter convenient to type of instrument grasp required.
F. Has handle with a finish which prevents slipping in the hand during operation.

TABLE 7.—COMPARISON OF THE PORTE POLISHER
AND THE PROPHYLAXIS ANGLE

Characteristic	Porte Polisher	Prophylaxis Angle
MASSAGING EFFECT	Provided for gingival margin and periodontal ligament.	No effect.
PROTECTION OF GINGIVA	Easy by use of slow, even strokes.	Difficult because of speed at which rubber cup is moving.
DANGER OF ABRADING ENAMEL AND CEMENTUM	Minimized.	Greater because of faster speed and decreased sense of touch.
STAIN REMOVAL	Removes all stains.	Time saved in the removal of gross stains but steady application of rubber cup could produce more heat than the patient could tolerate.
POLISH	High.	Superficial cleaning.
HEAT	None.	Much heat produced.
ACCESSIBILITY TO TOOTH SURFACE	Readily adapted to all surfaces.	Limited because of size and weight of handpiece.
OPERATOR'S SENSE OF TOUCH	Greater control of instrument is possible because sense of touch is present.	Sense of touch is decreased because of weight and size of handpiece.
COMFORT TO PATIENT	Increased because of quietness and lack of discomfort from heat.	Decreased because of noise, vibration and heat produced.
COMFORT TO OPERATOR	Light instrument, less tiring to trained hands.	Heavy instrument is tiring to hold.
POLISHING AGENT	Less damage from more abrasive powders; may mix fairly dry.	Only very fine grain powder should be used; must be applied very wet.
PORTABILITY	Is portable, therefore useful at any time (for example, bed-ridden patient).	Useful only in dental office, or with portable engine, with electricity.
CARE OF INSTRUMENT	Simple to sterilize.	More time required for cleaning, oiling, sterilizing.

III. SELECTION AND PREPARATION OF WOOD POINTS

Although several kinds of wood including cedar, maple and hard pine have been used for polishing points, orangewood is preferred because it is hard enough to withstand pressure without fraying readily, yet porous enough to hold polishing agents.

A supply of wood points of routinely used sizes and shapes should be cut, sterilized and stored in a sterile container in advance of patient appointments. Ready made woodpoints are available commercially in standard sizes and shapes.

A. Length
1. Short
   a. To maintain rigidity of wood.
   b. To prevent unnecessary retraction of cheek and tongue.
2. Long enough to gain access to tooth surfaces without interference of shank of the porte polisher.

B. Width
1. Narrow
   a. For adaptation to the variety of tooth surfaces and contours.
   b. To prevent damage to the gingival margins as the point is adapted to the curved tooth surfaces.
2. Wide enough for efficiency in polishing.
3. Recommended average width: equal to the diameter of the circular wood point holder of the porte polisher.

C. Shape
1. Wedge: for facial, lingual and proximal surfaces and inclined planes of cusps.
2. Cone (pointed): for occlusal pits and grooves.

D. Sterilization Procedure: Autoclave (see pages 45 and 47).

IV. TECHNIQUES FOR USE OF PORTE POLISHER

The principles of technique described in Chapter 14 are applied during hand polishing. A systematic order of procedure from one tooth surface to the next surface is prerequisite to thoroughness. Applications of the general principles are included here.

A. Instrument Grasps (see page 140)
1. Pen
   a. Recommended for all surfaces except maxillary anterior facial.
   b. Hold middle finger as near working end of instrument as possible as a guide and support.
2. Palm
   a. Recommended for maxillary anterior labial surfaces.
   b. Adapt to posterior maxillary facial surfaces when indicated by existing stains.

B. Fulcrum: Securely maintained on firm tooth.

C. **Strokes**
1. Circular: $\frac{1}{16}$ to $\frac{1}{8}''$ diameter; apply at cervical third and when adjacent to gingival margin.
2. Linear
   a. Horizontal: back and forth on buccal and lingual of posterior teeth and to proximal surfaces as applicable.
   b. Vertical: up and down over labial and lingual surfaces of anterior teeth.
3. Selection of type and size
   a. Provide greatest protection for gingiva.
   b. Provide greatest efficiency in technique in accord with the anatomy of the tooth and the nature and location of the plaques and stains.

D. **Manner of Operation**
1. Apply appropriate grasp and fulcrum and position wood point on the tooth surface.
2. Hand, wrist, and arm rotate to propel the porte polisher.
   a. Fulcrum finger remains positioned as hand pivots around it.
   b. Fingers remain immobile, grasping instrument.

E. **Pressure Applied**
1. Apply a directed, firm, moderate pressure with the use of slow deliberate strokes.
2. Apply increased pressure when circular stroke is directed away from free gingiva; decrease pressure when directed toward free gingiva.
3. Vary pressure with the tenacity of the deposit or stain to be removed.
4. Balance pressure applied to wood point with fulcrum pressure.
5. Effect of excess pressure
   a. Increases hazard of injury to the margin of the free gingiva.
   b. Decreases stability and control during stroke.

V. **TECHNICAL HINTS**
A. Edges of wood points should be trimmed and the wood grain smoothed to minimize splinters which may harm the gingival tissues.
B. Place wood point flush with porte polisher attachment to prevent possible irritation to cheek, lip, or tongue.
C. Change wood point frequently during polishing procedure as it becomes saturated with moisture and splintered.
   1. To prevent wood slivers from damaging free gingiva.
   2. To increase efficiency by having well-shaped wedge for polishing.
D. When more than one polishing agent is to be applied, use fresh woodpoints to prevent mixing the abrasives.
E. Use cotton roll or patient's partial removable denture in place for fulcrum when fulcrum teeth are missing.
F. Avoid pressure on pontics and mobile teeth.
G. Thorough flossing and patient rinsing following polishing is important as retained particles of polishing agent can be a source of irritation to the gingiva and increase postoperative discomfort.
H. An iodine disclosing solution applied to Green Stain prior to polishing tends to facilitate its removal.

VI. **FACTORS TO TEACH THE PATIENT**

A. The nature, occurrence, etiology and detrimental effects of plaques and stains.

B. Reasons for polishing the teeth.

C. Benefits of hand polishing.

D. Relationship of plaque and stain accumulation to the frequency and thoroughness of patient's personal oral care habits.

REFERENCE

1. Fones, A. C.: *Mouth Hygiene*, 4th ed. Philadelphia, Lea & Febiger, 1934, p. 277.

SUGGESTED READINGS

Beube, F. E.: *Periodontology*. New York, Macmillan, 1953, pp. 87–91.

Bunting, R. W.: *Oral Hygiene*, 3rd ed. Philadelphia, Lea & Febiger, 1957, pp. 255–258.

Fones, A. C: *Mouth Hygiene*, 4th ed. Philadelphia, Lea & Febiger, 1934, pp. 227–289.

Glickman, Irving: *Clinical Periodontology*, 2nd ed. Philadelphia, Saunders, 1958, p. 569.

Goldman, H. M., Schluger, Saul, Fox, Lewis, and Cohen, D. W.: *Periodontal Therapy*, 2nd ed. St. Louis, Mosby, 1960, p. 128.

Grant, Daniel, Stern, I. B., and Everett, F. G.: *Orban's Periodontics*, 2nd ed. St. Louis, Mosby, 1963, pp. 297–298.

Miller, S. C.: *Textbook of Periodontia*, 3rd ed. New York, Blakiston Division, McGraw-Hill, 1950, pp. 278–280.

Chapter 18

POLISHING WITH MOTOR-DRIVEN INSTRUMENTS

THE INSTRUMENTS

I. **HANDPIECE:** an instrument used to hold rotary instruments in the dental engine. It is connected by an arm, cable, belt, or tube to the source of power.

   A. **Slow Speed**
      The slow or conventional handpiece is constructed with sleeve-type bearings and has a typical range of from 1200 to 6500 r.p.m. (revolutions per minute). The lowest speed is that used for polishing teeth.

   B. **High Speed**
      These handpieces are constructed with ball bearings. Conventional handpieces have been outfitted with a high-speed motor and a large pulley to operate as high as 20,000 r.p.m. Many of the high speed handpieces can be adjusted to speeds from zero to their capacity, which make it possible to use them with the proper attachments, for the oral prophylaxis.

   C. **Ultra Speed**
      The three principal types of specially designed ultra-speed handpieces are water and air turbines and a high speed belt transmission type. Newer super-speed air-bearing turbines have speeds approximating 650,000 r.p.m.

II. **PROPHYLAXIS ANGLE:** contra or right-angle attachment for the handpiece to which polishing devices (rubber cup, bristle brush) are attached.

   A. **Characteristics**
      There are many types of prophylaxis angles available. They are generally made of stainless steel and may have hard chrome, carbon steel, or brass bearings. A few types are reversible in their action.

   B. **Service Life**
      The length of time which a prophylaxis angle is serviceable is related in part to the quality of materials used and the manner of construction. Primarily, however, *the length of life is directly proportional to the care provided in cleaning and lubricating after each use.* The care and sterilization of the prophylaxis angle are described on pages 26–27.

III. ATTACHMENTS FOR PROPHYLAXIS ANGLE

A. Rubber Polishing Cups

1. Types
   - a. Slip-on: with ribbed cup to aid in holding polishing agent.
   - b. Slip-on: with bristles inside cup.
   - c. Threaded (screw type): with plain ribbed cup or flange (webbed) type.
2. Materials
   - a. Natural rubber: more resilient and will not stain the teeth.
   - b. Synthetic: stiffer than natural rubber; white cups must be used since synthetic black may stain the teeth.

B. Bristle Brushes

1. Types
   - a. For prophylaxis angle: slip-on or screw type.
   - b. For handpiece: mandrel mounted.
2. Materials: nylon or natural bristles.

IV. USES OF MOTOR-DRIVEN INSTRUMENT ATTACHMENTS

A. Handpiece With Straight Mandrel

1. Dixon Bristle Brush (Type C, soft) for polishing removable dentures.
2. Mounted stone for sharpening scalers.
3. Rubber cup on mandrel for polishing labial surfaces of anterior teeth.

B. Prophylaxis Angle With Rubber Cup or Brush

1. Rubber cup for removal of gross plaques and stains from enamel surfaces.
2. Brush.
   - a. To remove stains from deep pits and fissures and tooth surfaces away from gingival margin.
   - b. To polish amalgam restorations.

USE OF THE PROPHYLAXIS ANGLE

In routine use, scaling is completed, gross stains and plaques are removed with the rubber cup, disclosing solution is applied, the fine, high polishing is accomplished with the wood point and fine abrasive, and the proximal surfaces are polished with dental tape.

I. PRECAUTIONS IN THE USE OF RUBBER POLISHING CUP AND BRISTLE BRUSH.

The use of motor-driven instruments can provide the patient with discomfort if care and consideration for the oral tissues are not exercised to prevent unnecessary trauma. The advantage in the use of the prophylaxis angle is in the conservation of time during the removal of gross stains. In saving time, awareness of the potential tissue damage which may result is important. The speed of the motor-driven rubber cups and brushes may abrade the thin covering of the dentin at the cervical area, may increase tooth sensitivity, and may denude the free margin of the gingiva. Frictional heat may cause pain or discomfort. Tactile sensitivity of the operator while using the thick, heavy handpiece, is diminished.

With these precautions in mind, damage to the oral tissues and patient discomfort can be minimized.

II. TECHNIQUE FOR USE OF THE PROPHYLAXIS ANGLE

As with all oral prophylaxis procedures, a systematic order of polishing should be followed. There are a number of differences in the manner of use of motor-driven instruments as compared to the use of the porte polisher. A variety of skills must be learned in using and caring for the equipment.

A. **Instrument Grasp:** Pen (see page 140)
   1. Hold middle finger as near working end of prophylaxis angle as possible to guide and support the handpiece. Use only the cushion of the middle finger, not the side of the first knuckle.
   2. Methods of relieving awkwardness in use of heavy handpiece.
      a. Use firm grasp to give support.
      b. Rest handpiece handle in the V between index finger and thumb when consistent with other positioning for accessibility to the field of operation.
      c. Adjust height of motor arm to relieve weight in hand.

B. **Fulcrum** (see page 141)
   1. Establish firmly on solid tooth structure.
   2. Use a wide fulcrum area when practical to aid in the balance of the heavy instrument. Example: place cushion of fulcrum finger across occlusal surfaces of bicuspids while polishing the molars.
   3. Avoid use of pontics or mobile teeth as fulcrums.

C. **Speed of Motor**
   1. Use slowest available speed to minimize frictional heat.
   2. Adjust r.p.m. by changing the position of the rheostat foot pedal.

D. **Use of Rheostat Pedal**
   1. Adjust screw clamps on top of rheostat to provide freedom for pedal movement so that motor will stop immediately upon release of foot pressure (all rheostats do not have such an attachment).
   2. Apply even pressure with foot to produce an even, slow speed.
   3. When seated during operation: keep sole of foot which activates rheostat pedal flat on the floor. Use toe to activate rheostat pedal.
   4. When standing: keep body weight distributed evenly on both feet, both feet flat on the floor. Use toe to activate rheostat pedal.

E. **Preparation of Polishing Agent**
   1. Agent is mixed as wet as possible but not so wet that it cannot be carried conveniently in the rubber cup from the dappen dish to the teeth (see pages 170–171).
   2. Wetness aids in alleviating the frictional heat produced.

F. **Stroke and Procedure**
   1. Rubber Cup
      a. Fill rubber cup with polishing agent, establish fulcrum, and bring rubber cup almost in contact with tooth surface before starting motor.
      b. Using slowest r.p.m., apply revolving cup lightly to tooth surface for two or three seconds.
      c. Move cup to adjacent area on tooth surface as in a patting action.
      d. Move cup from tooth to tooth, frequently replenishing supply of polishing agent.
      e. Turn handpiece to adapt rubber cup to fit each surface of the tooth, including proximal surfaces and gingival surfaces of fixed partial dentures.
      f. When two polishing agents of different abrasiveness are to be applied, use a separate rubber cup for each.
      g. Discard a rubber cup as it becomes less firm and before it wears on the edges. A rubber cup cannot be expected to serve for more than three to five oral prophylaxes.
   2. Bristle Brush
      a. Soak stiff brush in hot water to soften bristles.
      b. Distribute polishing agent over occlusal surfaces of teeth to be polished.
      c. Place fingers of left hand in a position which will both retract and protect cheek and tongue from the revolving brush.
      d. Establish a firm fulcrum and bring brush almost in contact with the tooth before starting motor.
      e. Using slowest r.p.m., apply revolving brush lightly to the occlusal surface only, avoiding contact of bristles with soft tissues.
      f. Use a short stroke in a brushing motion, following the inclined planes of the cusps.
      g. Move from tooth to tooth to prevent generation of excessive frictional heat. Replenish supply of polishing agent as necessary.

G. Flush teeth and interproximal areas thoroughly several times with water from the syringe to remove abrasive particles. The rotary movement of the rubber cup or bristle brush tends to force the abrasive into the gingival sulci, which may be a source of irritation to the soft tissues.

CLEANING THE REMOVABLE DENTURE

The complete oral prophylaxis includes the scaling and polishing of all natural teeth and their replacements. Complete and partial dentures may accumulate calculus, soft deposits, and stains which may affect the adaptation of the dentures in the mouth as well as afford a source of irritation to adjacent mucous membranes. A learning experience in the proper care of the dentures is provided for the patient as the dentures are cleaned professionally.

I. OBJECTIVES

A. Aids in preserving the natural teeth associated with a removable partial denture.
B. Removes calculus, soft deposits and stains, thereby smoothing the surfaces of the denture.
C. Improves the appearance of the denture.
D. Gives the patient a feeling of complete oral cleanliness.
E. Emphasizes to the patient the importance of routine personal and professional care of the denture.

II. CARE OF DENTURES DURING THE INTRA-ORAL PROPHYLAXIS

A. Provide the patient with a cleansing tissue as he may wish to cover his mouth when removing or inserting his denture.
B. Receive removable denture in paper cup or small basin.
C. Add water to cover. If calculus is present, add acetic acid (white vinegar) in the proportion of not more than one tablespoonful to one cup of water.
D. Place container in safe place away from working area to minimize hazard of breakage.

III. PROCEDURE FOR CLEANING THE REMOVABLE DENTURE

A. Grasps and Fulcrums

1. Denture
   a. Grasp firmly and securely in palm of left hand.
   b. Support clasp area with at least two fingers when working near the clasps.
   c. Avoid squeezing metal bar and clasps of a partial denture.
2. Scaler: pen grasp, ring finger fulcrum on denture, arm stabilized against body.
3. Handpiece with mandrel attached brush: palm grasp, thumb fulcrum on denture.
4. Prophylaxis angle with rubber polishing cup: pen grasp, ring finger fulcrum on denture.

B. Remove Calculus

1. Soak in dilute acetic acid (II., C., above).
2. Scaling: care must be taken not to scratch the denture surface.

C. Polish External Surface of Denture

1. Polishing at the dental chair.
   a. Preparation
      (1) Work over cuspidor beside patient.
      (2) Turn water off and line cuspidor with towel to prevent breakage if denture is dropped.

(3) Focus dental light on working area.
   b. Polish nonmetal parts with mounted brush (Dixon C in hand-piece) using wet flour of pumice.
   c. Polish metal parts with rubber polishing cup or wood point in porte polisher using whiting or other appropriate agent (see pages 169–170).
2. Polishing on dental lathe in laboratory.
   a. Use soft brush or rag wheel with fine abrasive for nonmetal parts and whiting or other agent for metal.
   b. Avoid clasps when polishing with the fast moving lathe. Use wood point in porte polisher or rubber cup for clasps.
   c. Run lathe at slowest r.p.m. and apply denture carefully, constantly changing surface position on wheel.
   d. Freely apply wet polishing agent to the denture and use short strokes to prevent overheating.
3. Rinse denture under faucet with warm (never hot) running water. Line sink with towel while rinsing.

D. **Brush Internal Surface of Denture**

1. Use only a denture brush with a detergent or soap on the inside of a denture to prevent alteration of its contour.
2. Hold denture over sink lined with towel.
3. Rinse thoroughly.

E. **Brush Internal Surfaces of Clasps with Clasp Brush.**

F. **Evaluate Cleanliness of Denture:** Examine under bright light, using compressed air stream to remove excess water which may mask small amounts of calculus or the colorless plaque-like film commonly found on dentures.

G. **Return Denture to Patient Wet so that Insertion Will Be Comfortable;** return denture on cleansing tissue or in paper cup.

POLISHING AMALGAM RESTORATIONS

All dentists do not request the dental hygienist to polish new amalgam restorations. Many prefer to do this themselves. The technique used by the dental hygienist needs to be adapted to the objectives of the dentist who has placed the restoration. The procedure suggested here is intended as a basic technique to provide understanding of principles.

I. **PURPOSES FOR POLISHING**

A. Provides a smooth restored tooth surface.
   1. Prevents retention of deposits.
   2. Prevents chronic irritation to the gingiva and tongue.
B. Prevents recurrent dental caries.
C. Prevents corrosion of the amalgam.[1]
D. Improves the appearance of the restoration.

II. **PRINCIPLES TO BE OBSERVED WHEN POLISHING**

A. Wait at least 24 hours after amalgam has been placed and carved before polishing. Amalgam must be completely "set."

B. Avoid overheating the restoration: use light intermittent contact of motor-driven polishing instruments.

C. Use care not to obliterate the anatomy carved by the dentist.

D. Use secure fulcrum and adequate retraction to protect soft oral tissues.

E. The contact area is not polished unless specific instructions are given by the dentist. Usually, the contact of the amalgam with the smooth matrix band during placement will result in an adequate finish.

F. Do not isolate routinely with cotton rolls.
1. Revolving polishing instruments catch the cotton rolls.
2. Repeated need for rinsing to clear away excess polishing agent for vision would necessitate use of considerable time in changing cotton rolls.

G. The abrasive agent can clog a saliva ejector if one is used. Clearing the saliva ejector after operation is essential.

III. **PROCEDURE FOR POLISHING**[2,3,4]

All margins of the restoration should be flush with enamel surface. If radiographic or instrumental examination reveals overhanging or excess amalgam, it should be called to the attention of the dentist.

A. **Removal of Irregularities in the Surface of the Amalgam**
1. Proximal: disks (fine garnet or coarse cuttle) mounted on mandrel.
2. Occlusal: mounted, small, fine-grained stones or plug finishing burs.

B. **Polishing:** instruments and polishing agents are used in the order given below.
1. Use wheel bristle brush (Dixon C).
   a. Soften brush with warm water by soaking for a few minutes before use.
   b. Use wet brush as carrier for moistened flour of pumice or the less abrasive lap emery.
   c. Apply brush to tooth with light intermittent "jabbing" motion. This permits the bristles to reach the bottom of the groove or pit without destroying the anatomy.
2. Use rubber polishing cup with same abrasive as used with bristle brush.
3. Rinse well.
4. Check for removal of all rough spots and scratches before applying finer polishing agent for high polish.
5. Use fresh rubber cup with moistened jeweler's white rouge, tin oxide or whiting to produce satin finish (high gloss).

TECHNICAL HINTS

I. Maintain several prophylaxis angles in practice to facilitate use during successive appointments. When this is done, care of the prophylaxis angles should be accomplished as soon as possible after use: within a few hours at the most.

II. Test staining potential of a black synthetic rubber cup by using it as an eraser on white paper. If black appears, the teeth can be stained.

III. Prevent rheostat from sliding on highly polished floor by placing 1 or 2 drops of carbon tetrachloride under the rheostat.

IV. To obtain proper tension of engine belt, test by hanging a $1\frac{1}{4}$ ounce weight on the middle of one side of belt. Tighten belt until it is $1\frac{1}{4}$ inches distant from other side of belt. (A paper clip bent to measure $1\frac{1}{4}$ inches, weighed to $1\frac{1}{4}$ ounces with attached wad of tinfoil is useful as a measuring device.)

V. A toothpaste or denture adhesive powder may be added to the polishing agent mixture to aid the mixture in adhering to an amalgam restoration during polishing.

FACTORS TO TEACH THE PATIENT

I. The purposes for use of both prophylaxis angle and porte polisher during the oral prophylaxis.

II. How plaques and stains form on the natural teeth and their replacements and why polishing in the dental office on a routine plan is necessary.

III. The relationship of the accumulation of deposits and stains to the patient's personal oral care habits.

IV. The need for adapting toothbrushing techniques to cleanse the abutment teeth.

V. The importance of regular cleansing of dentures with special attention to clasps.

VI. How to handle and cleanse the denture.

REFERENCES

1. SKINNER, E. W. and PHILLIPS, R. W.: *Science of Dental Materials*, 5th ed. Philadelphia, Saunders, 1960, pp. 397–398.
2. JACOBSON, F. L.: Seattle, School of Dentistry, University of Washington, personal communication.
3. STIBBS, G. D.: Seattle, School of Dentistry, University of Washington, personal communication.
4. SIMON, W. J.: *Clinical Operative Dentistry*. Philadelphia, Saunders, 1956, pp. 62–66.

SUGGESTED READINGS

KENNEDY, J. J., HANSEN, L. S., SCOFIELD, H. H., NIELSEN, A. G., and BUCKMAN, N.: Pulpae Response to Various High Speed Cutting Instruments, Dent. Prog., *3*, 6, October, 1962.
KILPATRICK, H. C.: *High Speed and Ultra Speed in Dentistry*. Philadelphia, Saunders, 1960, pp. 10–57.
SKINNER, E. W. and PHILLIPS, R. W.: *Science of Dental Materials*, 5th ed. Philadelphia, Saunders, 1960, pp. 352–365. (Dental Amalgam.)
STANLEY, H. R.: Traumatic Capacity of High-Speed and Ultrasonic Dental Instrumentation, Am. Dent. A. J., *63*, 749, December, 1961.
TAYLOR, D. F., PERKINS, R. R. and KUMPULA, J. W.: Characteristics of Some Air-Turbine Handpieces, Am. Dent. A. J., *64*, 794, June, 1962.

Chapter 19

POLISHING PROXIMAL SURFACES: DENTAL FLOSS, TAPE, AND POLISHING STRIPS

CONSIDERABLE care must be exercised in the use of dental floss, tape and polishing strips. Understanding the anatomy of the interdental papillæ and their relation to the contact areas and proximal surfaces of the teeth is prerequisite to the prevention of tissue damage.

As much polishing as possible of accessible proximal surfaces is accomplished during the use of the rubber cup in the prophylaxis angle and the porte polisher. This is followed routinely by the use of dental tape. Polishing strips are used only in selected instances when all other techniques fail to remove a stain.

DENTAL TAPE AND FLOSS

I. DESCRIPTION

Floss and tape are made of spun silk or nylon thread coated with wax. The wax covering affords some protection for the tissues, facilitates the movement of the floss or tape, prevents excessive absorption of moisture, and assists in the prevention of shredding. Dental floss is also available unwaxed, which is primarily useful in the preparation of teeth for a topical fluoride application. When waxed floss is used for this purpose there is the possibility of wax remaining on small areas of the tooth surface, thus preventing uniform contact of fluoride with the enamel.

Tape is flat and has relatively sharp edges whereas floss is round. Either floss or tape may injure the tissue when used incorrectly or carelessly.

II. USES

A. Tape for Polishing

1. Proximal tooth surfaces.
2. Gingival surface of fixed partial denture.

B. Floss for Removing

1. Gross debris and food particles
   a. At beginning of oral prophylaxis to facilitate proximal scaling.
   b. In preparation for topical fluoride applications.
2. Particles of polishing agents at completion of oral prophylaxis
   a. From interproximal areas and gingival sulci.
   b. From gingival surface of fixed partial dentures.
3. Retained abrasive particles after use of polishing strips.

III. TECHNIQUE FOR THE USE OF DENTAL FLOSS AND TAPE

A. Length

1. Approximately 12 inches.
2. Excessive length is awkward to handle in preventing the ends from sliding over the patient's face.
3. Insufficient length prevents adequate grasp.

B. For Interproximal Areas

1. Grasp
     Grasp floss or tape between index finger and thumb of each hand about ½ inch apart. Hold "tails" of floss or tape in a manner which will prevent them from sliding over the patient's face.
2. Fulcrum and retraction
     Establish fulcrum (tip of index finger) on facial surface of the tooth immediately adjacent to the area to be flossed or taped. Fulcrum finger and thumb serve to retract and protect lip and cheek.
3. Positioning
     Hold floss or tape at an oblique angle (Figure 40) and bring slowly through the contact area using a controlled moderate pressure. Retain a stationary fulcrum throughout the movement of the floss or tape. Direct floss or tape to the side of the interdental papilla.

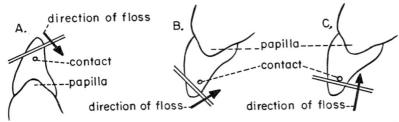

FIGURE 40.—Use of dental floss or tape. *A.* Floss at oblique angle for mandibular teeth. *B.* Floss at oblique angle for maxillary teeth. *C.* Incorrect: floss held horizontal. Danger of damage to papilla. (Modified from Beube, *Periodontology*, Macmillan Company.)

4. Polishing (tape)
     Apply moistened polishing agent to the tooth and press tape to the proximal surface. Move gently back and forth, rocking on established fulcrum. Raise tape over the tip of the interdental papilla and apply to adjacent proximal surface.
5. Removal of particles (floss)
     Guide floss through gingival sulcus about ½ inch, raise over the tip of the interdental papilla and slide through about ½ inch to clean sulcus of adjacent tooth.
6. Remove tape or floss at an oblique angle, slowly, still maintaining the fulcrum. The tape or floss is removed by returning through the contact area, or by sliding the floss through to the facial surface.
7. Move floss or tape through fingers to provide new section for the next interproximal area.
8. Request patient to rinse thoroughly.

C. **For Fixed Partial Denture**

1. Positioning

    The tape or floss is passed over the gingival border of the denture, pulled gently through, and used in a single strand. To slide the floss under the denture necessitates stiffening the end except when a space exists between the gingiva and the gingival border of the denture. Three ways of threading the floss are suggested here.

    a. Fold end of waxed tape or floss over approximately two inches and press together to make a firm end.

    b. Use commercial plastic threader (*Zon*, Johnson and Johnson).

    c. Prepare reinforced waxed ends by dipping in molten paraffin. Several lengths can be prepared in advance and stored in a clean, covered jar in the dental cabinet.

2. Polishing (tape)

    Apply moist polishing agent to the gingival surface of the denture and polish by drawing the tape gently back and forth in a $\frac{1}{4}$ inch arc in a lingual-facial direction. Position floss anteriorly and posteriorly to polish proximal surfaces of the abutment teeth. Slide tape through to an unused section to aid in the removal of abrasive particles.

3. Removal of particles (floss)

    Slide floss through in short sections until gingival surfaces and proximal surfaces of abutment teeth are free of particles. Apply compressed air to provide visibility for checking thoroughness.

4. Remove tape or floss by sliding through, taking care to protect lip, cheek, and gingival tissue under denture.

5. Flush under denture with water from syringe, and request patient to rinse thoroughly.

POLISHING STRIPS

I. **DESCRIPTION**

Polishing strips are also known as linen abrasive strips or finishing strips. They are usually made of linen and are available in four widths, extra narrow, narrow, medium and wide. The strips have one smooth side and one abrasive side which may be fine, medium or coarse grit. *Only extra narrow or narrow strips with fine grit are suggested for use during the oral prophylaxis and then only with discretion.*

II. **USE**

A. **For Stain Removal on Proximal Surfaces of Anterior Teeth:** when other polishing techniques are unsuccessful.

B. **Precautions for Use**

1. Edge of strip is sharp and may cut gingival tissue or lip.

2. Rough working side of strip is capable of removing tooth structure, and may make nicks or grooves, particularly in the cementum.

3. Polishing with polishing strip should be limited to enamel surfaces.

III. **TECHNIQUE FOR USE OF POLISHING STRIP**

A. **Grasp and Fulcrum**

Use a strip no longer than 6 inches. The grasp and fulcrum establishment are the same as for floss and tape. Protection of the lip by retraction with the thumb and index finger holding the strip is mandatory.

B. **Positioning**

1. Direct abrasive side of strip toward the proximal surface to be polished as the strip is worked slowly and gently between the teeth with a slightly sawing motion. Bring strip just through the contact area. If the strip breaks, immediately use floss to remove particles of abrasive.
2. When a space is clearly visible through an interproximal area and the interdental papilla is missing, a narrow polishing strip may be threaded through. Prepare strip by cutting the end on the diagonal to facilitate threading.

C. **Polishing**

1. Press abrasive side of strip against tooth. Draw back and forth in a $\frac{1}{8}$ inch arc 2 or 3 times, rocking on the established fulcrum.
2. Remove strip and insert for adjacent proximal surface. Do not attempt to turn the strip while it is in the interproximal area.

D. **Use Dental Floss:** follow each application of polishing strips with dental floss to remove abrasive particles.

TECHNICAL HINTS

I. Avoid hurrying through the contact area, causing sudden contact with and careless injury to the crest of interdental papilla.
II. Protect patient's lips at all times during use of floss, tape or polishing strip.

FACTORS TO TEACH THE PATIENT

I. The anatomical relationship of the contact area, interproximal area, interdental papilla, and the gingival sulcus.
II. The use of dental floss in personal oral care procedures as a supplement to toothbrushing (see pages 302–303).
III. The use of dental floss with thorough rinsing after meals when it is not possible to brush the teeth.
IV. The importance of daily use of dental floss for cleaning under fixed partial dentures.
V. Dangers in the use of floss or tape.
VI. The importance of having missing contact areas restored rather than using floss or tape repeatedly to alleviate the discomforts of food impaction.

SUGGESTED READINGS

BEUBE, F. E.: *Periodontology.* New York, Macmillan, 1953, pp. 243–244.
EVERETT, F. G. and KUNKEL, P. W.: Abrasion Through the Abuse of Dental Floss, J. Periodont., *24,* 186, July, 1953.
MILLER, S. C.: *Textbook of Periodontia,* 3rd ed. New York, Blakiston Division, McGraw-Hill, 1950, p. 280–281.

Chapter 20

EVALUATION OF THE COMPLETED ORAL PROPHYLAXIS AND POSTOPERATIVE PROCEDURES

USE OF DISCLOSING SOLUTION

A DISCLOSING solution is applied routinely following scaling and polishing procedures. The disclosing solution contains a dye or other coloring substance which imparts its color to calculus, plaques and films. When applied to the teeth it can be rinsed readily from clean tooth surfaces whereas deposits remain stained until removed by polishing. The removal is therefore facilitated because the deposits are distinctly seen. The coloring property of a disclosing solution provides a valuable aid in patient instruction since it dramatically indicates to the patient the presence of deposits and the areas needing special attention during routine personal oral care procedures.

The sequence of application during the techniques of the oral prophylaxis varies. For example, it may be preferable to apply disclosing solution before scaling, after scaling before polishing, after the general polishing with the prophylaxis angle and rubber cup before proceeding with the finer polishing of the porte polisher, or at more than one of these times. Whenever the solution is applied during the techniques, the most important time is for evaluation of the results at the completion of the oral prophylaxis.

I. PURPOSES FOR USE OF DISCLOSING SOLUTION

    A. Colors calculus, films, plaques or other foreign material on the surfaces of the teeth.
        1. Identifies deposits which are difficult to observe by direct vision.
        2. Aids in evaluating the completed oral prophylaxis.
        3. Aids in patient instruction.
    B. Conserves operating time by making inconspicuous deposits more visible.

II. FACTORS TO CONSIDER IN THE SELECTION OF A DISCLOSING SOLUTION

    A. **Intensity of Color**
        A distinct staining of deposits should be evident. The color should be in contrast to normal colors of the oral cavity.

    B. **Duration of Intensity**
        The color should not rinse off with ordinary rinsing methods, or be removable by the saliva for the period of time required to complete the polishing of a quadrant of the teeth. It is desirable for the

color to be removed from the gingival tissue by the completion of the appointment, as the patient may have a personal reaction to color retained for a period of time after leaving the dental office.

C. Taste

The patient should not be made uncomfortable by an unpleasant or highly flavored substance, since his cooperation may be decreased.

D. Irritation to the Mucous Membrane

The patient should be questioned concerning the possibility of an idiosyncrasy to an ingredient. When this information is obtained it should be entered on the patient's permanent history record. Because of the possibility of allergy, more than one type of disclosing solution should be available for use.

E. Diffusibility

The solution should be thin enough that it can be applied readily to the exposed surfaces of the teeth, yet thick enough to prevent its prompt diffusion over the gingival tissues to the mucobuccal folds and tongue.

F. Astringent and Antiseptic Properties

These properties may be highly desirable in that the disclosing solution will contribute other factors to the techniques. It is frequently recommended that an antiseptic be applied prior to scaling, and if an antiseptic disclosing solution is used, one solution serves a dual purpose.

III. FORMULÆ OF DISCLOSING SOLUTIONS

A wide variety of disclosing solutions has been used. Skinner's Iodine Solution has been perhaps the most classic and widely used. In general, iodine solutions are less desirable because of their unpleasant flavor.

The formulæ of a few of the more commonly used disclosing solutions are included in this chapter. Other well-known ones are Buckley's, Berwick's, Easlick's, Bender's, Talbot's Iodo-glycerol, and Metaphen solution.

A. Iodine Preparations

1. Skinner's Solution
   Iodine crystals . . . . 3.3 Gm.
   Potassium Iodide . . . 1.0 Gm.
   Zinc Iodide . . . . . 1.0 Gm.
   Distilled water . . . . 16.0 ml.
   Glycerin . . . . . 16.0 ml.

2. Iodine Disclosing Solution[1]
   Potassium Iodide . . . 1.6 Gm.
   Iodine crystals . . . . 1.6 Gm.
   Water . . . . . 13.4 ml.
   Glycerin . to make 30.0 ml.

3. Diluted Tincture of Iodine
   Tincture of Iodine . . . 21.0 ml.
   Water . . . . . . 15.0 ml.

B. **Mercurochrome Solution** (5%)

Mercurochrome	. . .	1.5 Gm.
Water to make	30.0 ml.

C. **Bismarck Brown**

Bismarck Brown	. . .	0.3 Gm.
Alcohol	10.0 ml.
Glycerin	.120.0 ml.
Anise (flavoring) . . .	1 drop

D. **Basic Fuchsin**

Basic Fuchsin	1.5 Gm.
Alcohol 95% . . .	.100.0 ml.
Distilled Water . .	1000.0 ml.

E. **Disclosing Tablets:** flavored tablets are available commercially. The patient is requested to chew the tablet and rinse.

IV. TECHNIQUE FOR APPLICATION OF DISCLOSING SOLUTION

Generally, applications are made to a quadrant of the teeth at one time in the order followed for instrumentation.

A. Dry the teeth with compressed air, retracting cheek or tongue.
B. Use very small cotton pellet with cotton pliers to carry the solution to the teeth.
C. Apply solution to the crowns of the teeth only.
D. Remove excess solution.
  1. Request the patient to rinse.
  2. When the flavor of the disclosing solution is unpleasant to the patient, it may be desirable to remove the excess solution by blotting with a cotton roll.
E. Apply compressed air and inspect.
F. Polish disclosed areas as required to remove visible deposits.

EVALUATION OF THE COMPLETED ORAL PROPHYLAXIS

At the completion of the polishing techniques, the results are appraised to determine that the objectives have been attained. Inspection includes consideration of the teeth and the gingival tissues.

The effects on the teeth are usually in immediate evidence whereas gingival changes need further evaluation a few days to a week after the oral prophylaxis. The objective at the time of the oral prophylaxis is to produce an environment in which the tissues may assume normal characteristics and appearance (see page 87) after being given time to respond.

Reevaluation at the succeeding appointment provides the opportunity to follow through with additional techniques and recommendations when needed. When the tissues have not responded favorably, particularly in isolated areas, it is essential to determine that all calculus definitely has been removed. Remaining particles, however small, are sufficient to prevent complete tissue healing. Because the detection of calculus in the gingival sulcus is an intricate and exacting procedure, even the most skilled operator must expect to recheck and complete the scaling as found necessary.

Demonstration of oral physical therapy measures by the patient at the succeeding appointment will determine whether cooperation in that phase of care has been obtained.   Learning is a slow process and many patients need repeated review of the correct manner in which to use the toothbrush and other implements.   This is especially true if a technique previously unfamiliar to the patient was introduced.

Notes concerning tissue response should be made on the patient's permanent record.   Reevaluation is a continuing process from one recall appointment to the next, and reference to previous records provides the opportunity for planning future dental hygiene care and instruction.

I. APPEARANCE OF THE TEETH AFTER THE ORAL PROPHYLAXIS

The experienced eye will recognize the bright luster of thoroughly clean teeth.   Polished enamel has a high gloss which reflects light.   All deposits have been removed and the surfaces are smooth to tactile examination.   The changes in appearance of the teeth after the oral prophylaxis are summarized in Table 8.

TABLE 8.—THE TEETH BEFORE AND AFTER THE ORAL PROPHYLAXIS

Characteristic	Before Scaling and Polishing	After Polishing
LUSTER	Dull	Bright
DEPOSITS	Particles visible; may be discolored	No visible irregularities
SURFACE TEXTURE DETECTED BY EXPLORER	Rough	Smooth
ANATOMY OF TEETH	May be masked at cingulum or on proximal surfaces	Clearly defined
PERCEPTION BY PATIENT'S TONGUE	Surface rough, filmy	Surface smooth and free of film

(Adapted from Beube, *Periodontology.*   Used by permission of the Macmillan Company.)

II. SUMMARY OF METHODS OF INSPECTION

Visual and tactile methods for inspection have been employed throughout the oral prophylaxis (see page 151).   The final evaluation to determine completeness of procedures involves all methods.

A. Tactile
1. Periodontal probe to supplement use of explorers in defining complete removal of submarginal deposits.
2. Explorers to assure smoothness of tooth surfaces.

B. Radiographic: Preparation of a second bite-wing radiographic survey is advisable at the completion of the oral prophylaxis to check extensive calculus cases.

C. **Visual**

1. *Compressed air* used in conjunction with mouth mirror and proper lighting to observe dry tooth surfaces and expose region just below gingival crest.
2. *Transillumination*
   a. An effective transillumination frequently may be accomplished by proper retraction of the lip, drying of the teeth with compressed air, adjustment of the light to allow it to shine through the anterior teeth, and adaptation of the mouth mirror at a proper angle. Opaque deposits such as calculus will appear as dark spots or shadows.
   b. The transilluminator: a mouth lamp designed for directing light through the teeth to reveal opaque deposits.
3. *Disclosing solution:* to color deposits not observable by direct vision.

POSTOPERATIVE PROCEDURES

I. THE GINGIVAL MASSAGE

A firm but gentle massage of the gingival tissue is recommended after completion of the oral prophylaxis. This procedure is soothing to the patient and stimulating to the circulation of the gingiva. It is performed prior to application of an antiseptic solution.

A. **Effects of Massage**

Massage is the systematic mechanical application and removal of pressure. The application of pressure forces stagnant blood from the tissues and produces a temporary ischemia; the removal of pressure allows arterial blood to enter the capillaries and produce a temporary hyperemia.

B. **Technique for Massage**

A flavored toothpaste may be applied to the gingiva as a lubricating agent, or the massage may be performed with the fingers moistened with water.

1. Follow the routine order of technique for the other procedures of the oral prophylaxis, or start from the midline to massage each quadrant.
2. Place the thumb and index finger over the teeth onto the attached gingiva.
3. Apply moderate, firm pressure, moving the fingers in the direction of the gingival papilla, toward the incisal or occlusal surfaces.
4. Release pressure at the tip of the papilla and return fingers to the attached gingiva above the adjacent tooth. Repeat rhythmically around the mouth.

II. THE APPLICATION OF AN ANTISEPTIC SOLUTION

Under the direction of the dentist, the dental hygienist may apply a soothing local antiseptic to the gingival sulcus at the completion of the oral prophylaxis. Application of an antiseptic solution is also recommended after scaling when more than one appointment is required to complete the oral prophylaxis.

Certain state laws governing practice do not permit the dental hygienist to apply "medicating" agents even under the direction of a dentist. The law must be followed meticulously.

The antiseptics usually employed for postoperative applications are iodine or mercury preparations in the proper dilutions for application to the oral mucous membrane. Merthiolate (1:1000) or Metaphen (1:200) are commonly used for this purpose.

A. **Purposes**

1. Reduces the possibility of infection.
2. Reduces postoperative discomfort.

B. **Technique for Application**

1. Hold small cotton pellet with cotton pliers and saturate in the antiseptic to be used. Express excess solution.
2. Provide adequate retraction of lip, cheek, and tongue, and apply solution to the crest of each interdental papilla on both facial and lingual surfaces.
3. Do not allow the patient to rinse.

III. **INSTRUCTION IN POSTOPERATIVE PROCEDURES FOR THE PATIENT**

Postoperative instruction is essential following scaling, particularly when the patient's gingiva have been hypersensitive or have hemorrhaged excessively, or when there has been extensive submarginal instrumentation. Directions for postoperative care include suggestions for rinsing and toothbrushing.

Dietary and nutritional factors may be discussed. The temporary use of bland foods lacking in strong, spicy seasonings, as well as nutritional foods to promote healing can be helpful.

Directions for postoperative care are best prepared in printed or mimeographed form to prevent incomplete or inaccurate interpretation of spoken directions.

A. **Rinsing**

A warm solution will be soothing to the tissue and improve the circulation for healing. A suggested solution should provide the appropriate concentration for osmotic balance of the salts of the solution with the salts of the oral tissue fluids.

1. Solutions suggested for use:[2]
   a. Mild hypertonic salt solution: level $\frac{1}{2}$ teaspoonful table salt in 8-ounce glass of warm water.
   b. Sodium bicarbonate solution: level $\frac{1}{2}$ teaspoonful baking soda in $\frac{3}{4}$ glass (8 oz.) warm water.
2. Directions for rinsing
   a. Every 2 hours; after eating; after toothbrushing; before retiring.
   b. Use the 8-ounce glass mouthful by mouthful, forcing the solution between the teeth (see page 311).

B. **Toothbrushing:** use of a soft multitufted brush may be advisable for the first few days after the oral prophylaxis. Careful instruction in the method of brushing recommended for the individual must be given (see pages 284–292).

TECHNICAL HINTS

I. Avoid using disclosing or antiseptic solutions on teeth which have silicate cement or resin restorations as these materials may be stained by coloring agent.

II. Purchase solutions in small quantities. Do not keep solutions containing alcohol longer than 2 or 3 months since the alcohol will evaporate and render the solution too highly concentrated.

III. Use small bottles with dropper caps for solutions. Transfer solution to a dappen dish for use. Do not contaminate the solution by dipping cotton pliers with pellet directly into the container bottle.

IV. Use only small, unsaturated cotton pellets with adequate retraction of cheeks and tongue to prevent staining of tongue and alveolar mucosa.

V. Maintain a list of methods for spot removal in case the dye-containing solutions are inadvertently spilled.

FACTORS TO TEACH THE PATIENT

I. Importance of meticulous inspection for completion of the oral prophylaxis.

II. Effects of incomplete removal of deposits.

III. Appearance and feeling of a clean mouth.

IV. Relationship of personal oral care habits to maintenance of cleanliness provided through the oral prophylaxis.

V. The effectiveness of the patient's personal care by applying disclosing solution before the oral prophylaxis.

VI. The effectiveness of the oral prophylaxis by applying disclosing solution at the completion of the oral prophylaxis.

VII. Purposes of postoperative care by the dental hygienist and the patient.

VIII. How to prepare solutions for postoperative rinsing.

IX. Directions for postoperative care.

X. Foods which promote healing because of their consistency or content of nutritional elements.

REFERENCES

1. American Dental Association, Council on Dental Therapeutics: *Accepted Dental Remedies*, 29th ed. Chicago, American Dental Association, 1964, p. 194.
2. Ibid., pp. 150, 151.

SUGGESTED READINGS

Disclosing Solutions

ARNIM, S. S.: Use of Disclosing Agents for Measuring Tooth Cleanliness, J. Periodont., *34*, 227, May, 1963.
BEUBE, F. E.: *Periodontology.* New York, Macmillan, 1953, p. 87.
BUNTING, R. W.: *Oral Hygiene*, 3rd ed. Philadelphia, Lea & Febiger, 1957, p. 275.
GLICKMAN, IRVING: *Clinical Periodontology*, 2nd ed. Philadelphia, Saunders, 1958, pp. 741–742.
MILLER, S. C.: *Textbook of Periodontia*, 3rd ed. New York, Blakiston Division, McGraw-Hill, 1950, pp. 280, 551.

Postoperative Procedures

American Dental Association, Council on Dental Therapeutics: *Accepted Dental Remedies*, 29th ed. Chicago, American Dental Association, 1964, pp. 106–121.
DOBBS, E. C.: *Pharmacology and Oral Therapeutics*, 12th ed. St. Louis, Mosby, 1961, pp. 519, 415–416.
GLICKMAN, IRVING: *Clinical Periodontology*, 2nd ed. Philadelphia, Saunders, 1958, pp. 944–945 (Gingival Massage); 792–793 (Antiseptics).

PART IV

Auxiliary Procedures of the Dental Hygiene Appointment

Chapter 21

THE TOPICAL APPLICATION OF FLUORIDE SOLUTION

The use of fluorides in preventive dental care is based on the principle that when the fluoride content of the teeth, particularly of the surface enamel, is increased, they are more resistant to dental caries. Fluoride is a nutrient essential to the formation of good teeth and bones. The four basic methods of use of fluorides are the fluoridation of the water supply, topical application of fluoride solution to erupted teeth, supplementation of fluoride in the daily dietary, and fluoride dentifrices. Patient instruction includes interpretation of current research in all four areas.

Fluoridation is the adjustment of the fluoride ion content of a communal water supply to the lowest level which will provide maximum prevention of dental caries. This has been established as the most efficient and effective means of giving teeth the benefits of fluorides.[1] One part per million (ppm.) has been determined as the optimum level for the water in temperate climates. For warmer and colder climates the amount can be adjusted from approximately 0.7 or 0.8 to 1.2 ppm. to accommodate for the quantity of water consumed.

Optimum benefits from fluoridation are an occurrence of an average of 60 to 65 per cent fewer new dental carious lesions in permanent teeth and about 50 per cent in primary teeth in individuals who have used the water since birth. Maximum benefits are derived when fluoridated water is consumed until 12 to 15 years of age, but there are also definite and significant reductions in dental caries prevalence in older children who already have erupted teeth when fluoridation is initiated.[2-4] Studies of adults in areas where water has contained natural fluoride for many years show the continuing benefits into adult life.[5,6]

Other means for obtaining fluoride are essential for persons who cannot have the benefits of controlled fluoridation. Dietary fluoride supplements are available for daily administration under professional supervision.[7,8] This method presents difficulties in that if substantial results are to be obtained, the supplements must be conscientiously and consistently used over the first 8 to 12 years of a child's life. Parents must be highly motivated to follow directions to the letter. Although research in this area is limited, results have been favorable.[9] There is little evidence that the administration of supplementary fluorides to pregnant women is of any benefit to the teeth of the children. Calcification of the entire permanent dentition and a large portion of the primary teeth is a postnatal process; therefore, in areas where there is no fluoridated water, dietary fluorides are best prescribed after birth for the child.[10]

Combining more than one fluoride procedure for dental caries prevention has shown multiple benefits. It has been demonstrated that when topical stannous fluoride applications are received by children who have consumed fluoridated water during the tooth development years, an additive effect results.[11] In another study it was shown that the daily use of a stannous fluoride dentifrice and the topical application of stannous fluoride solution every 6 months produced favorable results after 3 years.[12]

The characteristics of sodium fluoride and stannous fluoride are described in the succeeding sections of this chapter.

I. DEVELOPMENT OF THE USE OF TOPICAL FLUORIDE APPLICATIONS

Extensive research has been and continues to be conducted to evaluate the effectiveness of a variety of fluoride solutions. A summary of the reported research[13] shows that at least 20 studies on topical sodium fluoride solution had been made since the first project by Bibby using Brockton, Massachusetts school children in 1942[14] These studies and additional ones using fluoride compounds other than sodium, have attempted to clarify the factors relative to the most effective fluoride solution, the length of time it must be in contact with the enamel, the concentration and optimum pH of the solution, and the application procedure.

Sodium fluoride and stannous fluoride have been most widely used. Recent research has shown a superior effect of a sodium fluoride solution acidulated with orthophosphoric acid.[15,16] This solution has advantages in that it is recommended for single application, it does not have an unpleasant flavor, and its shelf life is indefinite when kept in a polyethylene container.

II. USE OF TOPICAL APPLICATION AS A SUPPLEMENT TO FLUORIDATION

Unfortunately, fluoridation cannot be made available to the total population at the present time. The groups listed below suggest the need for public health and private dental office programs for the topical application of fluoride solution. This procedure is more costly than fluoridation because individual application by a dental professional person is required.

A. For the nearly one-third of the population which cannot benefit from fluoridation because communal water supply is not available and private sources of water are used.
B. For children in communities where fluoridation is initiated, topical applications are used to protect the teeth of age groups too old to receive full benefit from fluoridation.

As a clinical operator, the dental hygienist contributes to the preventive care of the individual patient by making topical applications. In school and public health programs a multiple chair procedure is used.[17]   Although a few state laws governing dental hygiene practice are still not interpreted to include fluoride solution application as a service to be rendered by the dental hygienist, it is widely agreed that this service is one which can be delegated effectively by the dentist to the dental hygienist.

III. EFFECTS OF TOPICAL FLUORIDE SOLUTION ON THE TEETH

Maximum benefits of topically applied fluoride solution for dental caries prevention can be expected only as a result of a well-defined technique for the individual application as well as a carefully planned routine for appointment recall.   When a 2 per cent sodium fluoride solution is used, prevention of an average of 40 per cent new dental carious lesions can be expected.[13]   Stannous fluoride in an 8 per cent solution has been shown to be at least as effective.[18]   Studies using sodium fluoride acidulated with orthophosphoric acid show up to 70 per cent fewer new dental carious lesions over a two-year period.[15]

A. Factors Affecting Benefits to be Obtained
The effects of the topical applications are in proportion to the care taken during the procedure.   Whether a sodium or stannous fluoride solution is used, the essentials listed below are basic to obtaining a scientific result.

1. Application preceded by an oral prophylaxis to produce clean tooth surfaces: permits maximum contact of the solution with the enamel.
2. Exacting preparation and care of the solution in accord with its physical and chemical properties.
3. Isolation and drying of the teeth and maintenance of the isolated field during the required length of time for application.
4. Application of the solution to all tooth surfaces; repeated application as indicated by specific directions resulting from research.
5. Attention to keeping the solution in contact with the tooth surface for the proper length of time.
6. Repetition of applications at intervals in accord with the eruption pattern and dental caries susceptibility of the individual patient.

B. Characteristics of the Teeth After Application[19,20]
1. Teeth are less soluble in acids of the oral cavity.
2. Teeth have increased surface hardness.
3. Teeth with adsorbed fluorides inhibit acid formation from fermentable carbohydrate by oral microorganisms.

C. Mechanism of Action
1. Topical fluoride[21,22]
    The erupted tooth receives fluoride ions from the solution applied to the enamel surface.   A part of the surface hydroxyapa-

tite is changed to fluorapatite. Calcium fluoride, which is also formed, is partly washed away and what is left will be converted into hydroxyapatite. The depth of penetration into sound enamel is very slight, only 0.1 mm. Newly erupted teeth take up more fluoride than older teeth, and the partly decalcified areas of initial carious lesions take up 5 times as much fluoride as adjacent sound enamel.

Less fluoride is adsorbed from stannous fluoride than from sodium fluoride, but tin is also taken up which aids the effectiveness of the application. Tin phosphates and sulphides are formed. Tooth discoloration following stannous fluoride application is a result of the formation of tin sulphide.

2. Fluoridation[23]

For purposes of comparison with the mechanism of action of topical fluoride, a brief summary of the acquisition of fluoride from water consumption is included. Fluorapatite is formed during three stages in the life cycle of the tooth as follows:

a. Calcification: fluoride is distributed in the bulk of the enamel during the original formative period.

b. Pre-eruptive: after the enamel has been laid down, fluoride deposition continues in the surface of the enamel. During this stage the bulk of the enamel is inaccessible to the nutrient fluids. Nearly 3 times as much fluoride is deposited during this stage as during calcification.

c. Post-eruptive: the outer enamel surface has further pick-up of fluoride.

D. Effect on Adult Teeth

More research is available to show the benefits of sodium fluoride application to newly erupted teeth and to teeth up to 18 years of age, but there is evidence that teeth of adults over 18 may also benefit to a lesser degree.[24,25] Research using a 10 per cent solution of stannous fluoride shows favorable effects on adults.[27]

PRINCIPLES FOR APPLICATION

I. SODIUM FLUORIDE[27,28]

A series of 4 applications, spaced 2 days to a week apart, is made using a 2 per cent aqueous solution of sodium fluoride. The series of 4 applications is repeated at intervals throughout childhood in accord with the tooth eruption pattern of the individual child so that teeth may receive protection as soon after eruption as possible. Ages 3, 7, 10 and 13 are considered average and are generally used in public health programs. In addition, it has been recommended that a single application be made at 4 to 6 months intervals between the series of 4 in accord with routine dental office recall for the individual child's oral prophylaxis and dental inspection.[29]

A. Application

1. Oral prophylaxis precedes first application.
2. General removal of debris and materia alba precedes successive applications.

3. Teeth are isolated with cotton rolls and dried thoroughly immediately prior to each application.
4. Length of individual application: 3 minutes.

B. **Care of Solution**

The solution, generally obtained from a pharmacist, must be stored in a pyrex or polyethylene bottle to prevent changes in pH which occur in a plain glass container.[30,31] Fresh solution should be obtained every 2 to 3 weeks since even in a pyrex or polyethylene bottle hydrolysis can occur.

II. STANNOUS FLUORIDE[26,32,33]

A single application of an 8 per cent stannous fluoride solution is made for children at 6 or 12 months' intervals beginning at approximately age 3. A 10 per cent solution is used for adults at 6 or 12 months' intervals, depending on the dental caries susceptibility pattern of the individual patient. Because stannous fluoride can result in brown staining of cracks and decalcified areas of teeth and silicate cement restorations, it has been suggested that sodium fluoride may be applied in the anterior regions and stannous fluoride in the posterior.[34]

A. **Application**

1. Oral prophylaxis precedes application.
2. Teeth are isolated with cotton rolls and dried thoroughly immediately prior to application.
3. Length of individual application: 4 minutes.

B. **Preparation of Solution**

Stannous fluoride solution is unstable and so a fresh solution must be prepared for each patient. Clinical effectiveness of stannous fluoride depends on the maintenance of stannous tin in an active state. The solution oxidizes rapidly.

1. Obtain from pharmacist Lilly No. 0 gelatin capsules containing stannous fluoride powder.
   a. For 8 per cent: 0.8 Gm.
   b. For 10 per cent: 1.0 Gm.
2. Keep capsules in a tightly sealed container.
3. Immediately before use add the contents of one capsule to 10.0 ml. of distilled water and shake. Use a 25 ml. graduated cylinder for measuring the water and a 25 ml. polyethylene bottle for mixing the solution.
4. Add no flavoring or coloring agent as it decreases the anticariogenic effectiveness.
5. After contents have completely dissolved, transfer to a dappen dish and apply immediately to the clean, dry, isolated teeth.
6. Discard solution not used for the single appointment.

C. **Precautions for Use of Stannous Fluoride**

1. Use a coverall such as a plastic throw to protect the patient's clothing in case the solution is inadvertently spilled. Stannous fluoride reacts to discolor or remove color from certain materials.

2. Make necessary radiographs prior to stannous fluoride application to prevent contamination of the film either by solution in the patient's mouth or on the hands of the operator.[35]
3. Run a cupful of water through the saliva ejector after application on one side of the mouth because stannous fluoride deposits can clog the narrow tubing of the ejector.
4. Provide particular care for the equipment which has had contact with stannous fluoride solution because a whitish deposit is formed when the solution is left for a short time.
   a. Rinse the container in which the solution is mixed immediately after transfer to a dappen dish and wash thoroughly after completion of the application.
   b. At completion of the application: wash and scrub instruments and dappen dish thoroughly as the sterilizing equipment or disinfecting solution can become contaminated. Run at least a cupful of water through the saliva ejector.
   c. Each day remove the rubber end and screen of the saliva ejector and scrub thoroughly. When the deposit has dried on the screen, a metal instrument with a fine tip may be helpful to clean the mesh.

TECHNIQUE FOR TOPICAL APPLICATION OF FLUORIDE SOLUTION

The use of cotton roll holders permits two efficient applications, one for the right side, maxillary and mandibular, and one for the left side. Without cotton roll holders it is necessary to apply the solution to a quadrant at a time. With certain patients it may be possible to isolate the entire maxillary arch for one application, followed by the right and left mandibular quadrants separately.

I. PREPARATION OF COTTON ROLLS

Cotton rolls of various lengths are prepared in advance and a supply kept in the dental cabinet. The #2 cotton rolls are used for all patients except when a child with primary dentition and a small mouth requires #1. The ends are cut on the diagonal (at a 45° angle) to facilitate placement and retention in the proper position.

The objective in preparing cotton rolls is to use appropriate sizes and lengths to permit convenient positioning yet prevent absorption of the fluoride solution which should be on the enamel. When the cotton rolls are too short, inadequate isolation results and saliva may become mixed with the fluoride solution, rendering it less effective. In the case of stannous fluoride, the cotton rolls prevent the bitter-tasting solution from dispersing around the mouth. When the cotton rolls are too long they may become dislodged or may initiate gagging if they contact the tissues of the posterior region of the mouth.

A. Lengths for Primary Teeth and Mixed Dentition (Second permanent molars unerupted)

1. Facial cotton roll (5 to 6 inches long).
   a. Attach to buccal prong of cotton roll holder.
   b. Positioned to extend (in the mucobuccal folds) from the maxillary labial frenum to the mandibular labial frenum.

2. Lingual cotton roll ($1\frac{1}{2}$ inches long)
   a. Attach to lingual prong of cotton roll holder.
   b. Positioned to extend from cuspid area to just distal to the most posterior tooth.

B. **Lengths for Permanent Teeth** (Second permanent molar erupted)
   1. Maxillary cotton roll ($2\frac{1}{2}$ to 3 inches long): to extend from labial frenum to area distal to most posterior tooth and opening of Stenson's Duct.
   2. Mandibular cotton rolls.
   a. Facial ($2\frac{1}{2}$ to 3 inches long): attached to buccal prong of cotton roll holder; to extend from mandibular labial frenum to retromolar area.
   b. Lingual ($1\frac{1}{2}$ to 2 inches long): attach to lingual prong of cotton roll holder; to extend from cuspid area to just distal to the most posterior tooth.

II. PROCEDURE FOLLOWING ORAL PROPHYLAXIS

A. **Assemble Armamentarium**
   1. Cotton roll holders of proper size for patient.
   2. Cotton rolls of proper lengths attached to holders.
   3. Cotton pellets (6 to 8 medium size) and cotton pliers. Cotton applicators may be used.
   4. Dappen dish for fluoride solution.
   5. Saliva ejector connected and water control adjusted.
   6. Air tip connected.
   7. Timer (3 minute for sodium fluoride, 4 minute for stannous fluoride, 4 minute for sodium fluoride acidulated with orthophosphoric acid).

B. **Preparation of Patient**
   1. Chair position: upright to prevent solution from passing into throat.
   2. Place right cotton roll holder containing cotton rolls; adjust to proper position before tightening chin clamp.
   a. Cotton rolls should not touch the tooth surfaces.
   b. Lingual cotton roll attached to holder should be placed beside tongue, under the lateral margin, not pressing tongue down, to assure stability of holder. An extra $\frac{1}{4}$ to $\frac{1}{3}$ length of cotton roll frequently is required under the side of the tongue to balance the cotton roll holder and/or absorb excessive saliva.
   c. Cotton roll holder should be placed firmly to maintain its position without need for further stabilization.
   d. Facial cotton roll should extend only slightly distal to the most posterior tooth, and should be shortened if there is a tendency for it to curl up on the retromolar area. (This applies when separate maxillary and mandibular cotton rolls are used.)
   e. Check cotton roll holder to assure protection of oral tissues from any metal part.
   3. Place saliva ejector carefully, in region of cuspid opposite cotton roll holder.

    4. Maxillary
- *a.* Continuous cotton roll is twisted slightly (toward gingiva) as it is brought into position in the mucobuccal fold. End is fitted adjacent to labial frenum.
- *b.* Separate maxillary cotton roll is placed from the labial frenum, twisted slightly as it is inserted into the mucobuccal fold and the cheek is retracted.

    5. Retract cheek and hold maxillary cotton roll with index and middle fingers (on the left side the thumb and index fingers are used). Hold against the opening of Stenson's duct to absorb saliva.
- *a.* Thumb is kept distal to most posterior tooth (index finger on left side).
- *b.* Retraction is maintained throughout the application.

C. Application Procedure

1. Dry teeth thoroughly with compressed air.
   - *a.* Air pressure: adequate to dry all surfaces.
   - *b.* Routine order for increased efficiency.
     - (1) Maxillary buccal, occlusal, lingual.
     - (2) Mandibular buccal, occlusal, lingual.
2. Moisten all teeth with pellet saturated in fluoride solution (cotton applicator may be used). Apply slight pressure with wet pellet at each interproximal area to assure diffusion to contact area.
3. Start timer (patients may be instructed in this procedure).
4. *Continuous application:* maintain wet tooth surfaces by repeated application of solution throughout the 3- or 4-minute period.
5. *Single application*[6] solution is applied only once (sodium fluoride 2%).[27]

D. Completion of Application

1. Remove saliva ejector.
2. Release cotton roll holder clamp, and remove holder with cotton rolls attached.
3. Remove remaining cotton rolls with cotton pliers.
4. Instruct patient to postpone rinsing, eating or brushing as long as possible or at least one-half hour.[22]

E. Proceed to Opposite Side (repeat steps: II., B., C., D. above)

III. PROCEDURE FOR SUCCEEDING APPLICATIONS IN A SERIES (SODIUM FLUORIDE)

A. Assemble Armamentarium

1. Waste receiver, cotton pellets, gauze wipe.
2. Mouth mirror, explorer, cotton pliers.
3. Dappen dish containing 3 per cent hydrogen peroxide.
4. Dental floss: 10 to 12 inch length.
5. Topical fluoride equipment (II., A., page 203).

B. **Preparation of Patient**

1. General cleaning of teeth
   a. Request patient to demonstrate toothbrushing in his mouth.
      (1) To review previous patient instruction.
      (2) To remove soft deposits.
   b. Apply dental floss to all contact areas to remove debris.
   c. Scale teeth as indicated when calculus is present.
   d. Do not use an abrasive to clean the teeth because it is possible to remove the fluoride deposited during the previous application.[22]
   e. Check teeth for cleanliness with particular attention to areas where materia alba occurs most frequently (see Table 5, page 112.)
   f. Apply 3 per cent hydrogen peroxide for removal of remaining soft deposits.
      (1) Rub saturated pellet over tooth surfaces carefully, maintaining a fulcrum and keeping end of cotton pliers covered with cotton to prevent injury to the soft tissues.
      (2) Request patient to rinse thoroughly.
   g. Dry teeth and use explorer to inspect teeth for cleanliness.

C. **Application Procedure** (same as II., B., C., D., E. above)

TECHNICAL HINTS

I. **Adapt technique for small or unmanageable patient:** hold cotton rolls with fingers and apply solution to each of the four quadrants separately. Parent may be requested to assist in holding the cotton rolls.

II. **Record Keeping:** Particularly for the use of sodium fluoride, maintaining a record of the teeth present in the mouth at the time of application can aid in planning succeeding series in accord with the individual eruption pattern. Suggestions for accomplishing this are:

A. Record names or numbers of erupted teeth in the patient's permanent record along with the daily procedure.

B. Use a specially prepared diagrammatic chart which shows either a series of drawings of the complete dentition or a form with numbers for permanent teeth and letters for primary teeth (Fig. 41). Unerupted teeth can be marked and dated.

III. **Effect of Stannous Fluoride on Gingival Tissue:**[36,37] When the gingival tissue is inflamed at the time of the oral prophylaxis, or scaling has caused extensive tissue trauma and hemorrhage, it is advisable to postpone the application until the tissue has returned to normal. The solution may cause the irritated tissue to "burn" or "sting" and a blanching of the tissues may occur. At the second appointment the teeth need to be thoroughly polished again.[33]

UNIVERSITY OF WASHINGTON   DEPARTMENT OF DENTAL HYGIENE

TOPICAL FLUORIDE APPLICATION RECORD

Patient_____Birthdate __/__/__ Chart #_____

Residences, Birth to 10 yrs.(City, State, years)_____

_____

Natural Fluoride: Age_____ to _____ Fluoridation: Age _____ to _____.

Last Topical Fluoride: Date _____Series of 4_____Single_____

Dental Hygiene Clinic Record (Draw lines through missing and unerupted teeth)

1	2
Right **Left**	**Right** **Left**
E D C B A ┃A B C D E 8 7 6 5 4 3 2 1┃1 2 3 4 5 6 7 8 8 7 6 5 4 3 2 1┃1 2 3 4 5 6 7 8 E D C B A ┃A B C D E	E D C B A ┃A B C D E 8 7 6 5 4 3 2 1┃1 2 3 4 5 6 7 8 8 7 6 5 4 3 2 1┃1 2 3 4 5 6 7 8 E D C B A ┃A B C D E

Date_____ Age_____
                      yrs. mos.
Series   Single
	Date_____ Age_____
	                      yrs. mos.
	Series Single

3	4
Right **Left**	**Right** **Left**
E D C B A ┃A B C D E 8 7 6 5 4 3 2 1┃1 2 3 4 5 6 7 8 8 7 6 5 4 3 2 1┃1 2 3 4 5 6 7 8 E D C B A ┃A B C D E	E D C B A ┃A B C D E 8 7 6 5 4 3 2 1┃1 2 3 4 5 6 7 8 8 7 6 5 4 3 2 1┃1 2 3 4 5 6 7 8 E D C B A ┃A B C D E

Date_____ Age_____
                      yrs. mos.
Series   Single
	Date_____ Age_____
	                      yrs. mos.
	Series Single

5	6
Right **Left**	**Right** **Left**
E D C B A ┃A B C D E 8 7 6 5 4 3 2 1┃1 2 3 4 5 6 7 8 8 7 6 5 4 3 2 1┃1 2 3 4 5 6 7 8 E D C B A ┃A B C D E	E D C B A ┃A B C D E 8 7 6 5 4 3 2 1┃1 2 3 4 5 6 7 8 8 7 6 5 4 3 2 1┃1 2 3 4 5 6 7 8 E D C B A ┃A B C D E

Date_____ Age_____
                      yrs. mos.
Series   Single
	Date_____ Age_____
	                      yrs. mos.
	Series Single

FIGURE 41.—Topical fluoride application record. Unerupted teeth are marked when a fluoride application is made. Reference to the record provides information for determining the sequence and frequency of future applications as the teeth erupt.

FACTORS TO TEACH THE PATIENT*

    I. The importance of supplementing the topical applications with effective personal oral care procedures, dietary control of fermentable carbohydrates, and routine professional care by the dentist, if optimum prevention of dental caries is to be obtained.

   II. The need for four sodium fluoride applications in a series, or single application at a recall appointment, and how the appointments are planned.

  III. The relationship of the time of applications to the eruption pattern of the individual child.

  IV. How topical fluoride solution acts only to prevent new dental carious lesions but has no effect on existing lesions.

   V. The possible effect of fluoride solution in inhibiting pre-carious areas of decalcification such as may occur on the gingival third of teeth in dental caries susceptible patients. When stannous fluoride is applied such areas may become pigmented.

  VI. How fluorides affect the teeth to prevent dental caries.

 VII. The relative effectiveness of topical application of fluoride solution and fluoridation.

VIII. The significance of fluoridation to the community.

  IX. The effectiveness of the application of fluoride solution for desensitization of exposed cementum or dentin in certain cases (see page 210).

*The word "patient" means patient and parent when the patient is a child.

REFERENCES

1. AST, D. B. and FITZGERALD, B.: Effectiveness of Water Fluoridation, Am. Dent. A. J., *65*, 581, November, 1962.
2. ARNOLD, F. A., DEAN, H. T., JAY, P., and KNUTSON, J. W.: Effect of Fluoridated Water Supplies on Dental Caries Prevalence, Tenth Year of the Grand Rapids—Muskegon Study, Pub. Health Rep., *71*, 652, July, 1956.
3. HAYES, R. L., LITTLETON, N. W., and WHITE, C. L.: Posteruptive Effects of Fluoridation on First Permanent Molars of Children in Grand Rapids, Michigan, Am. J. Pub. Health, *47*, 192, February, 1957.
4. DIRKS, O. B., HOUWINK, B., and KWANT, G. W.: Some Special Features of the Caries Preventive Effect of Water Fluoridation, Arch. Oral Biol., *4*, 187, August, 1961.
5. RUSSELL, A. L. and ELVOVE, E.: Domestic Water and Dental Caries. VII. A Study of the Fluoride Dental Caries Relationship in an Adult Population, Pub. Health. Rep., *66*, 1389, October, 1951.
6. ENGLANDER, H. R., REUSS, R. C., and KESEL, R. G.: Dental Caries in Adults Who Consume Fluoridated Versus Fluoride-deficient Water, Am. Dent. A. J., *68*, 14, January, 1964.
7. American Dental Association: *Accepted Dental Remedies*, 29th ed. Chicago, American Dental Association, 1964, p. 131.
8. American Dental Association, Council on Dental Therapeutics: Prescribing Supplements of Dietary Fluorides, Am. Dent. A. J., *56*, 589, April, 1958.
9. ARNOLD, F. A., McCLURE, F. J., and WHITE, C. L.: Sodium Fluoride Tablets for Children, Dent. Prog., *1*, 8, October, 1960.
10. DALE, P. P.: Prenatal Fluorides: the Value of Fluoride During Pregnancy, Am. Dent. A. J., *68*, 530, April, 1964.
11. MUHLER, J. C.: Anticariogenic Effectiveness of a Single Application of Stannous Fluoride in Children Residing in an Optimal Communal Fluoride Area. II. Results at the End of 30 Months. Am. Dent. A. J., *61*, 431, October, 1960.
12. MUHLER, J. C.: A Practical Method for Reducing Dental Caries in Children Not Receiving the Established Benefits of Communal Fluoridation, J. Dent. Child., *28*, 5, 1st Quarter, 1961.
13. SHAW, J. H.: *Fluoridation as a Public Health Measure.* Washington, D. C., American Association for the Advancement of Science, 1954, pp. 152–154.

14. BIBBY, B. G.:   A New Approach to Caries Prophylaxis, a Preliminary Report on the Use of Fluoride Applications, Tufts Dental Outlook, *15*, 4, May, 1942.
15. WELLOCK, W. D. and BRUDEVOLD, F.:   Study of Acidulated Fluoride Solutions. II. The Caries Inhibiting Effect of Single Annual Topical Applications of an Acidic Fluoride and Phosphate Solution. A Two Year Experience. Arch. Oral Biol., *8*, 179, March-April, 1963.
16. PAMEIJER, J. H. N., BRUDEVOLD, F., and HUNT, E. E.:   Study of Acidulated Fluoride Solutions. III. Cariostatic Effect of Repeated Topical Sodium Fluoride Applications with and without Phosphate: a Pilot Study. Arch. Oral Biol., *8*, 183, March-April, 1963.
17. WARNER, E. M.:   Public Health, in Bunting, R. W.:   Oral Hygiene, 3rd ed. Philadelphia, Lea & Febiger, 1957, pp. 297–305.
18. MUHLER, J. C.:   Present Status of Topical Fluoride Therapy, J. Dent. Child., *26*, 173, 3rd Quarter, 1959.
19. SHAW: op. cit., pp. 167–171.
20. VOLKER, J. F. and CALDWELL, R. C.:   Prevention of Dental Caries with Fluoride, in Finn, S. B.:   *Clinical Pedodontics*, 2nd ed.   Philadelphia, Saunders, 1962, pp. 655–656.
21. BRUDEVOLD, F.:   Action of Topically Applied Fluoride, J. Dent. Child., *26*, 186, 3rd Quarter, 1959.
22. BRUDEVOLD, F.:   Fluorides in the Prevention of Dental Caries, Dental Clinics of North America, July, 1962, p. 397.
23. BRUDEVOLD, F., GARDNER, D. E., and SMITH, F. A.:   Distribution of Fluoride in Human Enamel, J. Dent. Res., *35*, 420, June, 1956.
24. SHAW: op. cit., p. 156.
25. MUHLER, J. C., HINE, M. K., and DAY, H. G.:   *Preventive Dentistry.* St. Louis, Mosby, 1954, pp. 256, 258–259.
26. MUHLER, J. C.:   Effect of a Single Topical Application of Stannous Fluoride on the Incidence of Dental Caries in Adults, J. Dent. Res., *37*, 415, June, 1958.
27. KNUTSON, J. W.:   Sodium Fluoride Solutions: Technic for Application to the Teeth, Am. Dent. A. J., *36*, 37, January, 1948.
28. McCAULEY, H. B.:   Topical Fluoride Solutions for Control of Dental Caries: Considerations Pertinent to Their Clinical Application, Am. Dent. A. J., *38*, 430, April, 1949.
29. BIBBY, B. G.:   Sensible Procedure for Topical Fluoride Applications (Editorial), Dental Survey, *28*, 820, June, 1952.
30. American Dental Association, Bureau of Chemistry and Council on Dental Therapeutics: Formulation and Packaging of Aqueous Solutions of Sodium Fluoride for Topical Application, Am. Dent. A. J., *38*, 142, January, 1949.
31. SAVCHUCK, W. B. and ARMSTRONG, W. D.:   The Stability of Aqueous Solutions of Sodium Fluoride, J. Dent. Res., *28*, 4, February, 1949.
32. MUHLER, J. C.:   Topical Application of Stannous Fluoride, Am. Dent. A. J., *54*, 352, March, 1957.
33. DAHL, L. O. and DUDDING, N. J.:   Single Stannous Fluoride Topical Treatments, Am. Dent. Hygienists' A. J., *33*, 112, July, 1959.
34. LAW, D. B.:   Present Status of Fluoride in Dental Practice, Am. Dent. Hygienists' A. J., *35*, 55, April, 1961.
35. DAHL, L. O. and MUHLER, J. C.:   Effect of Microconcentrations of Stannous Fluoride Solutions on Dental X-ray Films, Am. Dent. A. J., *58*, 24, February, 1959.
36. MUHLER, J. C.:   Effect on Gingiva and Occurrence of Pigmentation of Teeth Following the Topical Application of Stannous Fluoride or Stannous Chlorofluoride, J. Periodont., *28*, 281, October, 1957.
37. SWIETERMAN, R. P., MUHLER, J. C., and SWENSON, H. M.:   Effect of Highly Concentrated Solutions of Stannous Fluoride on Human Gingival Tissues, J. Periodont., *32*, 131, April, 1961.

SUGGESTED READINGS

American Dental Association, Council on Dental Therapeutics: *Accepted Dental Remedies*, 29th ed. Chicago, American Dental Association, 1964, pp. 129–137.
CAMPBELL, I. R.:   *Role of Fluoride in Public Health*, A Selected Bibliography. Cincinnati, Kettering Laboratory, College of Medicine, University of Cincinnati, 1963.
Fluoridation Issue (22 articles and 2 editorials), Am. Dent. A. J., *65*, 578–717, November, 1962.
LARGENT, E. J.:   *Fluorosis.* Columbus, Ohio State University Press, 1961, 140 pp.
McCLURE, F. J.:   *Fluoride Drinking Waters.* Bethesda, National Institute of Dental Research, United States Department of Health, Education and Welfare, Public Health Service Publication #825, 1962.
VOLKER, J. F. and CALDWELL, R. C.:   Prevention of Dental Caries with Fluoride, in Finn, S. B.: *Clinical Pedodontics*, 2nd ed.   Philadelphia, Saunders, 1962, pp. 635–659.

Chapter 22

THE CARE OF HYPERSENSITIVE TEETH

Areas of exposed tooth surface in the region of the cemento-enamel junction can produce considerable discomfort. Care must be taken during instrumentation and application of air to prevent a hypersensitive reaction. Since tooth sensitivity is frequently related to the accumulation of debris in the exposed cervical area, instruction in an exacting toothbrushing technique is indicated.

Patients are appreciative of clinical procedures directed at desensitizing the areas involved. A number of chemical and mechanical means have been used successfully to reduce or eliminate pain. Chemical desensitizers produce more effective results when applied to the clean tooth surface immediately following the oral prophylaxis. No known method is universally effective for desensitization.

I. FACTORS CONTRIBUTING TO HYPERSENSITIVITY

A. **Exposure of Cementum and Dentin**
1. Gingival Recession[1,2]
   a. Physiologic: related to aging.
   b. Pathologic (localized or generalized): inflammation which may stimulate proliferation of the epithelial attachment along the root surface.
   c. Traumatic: toothbrush or occlusion.
2. Periodontal Surgery: removal of gingival tissue.

B. **Anatomy of the Cemento-Enamel Junction[3,4]**
1. Zone of dentin occurs between the enamel and the cementum in 10 per cent of teeth.
2. Enamel meets cementum in 30 per cent of teeth.
3. Cementum overlaps enamel in 60 per cent of teeth.

C. **Loss of Cementum Denudes the Dentin:** Cementum is lost through abrasion, erosion, dental caries, scaling, curettage.

D. **Sensitivity of Dentin:** In most teeth the dentin is more sensitive on its outer surface.[5]

II. TYPES OF PAIN STIMULI[6,7]

A. **Mechanical:** toothbrush bristles, eating utensils, periodontal and dental hygiene instruments, friction from denture clasps or other appliances.

B. **Chemical:** acids formed from fermentable carbohydrates in debris and plaque, citrus fruit acids, or condiments.

C. **Thermal:** hot or cold foods or beverages; air entering the oral cavity.

14

III. **MODE OF ACTION OF DESENSITIZING AGENTS**[8]

Sensitivity is due to irritation of the organic matter or "nerve elements" in the dentinal tubules. Agents used for desensitization may be classified as those acting (1) by precipitation of the peripheral ends of the protoplasmic processes (Tomes' fibers), or (2) by an attempt to deposit an insoluble salt in the exposed dentinal tubules. The specific mode of action of most agents is not known.

IV. **METHODS OF DESENSITIZATION**

Dentists have used albumin precipitants such as 40 per cent formalin, 40 per cent zinc chloride, or 40 per cent silver nitrate to seal the dentinal tubules and hence reduce sensitivity. Cavity varnishes, thin mixes of crown and bridge cement, zinc oxide and eugenol packs or Gottlieb's solution have been used to protect the tooth surface against thermal shock.

Certain methods are used in the dental office whereas others are performed daily by the patient. A combination of professional and personal methods is recommended.

A. **Fluoride Preparations***

1. *Sodium Fluoride Aqueous Solution* (2 or 4 per cent): apply as in the topical application for the prevention of dental caries (see pages 200–201).
2. *Sodium Fluoride Desensitizing Paste:* 33 per cent sodium fluoride, 33 per cent kaolin, and 33 per cent glycerin.[9,10,11]
   a. Clean and isolate the sensitive tooth using cotton rolls, cotton roll holder for mandibular, and saliva ejector.
   b. Wipe exposed area with cotton pellet moistened in 2 per cent sodium fluoride solution.
   c. Dry area thoroughly using cotton pellets or cotton roll.
   d. Place small amount of desensitizing paste on area with tip of wood point in porte polisher. A narrow wood point fits the cervical area more effectively than a wide one.
   e. Massage paste on area gently but firmly with wood point, using small circular strokes. If patient suffers acute pain response at beginning of application, wipe off paste, have patient rinse with warm water, and begin again immediately.
   f. Continue massage for 3 minutes: use timer.
   g. Wipe off excess paste with cotton pellet.
   h. Remove cotton rolls and saliva ejector, and request patient to rinse with warm water.
   i. Repeat at future appointment if desensitization has not been accomplished.
3. *Sodium Silicofluoride Solution* (0.9 per cent).[12]
   a. Clean and isolate the sensitive tooth using cotton rolls, cotton roll holder for mandibular, and saliva ejector.

---

* Fluoride preparations are particularly adaptable to application by the dental hygienist because of familiarity with procedures of porte polishing tooth surfaces as well as the topical application of fluoride solutions for the prevention of dental caries. Desensitizing procedures are performed only under the direction of the dentist and in accord with laws governing the practice of dental hygienists in an individual state.

   b. Dry the area thoroughly using cotton pellets or cotton roll.
   c. Apply solution from dappen dish with cotton pellet or applicator.
   d. Keep area glistening (but not dripping) wet for 5 minutes.
   e. Remove excess solution with cotton pellets.
   f. Repeat weekly for maximum of 3 applications as needed: if desensitization is to occur, it will have occurred after 3 applications.

B. **Iontophoresis:**[13,14,15] impregnation of tissue with ions from dissolved salts with the aid of an electric current.
   1. Low-voltage batteries ($1\frac{1}{2}$ to 9 volts) supplies positive current to patient's tooth.
   2. Circuit completed by contact of brush applicator for negatively charged aqueous fluoride solution (1 to 2 per cent sodium fluoride used in dental office).
   3. Iontophoretic toothbrush available for home use with a commercial fluoride dentifrice: limited research with hopeful results.

C. **Personal Care by the Patient**
   1. Dietary control
      a. Effect: dietary limitation of foods such as excessive fermentable carbohydrates, citrus fruits or condiments which may cause pain stimulus.
      b. Case selection: questioning the patient may be sufficient to gain information concerning the diet. In certain instances, particularly when it is believed that fermentable carbohydrates are used in excess, a dietary survey will be required to impress the patient with the cause of his problem (see pages 356–361).
      c. Method: specific instruction in food selection.
   2. Toothbrushing
      a. Effect: removal of irritating substances and mild frictional action of the bristles against the tooth substance.
      b. Case selection: primarily effective when sensitivity is believed to be caused by acids from bacterial action in the materia alba and dental plaque and the patient does not cleanse the area adequately.
      c. Method: specific instruction in measures of oral physical therapy of choice for the patient (Table 11, page 286). A multitufted brush frequently is advisable during the period of sensitivity. Planned appointments for review of procedures are required.
   3. Dentifrices
      Dentifrices containing paraformaldehyde[16,17] or strontium chloride[18–20] have shown favorable results for certain patients after continued use.

V. **TECHNICAL HINTS**

A. Do not use compressed air on sensitive teeth. Dry only with cotton pellets or cotton roll.

B. Sodium silicofluoride solution and sodium fluoride desensitizing paste contain enough fluoride to cause nausea if swallowed in excess. Prevent by using only small amounts, wiping excess off with cotton pellets before removing cotton rolls, requesting the patient to rinse thoroughly, and using the saliva ejector to prevent the need for swallowing before the mouth can be rinsed.

C. Prepare solution of sodium silicofluoride weekly and store in polyethylene container. A chemical reaction results when a plain glass bottle is used.[12]

D. Keep jar containing sodium fluoride desensitizing paste tightly closed. Its shelf life can be indefinite because of its glycerin base.

VI. FACTORS TO TEACH THE PATIENT

A. Possible general causes of gingival recession.

B. Possible causes of hypersensitivity of teeth.

C. Limited probability of success of desensitization with fluorides, and that indefinite duration of results cannot be guaranteed.

D. Possibility that the hypersensitiveness will subside in time whether a desensitizer is applied or not.

E. Procedures of oral physical therapy as they apply to hypersensitive teeth.

F. Specific foods which should and should not be used in the diet if relief from sensitivity is to be obtained.

REFERENCES

1. GRANT, DANIEL, STERN, I. B., and EVERETT, F. G.: *Orban's Periodontics*, 2nd ed. St. Louis, Mosby, 1963, pp. 193–203.
2. GLICKMAN, IRVING: *Clinical Periodontology*, 2nd ed. Philadelphia, Saunders, 1958, pp. 115–117.
3. SICHER, HARRY: *Orban's Oral Histology and Embryology*, 5th ed. St. Louis, Mosby, 1962, pp. 174–175.
4. PERMAR, DOROTHY: *A Manual of Oral Embryology and Microscopic Anatomy*, 3rd ed. Philadelphia, Lea & Febiger, 1963, pp. 67, 74, 117, 141.
5. SICHER: op. cit., pp. 121, 132–133.
6. GRANT, STERN and EVERETT: op. cit., p. 323.
7. ABEL, IRWIN: Study of Hypersensitive Teeth and a New Therapeutic Aid, Oral Surg., Oral Med. & Oral Path., *11*, 491, May, 1958.
8. GRANT, STERN and EVERETT: op. cit., p. 325.
9. HOYT, W. H. and BIBBY, B. G.: Use of Sodium Fluoride for Desensitizing Dentin, Am. Dent. A. J., *30*, 1372, September, 1943.
10. American Dental Association, Council on Dental Therapeutics: Miscellaneous Therapeutic Applications for Sodium Fluoride in Dentistry, Am. Dent. A. J., *38*, 762, June, 1949.
11. American Dental Association: *Accepted Dental Remedies*, 29th ed. Chicago, American Dental Association, 1964, p. 135.
12. STOUT, W. C.: Sodium Silicofluoride as a Desensitizing Agent, J. Periodont., *26*, 208, July 1955.
13. SIEMON, W. H.: Iontophoretic Procedures in Dentistry, Dent. Dig., *68*, 172, April, 1962.
14. COLLINS, E. M.: Desensitization of Hypersensitive Teeth, Dent. Dig., *68*, 360, August, 1962.
15. JENSEN, A. L.: Hypersensitivity Controlled by Iontophoresis: Double Blind Clinical Investigation, Am. Dent. A. J., *68*, 217, February, 1964.
16. GRANT, STERN and EVERETT: op. cit., p. 326.
17. BURMAN, L. R. and GOLDSTEIN, ABRAHAM: Evaluation of a Desensitizing Agent by Response to a Controlled External Stimulus, J. Periodont., *32*, 257, July, 1961.
18. ROSS, M. R.: Hypersensitive Teeth: Effect of Strontium Chloride in a Compatible Dentifrice, J. Periodont., *32*, 49, January, 1961.

19. COHEN, ABRAM: Preliminary Study of the Effects of a Strontium Chloride Dentifrice for the Control of Hypersensitive Teeth, Oral Surg., Oral Med., & Oral Path., *14*, 1046, September, 1961.
20. SKURNIK, HARRY: Control of Dental Hypersensitivity. Preliminary Report on a Strontium-Containing Dentifrice, J. Periodont., *34*, 183, March, 1963.

SUGGESTED READINGS

BRANNSTROM, MARTIN: Dentin Sensitivity and Aspiration of Odontoblasts, Am. Dent. A. J., *66*, 366, March, 1963.
EVERETT, F. G.: Desensitization of Hypersensitive Exposed Root Surfaces, Dental Clinics of North America, March, 1964, p. 221.
FERRANTI, PALMYRO: Simple Technique for Treatment of Hypersensitive Exposed Dentin, Dent. Dig., *68*, 14, January, 1962.
MANNING, M. M.: New Approach to Desensitization of Cervical Dentin, D. Survey, *37*, 731, June, 1961.
MONICA, W. S.: Relief of Hypersensitivity to Temperature Change, D. Progress, *3*, 164, April, 1963.

Chapter 23

PREPARATION OF DENTAL RADIOGRAPHS

RADIOGRAPHS are an essential adjunct to other means of oral diagnosis for treatment planning in the dentist's complete care program for the patient. In the dental hygiene appointment, radiographs are used as a guide in oral prophylaxis procedures, as a source of information for charting existing conditions, and as an aid in patient instruction.

The objective in radiography is to use techniques which require the least amount of radiation possible to produce radiographs of the greatest interpretive value. This can be accomplished through routine application of known safety measures for the patient and operator, through analysis of techniques for prevention of repeated inadequacies, and through continuing study to keep informed of research developments.

Patients ask questions about safety factors and occasionally a patient may refuse to have any radiographs made. The patient must be reassured with confidence, be instructed in why radiographs are indispensable to oral care, and be informed in how modern equipment and techniques are in accord with minimum radiation. The Council on Dental Research of the American Dental Association has defined the need for radiographic examinations if complete dental care is to be provided, and stated that "the amount of radiation involved in making a complete roentgenographic survey of the entire mouth is far below the levels which would produce detectable damage to the body tissue."[1] Likewise, the American Academy of Oral Roentgenology indicates that "the benefits of the judicious use of x-rays in dentistry far outweigh any conceivable biologic consequences that might be involved."[2]

This chapter is designed to serve as a summary of terminology, fundamentals of x-ray production, techniques of exposure and processing, safety factors, analysis of the completed radiograph, and suggestions for patient instruction. A comprehensive bibliography is provided to allow for additional study.

TERMS USED IN RADIOGRAPHY*

I. **RADIOLOGY:** that branch of medicine dealing with the diagnostic and therapeutic applications of ionizing radiation.

II. **RADIOGRAPHY:** the art or science of making radiographs.

III. **RADIOGRAPH:** an image or picture produced on a radiation-sensitive film emulsion, by exposure to ionizing radiation directed through an area or region or substance of interest, followed by chemical processing of the film. (noun) To make a radiograph. (verb)

* All definitions in this chapter are taken from or adapted from and in accord with the *Glossary of Terms Used in Radiology* prepared by the Committee on Nomenclature, American Academy of Oral Roentgenology, 1962, and revised by John H. Barr, Simon Kinsman, and Albert G. Richards, 1963. Additional definitions to those included in this chapter may be found in the Glossary.

IV. TYPES OF RADIATION

A. **Primary:** radiation coming directly from the target of the x-ray tube. Except for the useful beam, most of this radiation is absorbed in the tube housing.

B. **Useful Beam:** that part of the primary radiation which is permitted to emerge from the tube housing as limited by the aperture, cone or other collimating devices.

C. **Leakage:** radiation other than the useful beam which escapes through the protective shielding of the x-ray tube housing.

D. **Secondary:** radiation emitted by any matter being irradiated with x-rays. It originates mainly in the irradiated soft tissues of the patient's face, the pointed plastic cone, and the filter.

E. **Scattered:** radiation that, during the passage through a substance has been deviated in direction and may have been modified with an increase in wave length. It is one form of secondary radiation.

F. **Stray:** a term used in a broad sense to include all radiation emitted in directions other than that of the useful beam, for example, leakage radiation, secondary radiation, scattered radiation.

V. IRRADIATION: the exposure of material to x-ray or other radiation. One speaks of radiation therapy but of irradiation of the patient.

ORIGIN AND CHARACTERISTICS OF X-RAY

X-rays were first discovered by Wilhelm C. Roentgen in 1895, who called them x-rays after the mathematical symbol "x" for an unknown. "Roentgen rays" is a term often applied to mechanically generated x-rays. Professor Roentgen used a Crookes Tube and it was not until 1913 that William D. Coolidge designed a tube in which electricity was used instead of gas. Modern x-ray tubes have the same principles of construction as the Coolidge Tube. The historical development of the science of radiology and radiography provides a realistic monument to the early researchers and their efforts.[3,4]

I. DEFINITION AND PROPERTIES OF X-RAY

A. **X-ray:** electromagnetic, ionizing radiation of very short wave length resulting from the bombardment of a material (usually tungsten) by highly accelerated electrons in a high vacuum.

B. **Properties**
   1. Short wave length
      a. Hard x-rays: shorter wave lengths, high penetrating power.
      b. Soft x-rays: relatively longer wave lengths, relatively less penetrating; more likely to be absorbed into the tissue through which the x-rays pass.
   2. Travel with the same speed as visible light.
   3. Power to penetrate opaque substances.
   4. Invisible.
   5. Ability to affect the emulsion of a photographic film.
   6. Ability to produce fluorescence on contact with certain crystals.
   7. Ability to stimulate or destroy living cells.

II. HOW X-RAYS ARE PRODUCED[5-10]

With reference to the definition of x-ray above, essential to x-ray production are (1) a source of electrons, (2) a high voltage to accelerate the electrons, and (3) a target to stop the electrons. The parts of the tube and the circuits within the machine are designed to provide these.

A. The X-ray Tube (Fig. 42).

    1. Protective tube housing: x-ray tube enclosure that reduces the primary radiation to permissible exposure levels; highly vacuated glass tube surrounded by a specially refined oil with high insulating powers.

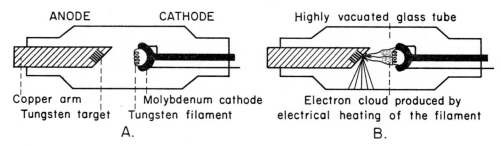

ANODE　　　CATHODE　　　Highly vacuated glass tube

Copper arm　　　Molybdenum cathode　　Electron cloud produced by
Tungsten target　Tungsten filament　　electrical heating of the filament

A.　　　　　　　　　　　　　　　B.

FIGURE 42.—*X-ray tube.* *A*. Inactive and *B*. In function. Highly accelerated electrons are propelled from the cathode to the anode. X-rays are produced as the electrons strike the tungsten target. (From Wuehrmann, *Radiation Protection and Dentistry*, Mosby.)

    2. Cathode:
        a. Tungsten filament: which is heated to give off a cloud of electrons.
        b. Molybdenum cup around the filament: to focus the electrons toward the anode.
    3. Anode:
        a. Copper arm containing a tungsten button, the target, positioned opposite the cathode.
        b. Focal Spot: that part of the target on the anode which is bombarded by the focused electron stream when the tube is energized.
    4. Aperture: where the useful beam emerges from the tube; is covered with a permanent seal of glass or aluminum.

B. Circuits

    1. Autotransformer: voltage compensator which adjusts variations in line voltage.
    2. High voltage transformer: step-up.
        a. Voltage of line current (110 volts) is increased to 65,000–90,000 volts.
        b. Purpose: give the electrons high speed.
    3. Filament circuit: step-down.
        a. Voltage of line current is decreased to approximately 3 volts.
        b. Purpose: heat the tungsten filament to produce electrons.
    4. Tube circuit: the flow of electrons from the cathode to the anode; activated when the timer button is depressed.

C. **Machine Control Devices**

   Machines vary, but in general in operating an x-ray machine there are four factors to control: the line switch (to electrical outlet), the kilovoltage, the milliamperage, and the time. Certain machines operate at a standard kilovoltage (usually 65 kVp) and milliamperage (10 mA.), whereas others permit a range of selection.

1. Voltage control (may be one or two meters, depending on the machine).
    a. Circuit voltmeter: registers line voltage before voltage is stepped up by the transformer (with alternating current this is 110 volts); or may register the kilovoltage that will result after step-up.
    b. KVp selector (kilovoltage peak): to change the line voltage to selected kilovoltage (65 to 90 kVp).
2. Milliamperage control: milliameter: to select the actual current through the tube circuit used during the time of exposure (10 to 20 mA.).
3. Time control
    a. X-ray timer: a time switch mechanism used to complete the electrical circuit so that x-rays will be produced for a predetermined time.
    b. Types of timers
        (1) Mechanical: spring-activated device; range from $\frac{1}{4}$ to 10 or 15 seconds; does not reset itself.
        (2) Electronic: vacuum tube device; range from $\frac{1}{30}$ second to 10 seconds; will reset itself automatically; meets needs of modern accelerated techniques.

D. **Steps in the Production of X-rays**[5]

1. Tungsten filament is heated and a cloud of electrons produced.
2. Difference in electrical potential (65–90 kVp) is developed between the anode and the cathode.
3. Electrons attracted to anode from cathode at high speed during the intervals of the alternating current when the anode is charged positive and the cathode negative. (During the alternating half of the cycle the electrons are attracted back into the filament in a self-rectifying tube.)
4. Curvature of the molybdenum cup controls the direction of the electrons and causes them to be projected on the focal spot.
5. Reaction of the electrons as they strike the tungsten target: loss of energy.
    a. Approximately 1 per cent of the energy of electrons is converted to electromagnetic energy of an x-ray. (Greater per cent at higher kilovoltages.)
    b. Approximately 99 per cent of the energy is converted to heat which is dissipated through the copper anode and oil of the protective tube housing.
6. X-rays leave tube through the aperture to form the useful beam.

TECHNICAL FACTORS WHICH INFLUENCE THE FINISHED RADIOGRAPH

As the beam leaves the x-ray tube it is collimated, filtered, and allowed to travel a designated source-film (or focal spot-film) distance before reaching the film of a selected speed.   The quality or diagnostic usefulness of the finished radiograph as well as the total exposure of the patient and operator are influenced by the collimation, filtration, source-film distance, film speed, kilovoltage, and milliampere seconds.   Film processing (see pages 243–247) also influences directly the quality of the radiograph, and indirectly the total exposure since re-exposure would be necessary should the film be rendered inadequate during processing.

I. CHARACTERISTICS OF AN ACCEPTABLE FINISHED RADIOGRAPH

    A. *All parts of the image are shown as close to their natural size and shape as possible with a minimum of distortion and superimposition.*

    B. *Area to be examined is shown completely with sufficient surrounding tissue included to provide for comparative interpretation.*

    C. *Highest film quality*

        1. *Density:* the degree of darkening of exposed and processed x-ray film.

        2. *Contrast:* the visual differences in density between adjacent areas on the radiograph.

        3. *Definition:* the property of the projected images relating to their sharpness, distinctness, or clarity of outline.

II. COLLIMATION:[11,12] technique or mechanism for reducing the spread of the bundle of radiation emitted through the aperture of the tube.

    A. **Purpose:** to eliminate peripheral or more divergent radiation.

        1. Minimize exposure to patient's face.

        2. Minimize secondary radiation which can fog the film and expose the bodies of patient and operator.

    B. **Method:** diaphragm, usually of lead, pierced with a central aperture of the smallest practical diameter for making radiographic exposure; located between the x-ray tube and cone.

        1. Recommended thickness of lead: $\frac{1}{8}$ inch.

        2. Recommended size of aperture: to permit a diameter of the bundle of radiation equal to $2\frac{3}{4}$ inches at the end of the plastic cone next to the patient's face.

          a. Spread of rays from the tube is in the form of a geometric cone, the diameter of which increases with distance; without a lead diaphragm the diameter varies with different machines from $3\frac{1}{2}$ to 5 inches at an 8-inch distance from the source.

          b. Example: a tissue exposure reduction of 50% results from narrowing the beam diameter from 4 to $2\frac{3}{4}$ inches, which is sufficient to expose a standard x-ray film.[12]

    C. **Relation to Techniques:** the dimensions of the largest periapical film are $1\frac{1}{4}$ by $1\frac{5}{8}$ inches.   Precise angulation techniques are required to eliminate cone-cut of film.

III. FILTRATION:[11,13] the use of absorbers for selective removal of x-rays of longer wave lengths from the primary beam.

    A. **Purpose:** to minimize exposure of the patient's skin to unnecessary radiation which will not reach and expose the film.

B. **Methods**

   1. Inherent filtration: accomplished by internal barriers built into the x-ray tube, including the glass wall of the tube and the insulating oil surrounding the tube.
   2. Added filtration: thin, commercially pure aluminum disks inserted between the lead diaphragm and the x-ray tube.
   3. Total filtration: the sum of the inherent and added filtration.
       a. Recommended total: equivalent of 2 to 2.25 mm. of aluminum.[14,15]
       b. Check the inherent filtration of the individual x-ray machine[14,16] then add a sufficient amount of commercially pure aluminum to bring the total to the recommended level.

C. **Disadvantage of Added Filtration:** some secondary radiation is produced which scatters in all directions.

IV. KILOVOLTAGE

   A. **Amount of Kilovoltage:** determines the quality of the x-radiation.

   1. Kilovoltage creates a difference in potential between the anode and the cathode for the production of x-rays.
   2. Higher the kilovoltage the greater acceleration of the electrons, the greater force with which they bombard the target; therefore, the shorter the wave length.
   3. The shorter the wave length, the greater the penetrating power.

   B. **Use of High Kilovoltage** *(90 kVp)*[11,17,18]

   1. Density of the finished radiograph increases with increased kilovoltage (other factors remaining constant).
   2. To maintain the proper film density, the milliampere seconds must be decreased as the kVp is increased.
   3. Variation in contrast[19]
       a. Low kilovoltage: high contrast, with sharp black-white differences in densities between adjacent areas, but small range of distinction between subject thicknesses recorded.
       b. High kilovoltage: low contrast, with wide range of subject thicknesses recorded: greater range of densities from black to white (more gray tones) which, when examined under proper viewing conditions, provide more interpretive details.
   4. Advantages in use of high kilovoltage
       a. Permit shorter exposure time.
       b. Reduce exposure to tissues lying in front of the film packet.
   5. Disadvantages
       a. Increased radiation to tissues outside the edges of the film.
       b. More scattered radiation at 90 kVp than at 65 kVp.

V. MILLIAMPERE SECONDS

   A. **Milliamperage:** the measure of the electron current passing through the x-ray tube: it regulates the heat of the filament which determines the number of available electrons to bombard the target.

B. **Quantity of Radiation** is expressed in milliampere seconds (mAs).
  1. MAs is the milliamperes multiplied by the time seconds of exposure.
  2. Example: at 10 milliamperes for $\frac{1}{2}$ second the exposure of the film is 5 mAs.

C. **Radiographic Density** increases with increased milliamperage and/or time of exposure (other factors remaining constant).

VI. **DISTANCE**[20,21]

Several distances are involved in x-ray film exposure. The source-surface, the source-film, and the object-film distances must be considered for film placement. In addition, there is the distance which the operator stands from the patient's head during film exposure which is outlined on pages 225–226 in connection with safety factors.

A. **Object-Film Distance**
In a technique where x-ray films are placed against the teeth being radiographed, the object-film distance would be negligible. Close adaptation of the film to the tooth is essential to obtain a sharp image when an 8-inch source-film distance is utilized.
With the paralleling or right-angle technique and use of a longer source-film distance (16–20 inches), there may be up to 1- or 2-inch object-film distance. A collimated beam and increased source-film distance compensate to preserve definition and film quality.

B. **Source-Film Distance**
The directing cone on the x-ray machine is designed to indicate the direction of the central axis of the x-ray beam and to serve as a guide in establishing a desired source-surface and source-film distance. Either an 8- or 16-inch source-film distance is commonly used. The source-film distance is the sum total of the distance from the source to the cone within the tube housing, the length of the directing cone, and the distance from the end of the cone (at face) to the film. Directions in technique call for touching the skin with the end of the cone to standardize the source-film distance.
  1. Principles related to source-film distance.
    a. The intensity of the x-ray beam varies inversely as the square of the source-film distance. Example: if a film of the same speed were used at a 16-inch source-film distance as at 8 inches, with all other factors such as kVp and mA remaining constant, the film at 16 inches would require 4 times the exposure (time) to maintain the same density in the finished radiograph.
    b. The exposure decreases as the distance increases: when the distance is made twice as great, the exposure is reduced to one-fourth.
    c. To maintain film density, an increase in mAs, kVp, or film speed is required when distance is increased.

C. **Advantages in the Use of an Extended Source-Film Distance**[22,23]
  1. Definition or distinctness and clarity of detail improves (because the image is produced by the more central rays).

2. Enlargement or magnification of image decreases (because at shorter distances the outer, more divergent rays tend to enlarge or magnify the image).
3. Skin exposure of the patient is reduced.
4. There is less tissue within the primary beam of radiation since there is less spreading of the x-ray beam.

VII. FILMS

The use of fast films reduces radiation of the patient more than any other single factor.[24] With optimum filtration, collimation and fast film, the skin dose to the face can be reduced as much as 89 per cent.[15] Within recent years the manufacture of very slow-speed films has been discontinued, the speed of many films has been doubled, and the use of higher speed films has gained increasing acceptance by the dental profession.[25]

Objection to the higher speed films in former years was related to their graininess but recent research has aided the manufacturers to improve their products to where little, if any, major difference can be detected between the images on medium or speed films. High-speed films have very sensitive emulsions, and the graininess which was believed to interfere with interpretation may well have been related to technical factors leading to film fog.[24]

A. **Film:** a thin, transparent sheet of cellulose acetate or similar material coated on one or both sides with an emulsion sensitive to radiation and light.

1. Emulsion: gelatin containing countless tiny crystals of silver halide.
2. Film Packet: small, light-proof, moisture resistant, sealed paper envelope containing an x-ray film (or two), and a thin sheet of lead foil.
   a. Two-film packet: useful for processing one film differently than the other to make diagnostic comparisons; for sending to specialist to whom patient may be referred; for legal evidence.
   b. Purpose of lead foil backing: prevent exposure of the film by scattered radiation that could enter from back of packet; protection of patient's tissues lying in path of x-ray, including the patient's finger if used to hold the film.

B. **Classification by Film Speed** (slow, medium, fast)

1. Factors in the determination of film speed.
   a. Grain size: smaller grain size the slower the film.
   b. Use of double or single emulsion: slower have single, on one side only. Nearly all present-day films have two emulsions.[26]
2. Film speeds: standards outlined by the American Dental Association, Council on Dental Research: classified from A (slowest) through F (fastest.)[27,28]

EFFECTS OF EXPOSURE TO RADIATION

A number of factors influence the biological effects of radiation including the quality of the radiation, the chemical composition of the absorbing medium, the tissues irradiated, the dose (total and rate per unit of time), the blood supply to the tissues, and the size of the area exposed.[29] Generally, radiation of a specific area would be less harmful than whole body radiation. Biological effects of radiation are either somatic (of the general body cells) or genetic (heritable changes, chiefly mutations, produced by the absorption of ionizing radiation by reproductive cells.)

I. IONIZATION

The phenomenon of separation of electrons from molecules which changes their chemical activity is called ionization. The organic and inorganic compounds which make up the human body may be altered by exposure to ionizing radiation. The biological effects following irradiation are secondary effects in that they result from physical, chemical, and biological actions set in motion by the absorption of energy from radiation.

II. PERMISSIBLE EXPOSURE

A. **Exposure:** a measure of the *x*-radiation to which a person or object, or a part of either, is exposed at a certain place, this measure being based on its ability to produce ionization.

   1. *Threshold exposure:* the minimum exposure that will produce a detectable degree of any given effect.

   2. *Entrance or surface exposure:* exposure measured at the surface of an irradiated body, part or object. It includes primary radiation and backscatter from the irradiated underlying tissue material. The term skin exposure is used with reference to the exposure measured at the center of an irradiated skin surface area.

   3. *Erythema exposure:* the radiation necessary to produce a temporary redness of the skin. The exposure required will vary with the quality of the radiation to which the skin is exposed.

B. **Exposure Units**

   1. Roentgen (R): unit of *x*-radiation exposure.

   2. Other units: *rad* (unit of absorbed dose); *rem* (unit of the RBE or Relative Biological Effectiveness).

C. **Dose:** the amount of energy absorbed per unit mass of tissue at a site of interest. The gonadal dose is the dose of radiation absorbed by the gonads.

D. **Permissible Dose:** the amount of radiation which may be received by an individual within a specified period without expectation of any significantly harmful result to himself.

   1. Assumptions on which permissible doses are calculated.[30]

     a. That no irradiation is beneficial.

     b. There is a dose below which no somatic change will be produced.

     c. Children are more susceptible than older people.

     d. There is a dose below which, even though it is delivered before the end of the reproductive period, the probability of genetic effects will be slight.

2. National Committee on Radiation Protection Specifications.[25]
   a. Limits for dentists and dental personnel (See Table 9).
   b. Limits for patients: exposure to *x*-ray radiation shall be kept to the minimum level consistent with clinical requirements. This limitation is determined by the professional judgment of the dentist.

TABLE 9.—MAXIMUM PERMISSIBLE EXPOSURES* TO WHOLE BODY, GONADS, BLOOD-FORMING ORGANS, OR LENS OF EYE[25]

Average Weekly Exposure†	Maximum 13-week Exposure	Maximum Yearly Exposure	Maximum Accumulated Exposure‡
0.1 R	3 R	5 R	5(N-18)R

* Exposure of persons for dental or medical purposes is not counted against their maximum permissible exposure limits.
† Used only for the purpose of designating radiation barriers.
‡ N = Age in years and is greater than 18. The unit for exposure is the roentgen (R).

III. SENSITIVITY OF CELLS

A. Factors Affecting

1. Maturity of cell: immature cells are most sensitive.
2. Reproductive capacity: rapidly reproducing are more sensitive; most sensitive when undergoing mitosis.
3. Metabolism: more sensitive in periods of increased metabolism.

B. Cells in Order of Their Sensitivity.[31-33]

1. Lymphocytes and Granulocytes (most radiosensitive).
2. Blood-forming.
3. Epithelial group (testis, ovary, skin).
4. Young bone.
5. Endothelial cells lining the closed cavities of the body such as the heart, intestines, and blood vessels.
6. Connective tissue.
7. Muscle cells including the heart.
8. Mature bone (not growth centers).
9. Nerve cells including brain (most radioresistant).

C. Tissue Reaction[31]

1. Latent period: lapse between the time of exposure and the time when effects are observed. (May be as long as 25 years, or relatively short as in the case of the production of a skin erythema.)
2. Cumulative effect.
   a. Amount of reaction depends on dose: less reaction when radiation is received in fractional doses than with one large dose.
   b. There will be partial or total repair as long as there is not complete destruction.
   c. There may be some irreparable damage which is cumulative as little by little more is added (examples: hair loss, skin lesions, falling blood count).

IV. **RELATIVE AMOUNTS OF EXPOSURE**

    A. **Machine Output:** a usual type of x-ray machine without added filtration, at 65 kVp, 10 mA, and at an 8-inch source-skin distance, produces approximately 2 R per second exposure.[34]

    B. **Average Skin Exposure for a Complete Oral Survey:** 5 to 315 R depending on kVp, beam collimation, number of exposures, amount of filtration, and film speed.[15,35,36]

    C. **Exposure to X-ray that Will Produce Threshold Erythema:** between 165 and 350 R; fewer R units when radiation of long wave lengths is used.[37]

    D. **Gonadal Dose per Specific Area Dose to the Face:** for each roentgen at the face, a maximum of approximately 0.001 R reaches the gonads of the adult male;[38] greater amount reaches the gonads of the male child because of physical nearness of the head of the machine to the child's lap. Approximately $\frac{1}{5}$ of the male gonadal dose is received by the female for each R produced at the face because of the increased depth of the organs within the body.[38] These measurements are without the protection of a lead apron.

RULES FOR RADIATION PROTECTION OF PATIENT AND OPERATOR

The Radiation Protection Committee of the American Academy of Oral Roentgenology has provided a concise outline designed for the effective use of x-rays in dentistry.[25] From this report are derived the lists included here for operator and patient protection. Information is not included relative to necessary radiation barriers within the dental office or clinic. The reader is referred to the comprehensive report[25] for this as well as pertinent lists of film speed group ratings, film badge service sources, and x-ray equipment data.

In the application of procedures for protecting the operator and the patient from excessive radiation, particular attention should be paid to unnecessary radiation which may result from the need for an unusual number of retakes due to inadequate technical procedures. Perfecting techniques contributes to the accomplishment of minimum exposure for maximum safety.

I. **PROCEDURES FOR PROTECTING THE OPERATOR**

    A. **Protection Against Exposure to Primary Radiation**

        1. Avoid the useful beam of radiation. When this is not possible, stand behind a protective barrier.
        2. Never hand-hold the film during exposure.
        3. Fluorescent mirrors shall not be used in dental examination.

    B. **Protection Against Exposure to Leakage Radiation**

        1. Do not hand-hold the tube housing or the directing cone of the machine during exposures.
        2. Test machine for leakage radiation. Sur-pak is a film device for surveying dental x-ray machines which can be obtained at no cost from a State Health Department. The survey determines

the size of the beam, the output of the machine, the total filtration, the beam symmetry, and the presence of leakage radiation occurring in a forward direction.

C. **Protection Against Exposure to Secondary Radiation**

The major sources of secondary radiation are the filter, the pointed plastic cone, and the irradiated soft tissues of the patient's face. The face produces the greatest amount. Methods of protection are related to these three sources.

1. Minimize total x-radiation
   a. Use high-speed films. When attempting to use high-speed films with older x-ray machines, the original mechanical timers may prove inadequate. Replacement timers are available.
   b. Replace ancient x-ray machines with modern shockproof equipment.
2. Use diaphragms or cones to collimate the useful beam to an area no larger than $2\frac{3}{4}$ inches in diameter when measured at the end of the directing cone.
3. Use an open-ended, shielded (lead lined) cone in place of the pointed plastic cone. The scattered secondary radiation from the filter and the plastic cone are controlled and eliminated respectively.[39]
4. Position of operator while making exposures.
   The operator shall stand behind the patient's head behind the three major sources of secondary radiation, where they cannot directly expose him.
   a. Exposure of the region of the central incisors: stand at a 45° angle to the path of the central ray. This position is approximately behind either the left or the right ear of the patient (Fig. 43).
   b. Exposure of other regions: stand behind the patient's head and at an angle of 45° to the path of the central ray of the x-ray beam.

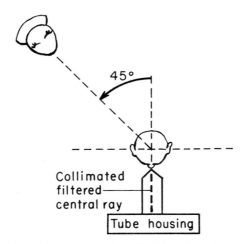

FIGURE 43.—Safer Position of Operator During Film Exposure. The operator stands behind the patient's head at a 45° angle to the path of the central ray. The irradiated tissues of the patient's face are the greatest source of secondary radiation.

5. Distance.
   a. Safety increases with distance. A long cord on the timer will permit greater freedom of movement.
   b. National Bureau of Standards recommends 6 feet.* However, safety depends primarily on workload.
   c. When space limitations within the dental office prevent occupying the safer positions listed above, the operator should step out of the room behind a wall.

E. **Film Badge Service**
   The amount of x-ray radiation that reaches the body of the dentist or dental personnel can be measured economically with a film badge. Badges can be obtained from one of several laboratories. The film badge is worn on the clothing for 1, 2 or 4 weeks and is then returned by mail to the laboratory where it was purchased. At the laboratory, the film in the badge is carefully processed and its exposure evaluated. The amount of radiation recorded by the film badge is a measure of the exposure of the wearer who is notified by mail of the amount of exposure.

II. PROCEDURES FOR PROTECTING THE PATIENT

A. **Films:** use high-speed films.

B. **Collimation:** use diaphragms or cones to collimate the useful beam.

C. **Filtration:** use filtration of the useful beam to a total of 2 to 2.25 mm. aluminum.

D. **Processing:** process films according to the manufacturer's directions. When a choice of two periods of development is offered, the exposure of the patient can be reduced if the longer development time is employed.

E. **Film Size:** use the largest intraoral film that can be skillfully placed in the mouth. Maximum coverage is provided in this manner with one exposure, whereas two exposures may be required if smaller films are used to examine the same area of the mouth. This factor is especially important when examining the mouths of children.

F. **Total Exposure:** do not expose the patient unnecessarily. There must be a good and valid reason for each exposure.

G. **Lead Apron:** use a lead apron, particularly for children and pregnant women. (Fig. 44.)

H. **High Voltage:** the use of high voltages has been overemphasized. High voltages permit shorter exposure times and reduce the exposure of tissues lying in front of the film packet, but the exposure of the gonads and the tissues lying behind the film packet increases with increased voltage.

* National Bureau of Standards: Medical X-ray Protection up to Three Million Volts, Handbook 76, Washington, D. C., 1961, Government Printing Office.

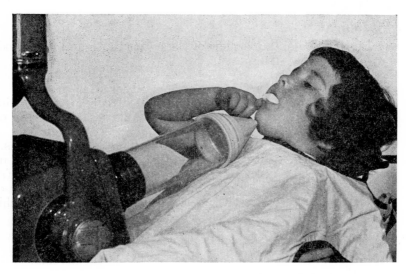

FIGURE 44.—Lead apron for a child patient. Note proximity of head of x-ray machine to the child's body when in position for the mandibular incisor film exposure. (Courtesy of Dr. Thompson M. Lewis.)

TECHNIQUES FOR FILM PLACEMENT AND ANGULATION OF THE RAY

The characteristics of the acceptable finished radiograph have been listed (page 218) and certain technical factors, including collimation, filtration, kilovoltage, milliampere seconds, distance and films have been described. For consideration next in the procedure for preparation of radiographs is the placement of the film and the angulation of the useful beam.

Intraoral techniques for periapical, bite-wing and occlusal radiographs are included in this chapter. A list of suggested readings is provided for extraoral radiography.

Two fundamental periapical techniques are used in practice, the *paralleling* or right-angle, and the *angle bisection*. The paralleling technique is sometimes referred to as the "long" or "extension cone" and the angle bisection as the "short cone" technique. However, the long cone may be employed with angle bisection procedures.

Operators vary in their application of the principles of the two techniques. At times it is necessary to adapt procedures in accord with the anatomy of the mouth of the patient. Basically, the primary ray should pass through the region to be examined and the film should be placed in relation to the ray so that all parts of the image are shown as close to their natural size and shape as possible with a minimum of distortion in the finished radiograph.

As with other techniques, the development of a systematic procedure is essential. A comfortable, smooth operation saves time and energy for both patient and operator, increases the confidence of the patient in the operator, and allows for consistency in technique which produces consistent results. A basic objective during radiographic technique is to minimize the length of time the film packet remains in the patient's mouth.

I. INTRAORAL SURVEYS

A. Periapical

1. Purpose: to obtain a view of the entire tooth and its periodontal supporting structures.
2. Films
   a. Standard ($1\frac{1}{4}'' \times 1\frac{5}{8}''$): may be used for all positions.
   b. Anterior ($\frac{15}{16}'' \times 1\frac{9}{16}''$): for anterior regions where width of arch makes positioning of standard film difficult or impossible.
   c. Child size ($\frac{7}{8}'' \times 1\frac{3}{8}''$): for primary teeth in small mouths.
3. Number of films used in a complete survey: for the adult mouth it will vary from 14 to 30 depending on the operator's preference, objectives for showing specific areas, anatomy of the patient's mouth, and the size of the films used. For children see pages 241–242.

B. Bite-wing (Interproximal)

1. Purpose: to show the crowns of the teeth, the alveolar crest and the interproximal area.
2. Films
   a. With tab attached.
      (1) For anterior teeth ($\frac{15}{16}'' \times 1\frac{9}{16}''$): three films are used.
      (2) For posterior teeth using standard size film.
         (a) Adult: four films, one for molar region and one for bicuspid, each side.
         (b) Child with first permanent molar erupted: one on each side.
      (3) For posterior teeth using longer, narrower film designated to include molars and bicuspids: one on each side. Not recommended for routine use because curvature of dental arch does not permit all proximal surfaces to be free from overlapping.
   b. Commercial tabs: to be attached to standard or child-size films: two types, one a loop to slide over the film packet and the other with an adhesive to attach directly to the film packet.

C. Occlusal

1. Purpose: to show large areas of the maxilla, mandible, or floor of the mouth.
2. Film: ($2\frac{1}{4}'' \times 3''$): for use in self packet or in intraoral casette.
3. Standard film ($1\frac{1}{4}'' \times 1\frac{5}{8}''$): for child or individual areas of adult.

II. PRELIMINARY PREPARATION

A. Equipment

1. Sanitization of patient surroundings (see page 57) includes wiping the parts of the x-ray machine which are handled in conjunction with oral contact (directing cone, handle of tube housing, timer).
2. Advanced readiness: the patient should not be kept waiting for procedures such as testing the x-ray machine or placing bite-wing tabs on film packets.

3. Timer: check automatic reset or adjust mechanical timer for exposure prior to film placement. Manufacturer's chart is consulted for exposure time at given source-film distance, kilovoltage, and milliamperes.

B. **Patient Preparation**
1. When films will be held in the mouth by the patient, invite him to wash his hands.
2. Remove eyeglasses, and removable dental appliances.

C. **Oral Inspection** (Table 4, pages 83–85).
1. Purpose: to determine necessary adaptations during film placement.
2. Factors of particular interest.
    a. Position of teeth and edentulous areas.
    b. Apparent length of teeth as compared to average length of teeth.
    c. Accessibility: height and shape of palate; flexibility of muscles of orifice, floor of the mouth; possible gag reflex, size of tongue.
    d. Unusual features: tori, sensitive areas of the mucous membranes.

III. **PATIENT COOPERATION: PREVENTION OF GAGGING**[40,41]

Gagging may be the result of psychological or physiological factors. It presents some problem in the placement of all films for molar radiographs, and may be initiated in the patient who ordinarily does not gag if techniques are not carried out efficiently. Many of the factors related to the prevention of gagging may be applied for the comfort and cooperation of all patients.

A. **Causes of Gagging**
1. Hypersensitive oral tissues, particularly of posterior region of oral cavity.
2. Anxiety and apprehension.
    a. Fear: of unknown, of the film touching a sensitive area.
    b. Previous unpleasant experiences with radiographic techniques.
    c. Failure to comprehend the operator's instructions.
    d. Lack of confidence in the operator.
3. Techniques: film moved over the oral tissues or retained in the mouth longer than necessary.

B. **Preventive Procedures**
1. Inspire confidence in ability to perform the service.
2. Alleviate anxiety: explain procedures carefully.
3. Film placement: firmly and positively without sliding the film over the tissue.
4. Film retention.
    a. Instruct patient to hold with positive pressure.
    b. Use a film holder on which the patient can bite (to distract him).

5. Instruct patient to breathe through the nose with quick, short breaths during film placement and to hold the breath during exposure.
6. Use of premedicating agent prescribed by the dentist.
7. Use of topical anesthetic.
   a. Cold water or ice cube held in the mouth for a short time before film placement dulls the sensory nerve endings.
   b. Salt: one-half teaspoonful dissolved on the tongue and swallowed has an anesthetic effect.
   c. Prepared topical anesthetics in the form of paste (applied with cotton swab), troche, spray or rinse give up to twenty minutes of anesthesia (see pages 159–160).

IV. **DEFINITIONS AND PRINCIPLES RELATED TO TECHNIQUES**

A. **Planes**

1. Sagittal or Median: the plane that divides the body in the midline into right and left sides.
2. Occlusal: the mean occlusal plane represents the mean curvature from the incisal edges of the central incisors to the tips of the occluding surfaces of the third molars. The occlusal plane of the bicuspids and first molar may be considered as the mean occlusal plane. When it is specified in techniques that the occlusal plane of the teeth being radiographed shall be parallel to the floor, at least three head positions are involved for the maxillary: for anterior teeth the head must be tipped forward, for bicuspids held at the mean occlusal plane, and for molars, tipped back.

B. **Angulation**

1. Horizontal: the angle at which the central ray of the useful beam is directed within a horizontal plane. Inadequate horizontal angulation results in overlapping or superimposition of parts of adjacent teeth in the radiograph.
2. Vertical: the plane at which the central ray of the useful beam is directed within a vertical plane. Inadequate vertical angulation results in elongation or foreshortening in the image.

C. **Long Axis of a Tooth:** an imaginary line passing longitudinally through the center of the tooth.

Because of marked variations in tooth position and root curvature[42] estimation of the long axis of a tooth is difficult. Clinically, it can be considered that the long axis of a posterior tooth is at right angles to the occlusal surface plane. For single-rooted teeth the long axis would ordinarily pass from the center of the incisal edge to the tip of the apex, but it is not possible to observe this in clinical inspection. It must be remembered that the line from the incisal to the cervical on the labial surface should not be confused with the long axis.

BITE-WING (INTERPROXIMAL) SURVEY

The bite-wing survey is used as an adjunct to the periapical survey. It has a special use at the time of periodic patient inspection at regular intervals between complete periapical surveys.   The complete survey is usually repeated every 2 to 3 years, depending on the oral problems of the individual patient.

When the angle bisection technique is used for the periapical radiographs, the bite-wing survey is essential, since an accurate view of all proximal surfaces cannot otherwise be obtained.

The angulation for the bite-wing radiographs is based on the same principle as that for periapical surveys made with the paralleling or right-angle technique. For this reason, dentists who use the paralleling technique do not always require a bite-wing survey at the time the periapical survey is prepared, since there would be duplicate sources of information for diagnosis. In fact, advocates of the paralleling procedure recommend the lack of need for the bite-wing survey as an additional means of minimizing patient exposure to radiation, since fewer films are used.

I. PREPARATION FOR FILM PLACEMENT

A. Position of Patient's Head

 1. Sagittal plane perpendicular to floor.
 2. Mean occlusal plane parallel with floor.

B. Vertical Angulation: set at +10 degrees.

C. Patient Instruction: request patient to practice closing on posterior teeth in centric relation (page 91) prior to positioning film for posterior bite-wings, and edge-to-edge (Fig. 25 page 92) for anterior.

II. FILM PLACEMENT AND CENTRAL RAY ANGULATION

Figure 45 shows in diagram form the position of the molar bite-wing film in relation to the teeth, the horizontal and vertical angulation and the image objective for both the bicuspid and molar completed radiographs when standard film is used.

A. Position of Film

 1. Molar (standard film): mesial border of film at mesial of maxillary second bicuspid or more distal as needed to include the distal surface of the third molar when it is erupted and in position.

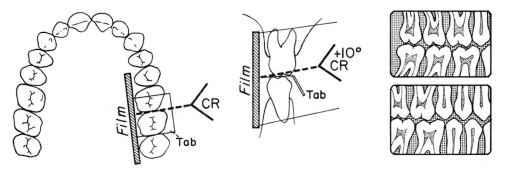

FIGURE 45.—Bite-wing radiograph.   Left, film position showing horizontal angulation for molar bite-wing; center, vertical angulation. Right, image objective for molar and bicuspid regions. (Adapted from Stafne, *Oral Roentgenographic Diagnosis*, Saunders.)

2. Bicuspid (standard film): mesial border of film at center or mesial of maxillary cuspid.

3. Anterior: center of film at mesial of maxillary cuspid for the two lateral bite-wings; center of film at midline for central bite-wing.

B. **Position of Directing Cone:** with the vertical angulation at +10 degrees, the horizontal angulation is adjusted to direct the central ray to the center of the film. The ray must pass through the interproximals or parallel to a line through the interproximals.

C. **Maintain Film Flat During Exposure:** although slight curving of the film may be needed for certain patients depending on the oral anatomy and tissue sensitivity, the basic rule is to keep the film as flat as possible to prevent distortion.

PERIAPICAL SURVEY: PARALLELING OR RIGHT-ANGLE TECHNIQUE

The paralleling or right-angle technique is based on the principles that the film is placed as nearly parallel to the long axis of the teeth as the anatomy of the oral cavity will permit and the central ray is directed at right angles to the film. In Figure 46 *A* the parallel relationship of the film with the long axis of the tooth and the right-angle direction of the central ray are shown. This technique has been called the Fitzgerald technique because of the study and development of specific procedures by Dr. Gordon Fitzgerald.[43,44]

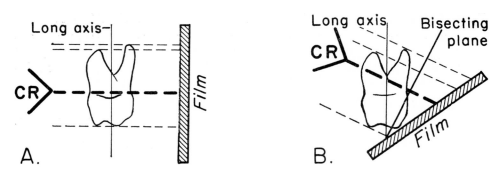

FIGURE 46.—Comparison of paralleling with angle bisection technique. Note comparative projection of the parts of the tooth on the film.

The distance between the crown of the tooth and the film is increased to attain parallelism. In the majority of positions for individual films, the edge of the film against the soft tissues is approximately in the same position on the palate or the floor of the mouth as when the film is placed against and close to the tooth in, for example, the angle bisection technique. In other words, the distance between the root apex and the film is not materially different from that in the angle bisection technique. Figures 46*A* and *B* show the comparative projection of the parts of the tooth on the film to produce the image in the radiograph when a source-film distance of 16 to 20 inches is used. The distance factor has been described on page 220.

I. POSITION OF PATIENT'S HEAD

As long as the film is parallel to the long axis of the tooth and the central ray is directed at right angles to the film, the head may be in any position convenient to the operator and comfortable for the patient.[45] The use of film holders facilitates angulating the ray, since the directing cone for the central ray may be lined up with the part of the film holder which extends from between the teeth and which is designed to be at right angles to the film.

For the inexperienced operator, horizontal angulation may be visualized more readily when the occlusal plane of the teeth being radiographed is parallel with the floor and the sagittal plane is perpendicular to the floor.

II. FILM PLACEMENT TO OBTAIN PARALLELISM

The anatomy of the patient's mouth, such as a low palatal vault, will not always allow absolute parallelism. Research has shown that as long as the film-to-tooth relationship is within 20° of being parallel, the resultant image is acceptably free from distortion.[46]

A. Film Position and Angulation of the Central Ray

Only the general instructions for film placement and angulation are included in this section. In addition to the references associated with specific parts of this section, other references will be helpful in studying and perfecting techniques.[45,47-50]

1. Basic principles for film placement and angulation of the central ray are shown in Figures 47 through 54. The image objective in the completed radiograph is also illustrated.
2. Horizontal angulation: the ray is directed approximately at the center of the film and through the interproximal area.
3. Vertical angulation: the ray is directed at right angles to the film.

B. Film Positioning Devices (Fig. 55).

Except for the mandibular molar radiograph where parallelism generally may be obtained by placing the film directly beside the teeth, some type of film holder is a necessity. A variety of these have been developed. In selecting a film holder for use, some of the factors which should be considered are its ability to attain the proper position of the film in both the maxillary and the mandibular, the maintenance of stability of the film during exposure, patient comfort, simplicity of use, and the ease of sterilization of the holder.[51]

Cotton rolls may suffice in certain areas. Any device which requires the patient to hold the film increases the time spent in instruction to gain patient cooperation, increases the possibility of film movement, as well as increases irradiation of the patient's finger or thumb.

1. Cotton rolls: held in place with the film by the patient; may be taped to the film.
2. Hemostat with rubber bite block or tubing around the shank; patient bites on the rubber to hold the hemostat and hence the film.
3. Bite blocks: plastic (short and long for different areas of the mouth), wooden, thumb screw.[51]

PARALLELING TECHNIQUE

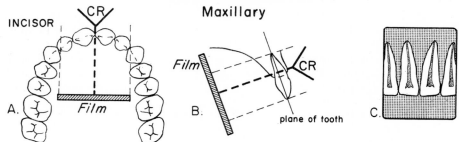

FIGURE 47.—Paralleling technique, maxillary incisor region.* *A*. Film placed parallel to long axes of teeth. *B*. Central Ray (CR) directed perpendicular to film. *C*. Image objective.

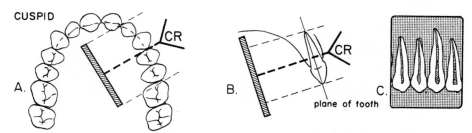

FIGURE 48.—Paralleling technique, maxillary cuspid region. *A*. Film placed parallel to long axes of teeth. *B*. Central Ray (CR) directed perpendicular to film. *C*. Image objective.

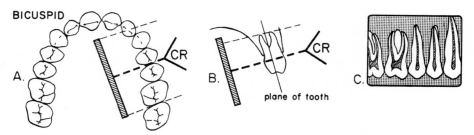

FIGURE 49.—Paralleling technique, maxillary biscuspid region. *A*. Film placed parallel to long axes of teeth. *B*. Central Ray (CR) directed perpendicular to film. *C*. Image objective.

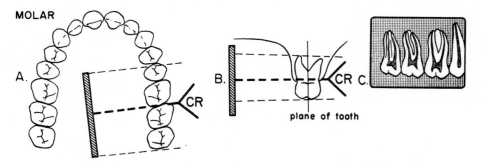

FIGURE 50.—Paralleling technique, maxillary molar region. *A*. Film placed parallel to long axes of teeth. *B*. Central Ray (CR) directed perpendicular to film. *C*. Image objective.

* Figures 47 to 54 adapted from Stafne, *Oral Roentgenographic Diagnosis*, Saunders.

PARALLELING TECHNIQUE
Mandibular

INCISOR

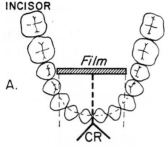

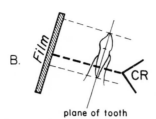

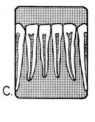

FIGURE 51.—Paralleling Technique, Mandibular Incisor Region. *A*. Film placed parallel to long axes of teeth. *B*. Central Ray (CR) directed perpendicular to film. *C*. Image objective.

CUSPID

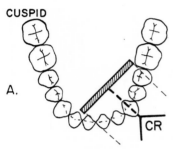

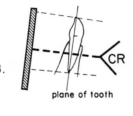

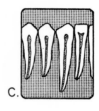

FIGURE 52.—Paralleling Technique, Mandibular Cuspid Region. *A*. Film placed parallel to long axes of teeth. *B*. Central Ray (CR) directed perpendicular to film. *C*. Image objective.

BICUSPID

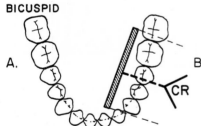

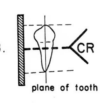

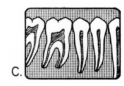

FIGURE 53.—Paralleling Technique, Mandibular Bicuspid Region. *A*. Film placed parallel to long axes of teeth. *B*. Central Ray (CR) directed perpendicular to film. *C*. Image objective.

MOLAR

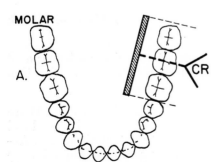

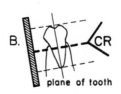

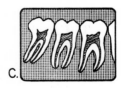

FIGURE 54.—Paralleling Technique, Mandibular Molar Region. *A*. Film placed parallel to long axes of teeth. *B*. Central Ray (CR) directed perpendicular to film. *C*. Image objective.

(235)

4. Plastic film holders (Rinn).
5. Supplements.
   a. Removable denture may be needed in place in opposite jaw to stabilize the film holder.
   b. A cotton roll between the film holder or bite block and the biting surface can aid in paralleling when the teeth are short and/or the palatal vault is low.

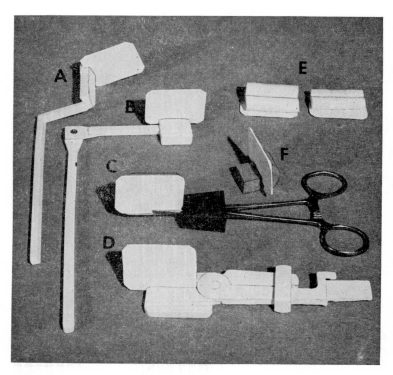

FIGURE 55.—Film positioning devices. *A* and *B*, Rinn XCP instruments for paralleling technique, *A* for anterior films and *B* for posterior. Indicator rod permits convenient positioning of the central ray at right angles to the film. *C*. Hemostat with rubber bite block. A metal plate backs the film and holds it rigid. *D*. Rinn Film Holder. Film is in horizontal position for posterior teeth on left end. For anterior teeth the right end is used to hold the film in a vertical position. *E*. Cotton rolls affixed to film with scotch tape. *F*. Wooden bite block with film in position.

III. ADVANTAGES OF THE PARALLELING OR RIGHT-ANGLE TECHNIQUE[22,52,53]

A. **Technically Superior Radiographs:** truer size and shape of dental structures with less distortion than when angle bisection technique is used.

B. **Anatomic Relationship of One Structure to Another is More Accurately Shown:** for example, buccal and lingual bone level is normally the same, but in angle bisection technique one frequently appears higher than the other; buccal and lingual cusp length of a particular tooth shows them in normal relation in paralleling technique; position of the zygomatic bone is normally above the root apices of the molars and bicuspids as shown in paralleling technique.

PERIAPICAL SURVEY: ANGLE BISECTION TECHNIQUE

The angle bisection technique is based on the geometric principle that the central ray is directed perpendicular to an imaginary line which is the bisector of the angle formed by the long axis of the tooth and the plane of the film. Figure 46*B* illustrates in diagram form the relationship of the long axis of the tooth, the film, and the bisector of the angle formed by these two.

I. POSITION OF PATIENT'S HEAD

A. **Sagittal Plane:** perpendicular to the floor.

B. **Occlusal Plane:** parallel to the floor (page 230).

II. FILM PLACEMENT AND POSITION

Only general instructions are included in this section. Additional references will be helpful in studying and perfecting techniques.[54-57]

A. **Basic Considerations**
   1. Center of film: at center of teeth being radiographed. The exception to this rule is the maxillary cuspid film which is placed slightly distal to accommodate film positioning.
   2. Border of film: $\frac{1}{8}$ to $\frac{1}{4}$ inches beyond occlusal or incisal.
   3. Film must be kept as flat as possible. A cotton roll may be used with the anterior and maxillary molar films to aid in accomplishing this.

B. **Film Position in Relation to Angulation of the Central Ray**
   Figures 56 through 63 show the position of the individual films, the horizontal and vertical angulations, and the image objective in the completed radiograph.

III. DIRECTION OF THE CENTRAL RAY

A. **Direct the ray through the apical $\frac{1}{3}$ of the teeth being radiographed.**
   1. Maxillary: to determine location of the apices of the teeth draw an imaginary line from the ala of the nose to the tragus of the ear, and the apices will be approximately at that level.
   2. Mandibular: apices are located approximately $\frac{1}{2}$ inch above the lower border of the mandible.

B. **Horizontal Angulation:** the ray should pass through the interproximal or parallel to a line through the interproximal, at approximately the center of the area being radiographed.

C. **Vertical Angulation:** bisect the angle formed by the film and the long axis of the teeth, and direct the ray perpendicular to this line.

ANGLE BISECTION TECHNIQUE

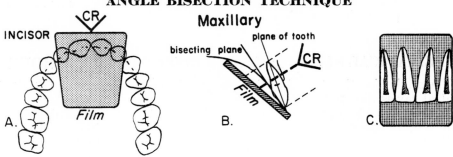

FIGURE 56.—Angle Bisection Technique, Maxillary Incisor Region.* *A.* Film placed against teeth. *B.* Central Ray (CR) directed perpendicular to the bisector of the angle formed by the film and the long axes of the teeth. *C.* Image objective.

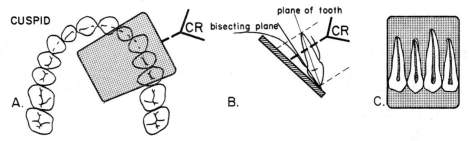

FIGURE 57.—Angle Bisection Technique, Maxillary Cuspid Region. *A.* Film placed against teeth. *B.* Central Ray (CR) directed perpendicular to the bisector of the angle formed by the film and the long axes of the teeth. *C.* Image objective.

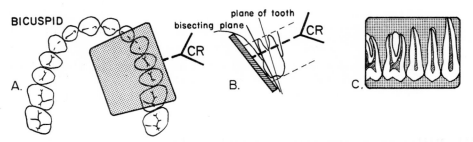

FIGURE 58.—Angle Bisection Technique, Maxillary Biscuspid Region. *A.* Film placed against teeth. *B.* Central Ray (CR) directed perpendicular to the bisector of the angle formed by the film and the long axes of the teeth. *C.* Image objective.

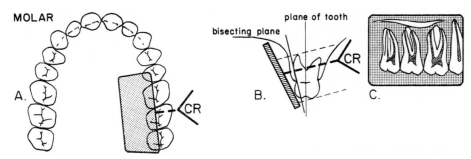

FIGURE 59.—Angle Bisection Technique, Maxillary Molar Region. *A.* Film placed against teeth. *B.* Central Ray (CR) directed perpendicular to the bisector of the angle formed by the film and the long axes of the teeth. *C.* Image objective.

* Figures 56 to 63 adapted from Stafne, *One Roentgenographic Diagnosis*, Saunders.

ANGLE BISECTION TECHNIQUE
Mandibular

INCISOR

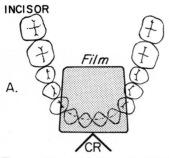

A.

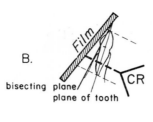

B.

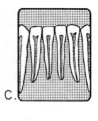

C.

bisecting plane
plane of tooth

FIGURE 60.—Angle Bisection Technique, Mandibular Incisor Region.   *A.* Film placed against teeth. *B.* Central Ray (CR) directed perpendicular to the bisector of the angle formed by the film and the long axes of the teeth. *C.* Image objective.

CUSPID

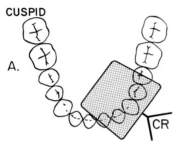

A.

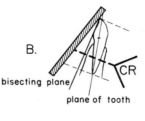

B.

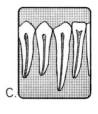

C.

bisecting plane
plane of tooth

FIGURE 61.—Angle Bisection Technique, Mandibular Cuspid Region.   *A.* Film placed against teeth. *B.* Central Ray (CR) directed perpendicular to the bisector of the angle formed by the film and the long axes of the teeth. *C.* Image objective.

BICUSPID

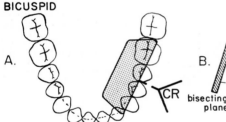

A.

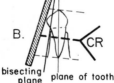

B.

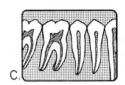

C.

bisecting plane   plane of tooth

FIGURE 62.—Angle Bisection Technique, Mandibular Bicuspid Region.   *A.* Film placed against teeth. *B.* Central Ray (CR) directed perpendicular to the bisector of the angle formed by the film and the long axes of the teeth. *C.* Image objective.

MOLAR

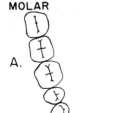

A.

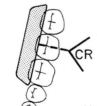

B.

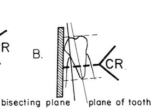

C.

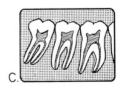

bisecting plane   plane of tooth

FIGURE 63.—Angle Bisection Technique, Mandibular Molar Region.   *A.* Film placed against teeth. *B.* Central Ray (CR) directed perpendicular to the bisector of the angle formed by the film and the long axes of the teeth. *C.* Image objective.

D. **Average Angles for Vertical Angulation**
1. Uses
   a. For the anatomically ideal mouth: a check on the average angle by applying the bisection principle would not require any changes.
   b. As a point from which to begin when bisecting the angle: usually the angle of the bisection would be within 5 to 10° of the average angle.
   c. As a time saver in angle bisection technique: prior to placing the film in the patient's mouth the cone is positioned at the average angle to facilitate angulation and prevent undue discomfort on the part of the patient.
   d. For the beginner, as a first technique, while he is developing concepts of angle bisection.
2. The average angles

Maxillary		*Mandibular*	
Central	+ 40–45	Central	− 15–20
Cuspid	+ 45–50	Cuspid	− 20–25
Biscuspid	+ 30–35	Biscuspid	− 10–15
Molar	+ 20–25	Molar	− 5–0

OCCLUSAL SURVEY

The use of occlusal films is particularly important in observing areas which cannot be completely or conveniently shown on other film, in cases where positioning periapical films is difficult or impossible, to supplement the angulation provided by other films in such conditions as fractures, impacted teeth, or salivary duct calculi, and as a specific part of the complete survey for edentulous and very young patients (see pages 241 and 242).

In this section only the central midline films for maxillary and mandibular are described. A variety of positions for the occlusal films is possible, depending on the area to be examined. Additional references will be helpful as a guide.[58–60]

I. **MAXILLARY CENTRAL (MIDLINE) OCCLUSAL RADIOGRAPH**

A. **Position of Patient's Head:** line from tragus of the ear to ala of the nose is parallel with the floor.

B. **Film Position:** emulsion side toward the palate; posterior border of film brought back close to third molar region; film held between the teeth with edge-to-edge closure.

C. **Angulation:** the cone is directed toward the bridge of the nose at an angle of 65 degrees.

D. **Exposure:** consult chart of film manufacturer's specifications for exposure related to source-film distance, kilovoltage and milliamperage. When a cassette is used, exposure time is reduced, an advantage in the prevention of movement of the film.

II. MANDIBULAR CENTRAL (MIDLINE) OCCLUSAL RADIOGRAPH

A. **Position of Patient's Head:** tilted directly back.

B. **Film Position:** emulsion side toward floor of mouth, posterior border of film in contact with soft tissues of retromolar area; film held between teeth in edge-to-edge bite.

C. **Angulation:** for incisal region the cone is pointed at the tip of the chin at an angle of approximately 55°. For the floor of the mouth, the cone is directed from under the chin, at a right angle to the film.

D. **Exposure:** consult chart of film manufacturer's specifications.

SURVEY FOR THE CHILD PATIENT

The frequency for making a radiographic survey for a child, the size and number of films used, and the techniques of film placement, depend on a number of factors. These include primarily the information sought by the dentist to fulfill his responsibility for oral care of the patient, and the age and cooperation of the patient.

Aside from the need for radiographs at an early age for accidents or anomalies, the initial survey in the child's life may be made soon after all of the primary teeth are erupted. Adequate oral supervision would suggest a second survey at approximately age 6 and the third at approximately age 9. Bite-wing surveys at appropriate intervals between complete surveys would be made primarily for dental caries detection.

By the age of 9 or 10 the size and number of films used for an intraoral survey approximates the adult survey. This section is devoted to a brief consideration of the surveys for the pre-school (primary dentition) and the child of 6 to 7 years (initial stage of mixed dentition).

The first aim in the survey for the young child is to make a thorough examination of the teeth and their surrounding structures. The fewer exposures required to accomplish this with the least discomfort on the part of the patient are second aims.

I. PRIMARY DENTITION (CHILD 3 TO 6 YEARS)

Various combinations of periapical, bite-wing, occlusal and extraoral films are recommended by the specialists. Film size is suggested which will be consistent with the size of the mouth, the cooperation of the patient, and the ability of the operator. Examples of number and size of films for four effective surveys are listed here.

A. Occlusal views of anterior maxillary and mandibular (standard film) and posterior bite-wings (child or adult anterior film); total of 4 films.[61]

B. Occlusal views of anterior maxillary and mandibular and maxillary posterior (standard film), posterior bite-wings (child or standard film) and extraoral lateral jaw films (5 × 7″); total of 8 films.[62]

  C. Occlusal views of anterior maxillary and mandibular (standard film), posterior bite-wings (2 or 4, child or standard film), and 4 extraoral lateral jaw films (8 × 10"); total of 8 or 10 films.[63]

  D. Periapical views for each posterior quadrant and one each for anterior (child size film); total 6 films.[64]

II. MIXED DENTITION (Child 6 to 9 Years)

Twelve to 14 exposures using standard film are recommended. These include 2 posterior bite-wings, 4 molar (to include first permanent and primary molars), 4 cuspid, and 2 or 4 incisor periapical views.[61,64,65]

III. SUGGESTIONS FOR TECHNIQUE WITH CHILDREN

A. Orientation to Lessen Apprehension

1. For young child's first visit to the dental office: making the radiographic survey may be an excellent first procedure;[61] when the child is not cooperative the survey should be delayed until the second or even the third visit.[65]
2. Explain procedures carefully; rehearse to show what is to be done; repeat instructions with each film placement.

B. Sequence: make the easiest, most comfortable exposures first (extraoral, occlusal).

C. Periapical Films

1. Cotton rolls, bite blocks or other film holders are used.
2. Film held by the child: aid the child in placing finger or thumb in proper place.
3. Parent may hold film when child cannot cooperate.

D. Use a Lead Apron over the body of the child. Because of the size of the child, the gonads are closer to the sources of secondary radiation than with an adult.[66] (Fig. 44.)

SURVEY FOR THE EDENTULOUS PATIENT

I. TYPES AND NUMBER OF FILMS USED

A. Routine 14 Film Survey preferred by certain dentists.

B. Use of Occlusal Films with periapicals: 7 exposures:[67,68]

1. Two occlusal views: one of entire maxillary and one entire mandibular.
2. Five periapicals: one each in the 4 molar areas and one for mandibular incisors.

II. VARIATION IN EXPOSURE TIME: usually reduced by approximately 25 per cent.[69]

III. FILM PLACEMENT

A. Parallel or Right-Angle Technique

1. Use of film holder: it is necessary to provide a wider biting area

for the patient. The rubber bite block on a hemostat may be turned around so that the broader dimension is in a vertical plane. Padding or cotton rolls may be an aid in the retention of certain holders.

   2. Cotton rolls may provide sufficient paralleling in some areas.

B. **Angle Bisection Technique**

   1. Cotton rolls are indicated to aid in positioning films.

   2. Angulation increased to accommodate flattened film position.

C. **Occlusal Films:** film retention is accomplished by having the patient hold the maxillary film with the two thumbs placed one on each side under the maxillary arch. Likewise, the index fingers hold the mandibular film down.

FILM PROCESSING

Film processing is the chemical transformation of the latent image, produced in a film emulsion by exposure to radiation, into a stable image visible by transmitted light. The usual procedure is basically a selective reduction of affected silver halide salts to metallic silver grains (development), followed by the selective removal of unaffected silver halide (fixation), washing to remove the processing chemicals, and drying.

Standardization of processing procedures goes hand in hand with standardized exposure techniques if consistently acceptable radiographs are to be prepared. Processing should be treated as an exacting chemical operation in which each step has specific objectives for the finished product. Fast and extra-fast film are even more sensitive to variations in temperature, light, and processing chemicals than medium and slow film formerly in general use, hence the need for fastidious attention to detail.

I. **ESSENTIALS OF AN ADEQUATE DARKROOM**

   Cleanliness and orderliness are mandatory. Since the films are handled in near darkness, materials must be available at the finger tips and each piece of equipment kept in its own place. The work area must be free from chemicals, water, dust, and other substances which can contaminate the film either by splashing or direct contact should a film touch the bench. The processing room should not be used as a storage room or for other dental procedures in which dust or fumes might be produced.

   Convenience and ease in carrying out precision techniques can be provided through good planning for the location and arrangement of equipment.

A. **Lighting**

   1. Darkroom completely void of white light.
      a. All possible light leaks found and eliminated.
      b. Overhead light not fluorescent because of after-glow.
   2. Safelight
      a. Filter: Wratten Series 6 *B*
      b. Light bulb: $7\frac{1}{2}$ watts at 4 feet; 10 watts at 5 feet; 15 watts at 6 feet from bench top.[70]

3. Safe lighting test[71]
    a. Expose a periapical film under usual clinical circumstances.
    b. Unwrap film in totally dark darkroom.
    c. Place film on work table top and place a coin on the film.
    d. Turn on safelight and leave for maximum amount of time (such as 20 to 25 minutes) typical of that required when preparing several surveys to be processed together.
    e. Turn off safelight, remove coin, process film.
    f. Observe radiograph: if any evidence of light circle where coin was placed, the darkroom safelight is excessive.
4. Lock on door of darkroom; signal light on outside to show room in use.

B. **Basic Equipment and Facilities**
    1. Tanks for developer and fixer with water bath between.
        a. Removable tanks made of stainless steel with joints welded and polished to prevent reactions with the processing chemicals.[71]
        b. Close-fitting light-proof cover for tank.
        c. Stirring paddles identified for developer and fixer.
        d. Water bath with connecting water flow and temperature control indicator.
        e. Floating tank thermometer (kept in developer tank).
    2. Work bench: covered with linoleum or formica for easy cleaning.
    3. Drying facilities: rod to hold hangers over drip pan; electric fan to facilitate drying.
    4. Utility sink.
    5. Interval timing clock.
    6. Storage area beneath workbench for materials to change solutions.
    7. Waste receiver: conveniently located for ready disposal of film wrappers to prevent losing films in midst of paper wrappers.

C. **Care of Solution**
    1. Factors affecting life of solution.
        a. Original quality (care in preparation).
        b. Age.
        c. Care received (temperature, whether kept covered, contamination).
        d. Number of films processed.
    2. Changing solutions: at least every 3 weeks.
    3. Preparation of new solution.
        a. Tanks must be thoroughly scrubbed with water and a soft brush and then thoroughly rinsed.
        b. Label tanks as well as stirrers and mixing jars to prevent possibility of interchange.
        c. Follow manufacturer's specifications and directions precisely.
    4. Keep tanks covered.
        a. Use same position for tank cover so that same side routinely covers the same solution.
        b. Purposes for covering tanks
            (1) Prevent evaporation: changes concentration of the solutions and lowers level so top film on rack is not covered during processing.

(2) Prevent oxidation: reduces useful life of solution.
(3) Prevent contamination: dust, drippings.
5. Temperature: keep cool when not in use: heated solutions can oxidize rapidly.
6. Replenisher: between changing of solutions freshness may be maintained by replenishment according to manufacturer's specifications.

II. PROCEDURE FOR PROCESSING

A. Preparation

1. Stir solutions and check temperature of solutions and water bath: all should be 68° F. (within 2°).
   a. Lower temperatures: chemical reactions too slow.
   b. High temperatures: cause fogging and may soften the emulsion.
2. Check cleanliness of workbench and film racks; wash hands to prevent film contamination.
3. Plan number of films to be processed so that facilities will not be overcrowded: films must hang individually out of possible contact with other films, sides of tanks or wall in drying area.
4. Prepare labels for identification of radiographs.
5. Extinguish white lights; turn on safelight; lock door.
6. Load film hangers.
   a. Hold film by edges to avoid finger marks, scratches or bending.
   b. Clip firmly: test by pulling gently on film.

B. Developing

1. Set timer. (Refer to Time-temperature Chart provided by the film manufacturer.*)
2. Completely immerse rack with films in developer; turn on timer.
3. Agitate racks (without splashing) to eliminate air bubbles and assure contact of solution with all film surfaces.
4. When timer rings, remove racks to water or stop bath.

C. Rinsing

1. Immerse in freely running water for at least 30 seconds: agitate to provide contact of water with film.
2. Stop bath: a 10 per cent acetic acid may be preferred in place of running water: immerse for 30 to 45 seconds.
3. Remove and drain for several seconds to prevent carrying an excess of water or acetic acid to fixing bath.

D. Fixing

1. Immerse completely; set and start timer.
2. Agitate racks to remove air bubbles and assure contact of the solution with all parts of the film surfaces.

---

* The time-temperature method of processing is the only way to be assured of dependable results. Processing by the "visual inspection" method is not recommended because of the guesswork factor.

3. Time.
  a. Clearing time: time needed for complete disappearance of white or milky opaqueness.
  b. Total fixing time: minimum of twice clearing time.
    (1) Check manufacturer's specifications.
    (2) Minimum of 10 minutes and maximum one hour are safe; excess time will produce a light radiograph.
  c. Negatives may be viewed for limited time after clearing when needed for immediate use; return to fixer promptly for completion of fixing process.

E. Washing

1. Place in running water bath for minimum of 20 minutes.
2. Temperature: 68° F.
  a. Too warm: gelatin will swell, thus hindering diffusion.
  b. Drastic temperature changes cause reticulation (network of wrinkles or corrugations in the emulsion); retake necessary.

F. Drying

1. Drain off water and place in dryer.
2. Radiographs become brittle when left in heated drying cabinet too long.

III. HOW THE IMAGE IS PRODUCED

A. Outline of the Chemistry of Processing

1. Film emulsion contains crystals of silver halides (bromine and iodine).
2. X-ray exposure changes the silver halides to silver and halide ions.
3. Developer reacts with the halide ions leaving only the metallic silver in a specific arrangement corresponding with the radiolucency and radiopacity of the tissue being radiographed.
4. Fixer removes only those crystals of silver halide which were not affected by the action of the x-rays. Fixer has no effect on the black metallic silver produced by the developer.
5. End result: negative showing various degrees of lightness and darkness (microscopic grains of black metallic silver).

B. Developer Action

1. Purpose: to remove the halides from the metallic silver.
2. Constituents
  a. Developing agents (reducers).
    (1) Elon: brings out detail.
    (2) Hydroquinone: reacts slowly and brings out contrast.
  b. Preservative: sodium sulfite: to protect the developing agents from oxidizing rapidly in air.
  c. Restrainer: potassium bromide: inhibits the fogging tendency of the solution and slows the reaction of the reducers.
  d. Activator (alkali): sodium carbonate: initiates the action of the reducers with the halides.
3. Transfer to water bath at completion of developing time: if racks are shaken or allowed to drip over the developer, the solution falling back into the tank will be highly oxidized which will shorten the life of the solution.

C. **Rinsing Purposes.**

    1. To stop the developing process.

    2. To remove the developing solution from the emulsion to reduce carry-over of alkaline developer to the acid fixing bath.

    3. To preserve the acidity of the fixer and hence make a more efficient, longer-lasting fixing bath.

D. **Fixer Action**

    1. Purpose: to remove the undeveloped halide salts.

    2. Constituents

        a. Fixing agent: sodium thiosulfate ("hypo"): to dissolve the silver halides.

        b. Acidifier: acetic acid: to neutralize the alkali from the developer.

        c. Hardener: potassium alum: to shrink and harden the emulsion.

        d. Preservative: sodium sulfite: to counteract surface oxidation and stabilize the solution.

E. **Washing Purpose:** to remove residual chemicals from the negative.

ANALYSIS OF COMPLETED RADIOGRAPHS

The completed radiographs are mounted and examined at a viewbox or other adequate light source. The characteristics of the acceptable finished radiograph (page 218) serve as a basis for analysis. Nothing less than the ideal should satisfy, and errors must be studied in order to improve techniques for future surveys. Interpretation of radiographs is difficult for the dentist and the determination of pathology takes complex scientific skill, but to attempt to base interpretation on inadequate, insufficient radiographs is guesswork rather than true, timely diagnosis.

I. **Mounting**

    A. Legibly mark the mount with the name of patient, date, name of dentist: printing preferred.

    B. Handle radiographs only by the edges with clean, dry hands or wear clean cotton gloves.

    C. Keep films clean, free from dust, liquids or other contaminants.

    D. Place a clean, dry towel or paper in front of the illuminator where mounting is to be done; arrange radiographs on this, or mount one by one directly as they are removed from the rack.

    E. The embossed dot near the edge of the negative is the guide to mounting: the depressed side of the dot is on the lingual.

    F. Identify individual negatives by the teeth and other anatomical landmarks.

II. **ANATOMICAL LANDMARKS**

    A. **Definition:** an anatomical structure whose image may serve as an aid in the localization and identification of the regions portrayed by a radiograph.

B. **Landmarks Which May be Seen in the Individual Radiographs**

1. Maxillary molar: maxillary sinus, zygomatic process, malar bone, hamular process, coronoid process of the mandible, maxillary tuberosity.
2. Maxillary bicuspid: maxillary sinus.
3. Maxillary cuspid: maxillary sinus.
4. Maxillary incisors: incisive foramen, nasal septum and fossae, median palatine suture, symphysis of the maxillae.
5. Mandibular molar: mandibular canal, external oblique ridge, mylohyoid ridge.
6. Mandibular bicuspid: mental foramen.
7. Mandibular incisors: lingual foramen, mental ridge, genial tubercles, symphysis of the mandible; nutrient canals seen most frequently in this radiograph.

III. IDENTIFICATION OF INADEQUACIES IN RADIOGRAPHS

Inadequacies are related to film placement, angulation, exposure, processing, care and handling of the film, and, indeed, any step in the entire procedure. Errors appear as problems of inadequate density, contrast, incomplete or distorted images, fogging, artifacts, or stains. Table 10 outlines the more common inadequacies and their causes, the keys to correction.

TABLE 10.—ANALYSIS OF RADIOGRAPHS: CAUSES OF INADEQUACIES

Inadequacy	Cause: Factors in Correction
Image	
Elongation	Insufficient vertical angulation.
Foreshortening	Excessive vertical angulation.
Superimposition (overlapping)	Incorrect horizontal angulation (central ray not directed through interproximal).
Partial Image	Cone-cut (incorrect direction of central ray or incorrect film placement). Incompletely immersed in processing tank. Film touched other film or side of tank during processing.
Blurred or Double Image	Patient, tube or packet movement during exposure. Film exposed twice.
Stretched Appearance of Trabeculae or Apices	Bent film.
No Image	Machine misfunction from time switch to wall plug. Failure to turn on the machine. Film placed in fixer before developer.
Density	
Too Dark	Excessive exposure. Excessive developing. Developer too warm. Unsafe safelight. Accidental exposure to white light (may be completely black).

TABLE 10.—ANALYSIS OF RADIOGRAPHS: CAUSES OF INADEQUACIES (*Continued*)

Inadequacy	*Cause: Factors in Correction*
Density (*continued*)	
Too Light	Insufficient exposure.
	Insufficient development or excessive fixation.
	Too cool solutions.
	Use of old, contaminated, or poorly mixed solutions.
	Film placement: leaded side toward teeth.
	Films used beyond expiration date.
Fog	
Chemical Fog	Imbalance or deterioration of processing solutions.
Light Fog	Unintentional exposure to light to which the emulsion is sensitive, either before or during processing.
	(*a*) unsafe safelight
	b) darkroom leak
Radiation Fog	Improper film storage of unused film and exposed film prior to processing.
Reticulation	
(puckered or pebbly surface)	Sudden temperature changes during processing, particularly from warm solutions to very cold water.
Artifacts	
Dark Lines	Bent or creased film.
	Static electricity.
	(1) Film removed from wrapper with excessive force.
	(2) Wrapper sticking to film when opened with wet fingers or if there was excessive moisture from patient's mouth.
	Fingernail used to grasp film during opening.
Herringbone Pattern (light film)	Packet placed in mouth backwards with foil next to teeth.
Stains and Spots	Foreign bodies in cone of machine.
	Unclean film hanger.
	Splatterings of developer, fixer, dust.
	Finger marks.
	Insufficient rinsing after developing before fixing.
	Splashing dry negatives with water or solutions.
	Air bubbles adhering to surface during processing (insufficient agitation)
	Overlap of film on film in tanks or while drying.
	Paper wrapper stuck to film (film not dried when removed from patient's mouth).
Discoloration at later date after storage of completed radiographs	Incomplete processing or rinsing.
	Storage in too warm a place.
	Storage near chemicals.

TECHNICAL HINTS

I. **NEVER** hold a film in a patient's mouth during exposure.

II. **INQUIRE** as to whether the patient is receiving radiation treatment. It may be necessary to minimize the number of exposures. The patient's physician should be consulted.

III. **FILM PLACEMENT:** Embossed dot on film is placed toward the occlusal or incisal to prevent its superimposition over image.

IV. **CHECK STATE RADIATION PROTECTION LAWS.** Many states have regulations concerning x-ray unit registration, inspection, safety requirements and limitations for use of x-rays.[72]

V. **RECORD IN PATIENT'S PERMANENT RECORD** when a patient refuses to have radiographs made. Obtain patient's signature to a statement indicating such refusal in the event a legal issue should arise related to the operation performed.

VI. **WHO OWNS DENTAL RADIOGRAPHS?** They are part of the dentist's record and remain his property the same as other parts of the case record.[73]

VII. **FILM STORAGE:** always in a clean, dry place. Keep in lead lined container. Watch expiration dates. Store oldest film in front for next use. Purchase as needed, not in quantity.

VIII. **STUDY INFORMATIONAL SHEETS** provided in package of film. This applies particularly when a new brand of film is being used.

IX. **STAIN REMOVAL FROM CLOTHES:**[74] Do not launder before spot removal.

   A. **Developer**
   1. Apply Solution A (2 Gm. potassium permanganate, 4 ml. concentrated sulfuric acid in water to make one liter) until a dark stain is produced over and around the original area.
   2. Wash out excess Solution A with water.
   3. Apply Solution B (30 Gm. sodium bisulfite, 30 Gm. sodium sulfite in water to make 1 liter).
   4. Wash with water.

   B. **Fixer**
   1. Swab with fixer to which a small amount of citric acid has been added, or apply tincture of iodine, then fixer.
   2. Soak overnight for stubborn silver stains.
   3. Wash with water.

   C. **Launder** soon after spot removal.

   D. **Commercially** prepared spot removers are available from dental supply companies.

FACTORS TO TEACH THE PATIENT

I. **WHEN THE PATIENT ASKS ABOUT THE SAFETY OF RADIATION**

   A. Adapt the answer to the patient. Certain patients will have more fear; others will have more knowledge about x-rays. Expression of confidence will aid in allaying fears. Hesitation will increase the patient's doubt.

B. Radiographs are essential to diagnosis and treatment. Without the information provided, the dentist can only guess at conditions not visible to him.

C. The benefits resulting from the intelligent use of x-rays outweigh any possible negative effects.

D. Modern x-ray machines are equipped for safety. For the patient who will understand, details about filtration, collimation, film speed and short exposure times can be explained.

E. It has never been shown that any harm has resulted from the small amount of x-ray from dental sources. Exposure is distributed to different areas and the amount to any one area is small.

F. When the patient understands ionizing radiation, it may be important to explain more concerning the effects.

II. EDUCATIONAL FEATURES IN DENTAL RADIOGRAPHS

(Avoid diagnosis. For teaching, it may be advisable to use radiographs of someone other than the patient.)

A. Position of unerupted permanent teeth in relation to primary teeth.

B. Detection of early carious lesions not visible in clinical examination.

C. Effects of loss of teeth and the importance of having replacements.

D. Observation of submarginal, proximal calculus deposits to explain need for complete scaling and personal care procedures.

E. Periodontal changes and other pathology appropriate to education of individual patient.

REFERENCES

1. American Dental Association, Council on Dental Research: Council Reaffirms Policy on Radiation Hygiene, Am. Dent. A. J., *61*, 275, August, 1960.
2. Statement of the American Academy of Oral Roentgenology's Stand Regarding the Use of X-rays in Dentistry, Oral Surg., Oral Med., & Oral Path., *15*, 1350, November, 1962.
3. ENNIS, L. M.: Highlights of American Dentistry in the Field of Roentgenology, Internat. D. J., *10*, 139, June, 1960.
4. ENNIS, L. M.: Resumé of Roentgenology (Henry Cline Fixott, Sr. Memorial Lecture), Oral Surg., Oral Med., & Oral Path., *15*, 680, June, 1962.
5. WUEHRMANN, A. H.: *Radiation Protection and Dentistry.* St. Louis, Mosby, 1960, pp. 44–52.
6. ENNIS, L. M. and BERRY, H. M.: *Dental Roentgenology,* 5th ed. Philadelphia, Lea & Febiger, 1959, pp. 47–66.
7. JACOBSON, F. L.: *Oral Roentgenology Syllabus.* Seattle, University of Washington, School of Dentistry, 1962–63, pp. A1–A10.
8. McCALL, J. O. and WALD, S. S.: *Clinical Dental Roentgenology,* 4th ed. Philadelphia, Saunders, 1957, pp. 5–12.
9. BERRY, H. M.: An Introduction to Dental Roentgenology, in Peterson, Shailer: *Clinical Dental Hygiene,* 2nd ed. St. Louis, Mosby, 1963, pp. 207–218.
10. General Electric, Technical Services X-ray Department: X-ray Generation and Radiographic Principles in Dentistry. Milwaukee, Pub. 13–3549*B*.
11. RICHARDS, A. G.: Technical Factors that Control Radiographic Density, Dental Clinics of North America, July, 1961, p. 371.
12. WUEHRMANN: op cit., pp. 136–144.
13. WUEHRMANN: op cit., pp. 128–136.
14. RICHARDS, A. G., NELSON, R. J., FITZGERALD, G. M., WALD, S. S., and SPANGENBERG, H. D.: X-ray Protection in the Dental Office, Am. Dent. A. J., *56*, 514, April, 1958.
15. RICHARDS, A. G.: Roentgen-ray Doses in Dental Roentgenography, Am. Dent. A. J., *56*, 351, March, 1958.
16. BARR, J. H. and BROCKMAN, M. K.: Radiation Dosage in Dental Offices, Oral Surg., Ora Med., & Oral Path., *13*, 696, June, 1960.
17. WUEHRMANN: op. cit., pp. 167–175.

18. SPANGENBERG, H. D., JR. and POOL, M. L.: 65 or a 90 Kilovolt X-ray Machine? Oral Surg. Oral Path., & Oral Med., *13*, 552, May, 1960.
19. UPDEGRAVE, W. J.: High or Low Kilovoltage, Dent. Radiog. & Photog., *33*, 71, #4, 1960.
20. WUEHRMANN: op. cit., pp. 72–75, 145–149, 156–157.
21. ENNIS: op. cit., pp. 39, 70–71, 137–138.
22. WAGGENER, D. T.: Roentgenographic Techniques. The Right-Angle Technique Using the Extension Cone, Dental Clinics of North America, November, 1960, p. 783.
23. Roentgeno-Questions, What Are the Advantages of a "Long Cone" on a Dental Machine? Oral Surg., Oral Med., & Oral Path., *14*, 961, August, 1961.
24. WUEHRMANN: op. cit., p. 155.
25. American Academy of Oral Roentgenology, Radiation Protection Committee: Effective Use of X-ray Radiation in Dentistry, Oral Surg., Oral Med., & Oral Path., *16*, 294, March, 1963.
26. VAN AKEN, J.: Study of Some Properties of Twenty-three Different Dental X-ray Films, Oral Surg., Oral Med., & Oral Path., *15*, 1330, November, 1962.
27. American Dental Association, Council on Dental Research: Council Adopts American Standard Speed Classifications for Intraoral Dental Radiographic Film. Diagnostic Grade, Am. Dent. A. J., *65*, 280, August, 1962.
28. PAFFENBARGER, G. C., FORZIATI, A. F., and KUMPULA, M. P.: Discussion of Federal Specifications GG-X-620 and L-F-310 for Dental X-ray Apparatus and Dental X-ray Film, Am. Dent. A. J., *59*, 472, September, 1959.
29. STAFNE, E. C.: *Oral Roentgenographic Diagnosis*, 2nd ed. Philadelphia, Saunders, 1963, pp. 398–399.
30. Ibid., p. 403.
31. MANSON-HING, L. R.: Fundamental Biologic Effects of X-rays in Dentistry, Oral Surg., Oral Med., & Oral Path., *12*, 562, May, 1959.
32. WUEHRMANN: op. cit., p. 81.
33. SEARS, T. P.: Biological Reaction to Ionizing Radiation Atomic Structure, J. Periodont., *34*, 174, March, 1963.
34. WUEHRMANN: op. cit., p. 84.
35. NOLAN, W. E.: Radiation Hazards to the Patient from Oral Roentgenography, Am. Dent. A. J., *47*, 681, December, 1953.
36. BUDOWSKY, JACK, PIRO, J. D., ZEGARELLI, E. V., KUTSCHER, A. H., and BARNETT, ALICE: Radiation Exposure to the Head and Abdomen During Oral Roentgenography, Am. Dent. A. J., *52*, 555, May, 1956.
37. RICHARDS, A. G.: Production of Erythema of the Skin by Exposure to X-ray Radiation, J. Dent. Res., *34*, 100, February, 1955.
38. STANFORD, R. W. and VANCE, J.: Quantity of Radiation Received by the Reproductive Organs of Patients During Routine Diagnostic X-ray Examinations, Brit. J. Radiol., *28*, 266, May, 1955.
39. RICHARDS, A. G.: New Method for Reduction of Gonadal Irradiation of Dental Patients, Am. Dent. A. J., *65*, 1, July, 1962.
40. ENNIS: op. cit., pp. 104–105.
41. SILHA, R. E.: Roentgenographic Service for the Gagging Patient, Oral Surg., Oral Med., & Oral Path., *15*, 62, January, 1962.
42. DEMPSTER, W. T., ADAMS, W. J., and DUDDLES, R. A.: Arrangement in the Jaws of the Roots of the Teeth, Am. Dent. A. J., *67*, 779, December, 1963.
43. FITZGERALD, G. M.: Dental Roentgenography. I. An Investigation in Adumbration, or the Factors that Control Geometric Unsharpness, Am. Dent. A. J., *34*, 1, January 1, 1947.
44. FITZGERALD, G. M.: Dental Roentgenography. II. Vertical Angulation, Film Placement and Increased Object-Film Distance, Am. Dent. A. J., *34*, 160, February 1, 1947.
45. UPDEGRAVE, W. J.: Higher Fidelity in Intraoral Roentgenography, Am. Dent. A. J., *62*, 1, January, 1961.
46. BARR, J. H. and GRØN, Paul: Palate Contour as a Limiting Factor in Intraoral X-ray Technique, Oral Surg., Oral Med., & Oral Path., *12*, 459, April, 1959.
47. FITZGERALD, G. M.: Dental Roentgenography. III. The Roentgenographic Periapical Survey of the Upper Molar Region, Am. Dent. A. J., *38*, 293, March, 1949.
48. SILHA, R. E.: Horizontal Angulation in Maxillary Cuspid Roentgenography, Oral Surg., Oral Med., & Oral Path., *13*, 710, June, 1960.
49. UPDEGRAVE, W. J.: Paralleling Extension-Cone Technique in Intraoral Dental Radiography, Oral Surg., Oral Med., & Oral Path., *4*, 1250, October, 1951.
50. UPDEGRAVE, W. J.: Simplifying and Improving Intraoral Dental Roentgenography, Oral Surg., Oral Med., & Oral Path., *12*, 704, June, 1959.
51. CARR, J. D.: Universal U and L Bite-block Film Holder. A Method of Positioning and Holding Intraoral X-ray Films for Both Maxillary and Mandibular Exposures, Oral Surg., Oral Med., & Oral Path., *14*, 954, August, 1961.

52. WILLIAMS, S. W.:   Paralleling Technic for Intraoral Roentgenology, Am. Dent. A. J., *43*, 419, October, 1951.
53. WUEHRMANN, A. H.:   The Long Cone Technic, Practical Dental Monographs, July, 1957, p. 8.
54. McCALL and WALD: op. cit., pp. 23–44.
55. ENNIS: op. cit., pp. 75–95.
56. BERRY: op. cit., pp. 228–241.
57. Eastman Kodak Company, X-ray Division: X-rays in Dentistry, pp. 26–39.
58. ENNIS: op. cit., pp. 109–117.
59. STAFNE: op. cit., pp. 381–386.
60. Eastman Kodak: op. cit., pp. 44–52.
61. WAGGENER, D. T. and IRELAND, R. L.:   Intraoral Roentgenography for Children, Am. Dent. A. J., *47*, 133, August, 1953.
62. HAYDEN, JESS, JR., and RICHARDS, A. G.:   Procedures for Adequate Radiographs of Pre-school Children, J. Dent. Child., *22*, 70, 2nd Quarter, 1955.
63. UPDEGRAVE, W. J.:   Supplementary Radiographic Examination for Children, Pennsyl. D. J., *27*, 3, January, 1960.
64. BARBER, T. K.:   Roentgenographic Techniques for Children, Dental Clinics of North America, November, 1961, p. 549.
65. LEWIS, T. M., TIDSWELL, B. A., and McQUILLAN, K. A.:   Pedodontic Roentgenology—A Practical Technique, Austral. D. J., *8*, 97, April, 1963.
66. YALE, S. H., MOOS, W. S. and VIDEKA, M. A.:   Measurement of Gonadal Dose in Children During Intraoral Radiography, Oral Surg., Oral Med., & Oral Path., *13*, 1081, September, 1960.
67. CRANDELL, C. E.:   Cause and Frequency of Intraoral X-ray Errors by Dental and Dental Hygiene Students, J. Dent. Educ., *22*, 189, May, 1958.
68. ENNIS: op. cit., pp. 223–252.
69. Eastman Kodak Company: Exposure and Processing Chart.
70. SWEET, A. P. S.:   Safelights Reconsidered, Dent. Radiog. & Photog., *35*, 39, #2, 1962.
71. WUEHRMANN: op. cit., pp. 159–161.
72. American Dental Association, Council on Legislation: State "Radiation Protection" Laws, Am. Dent. A. J., *60*, 126, January, 1960.
73. ENNIS: op. cit., p. 217.
74. CARR, J. D., and NORMAN, R. D.:   Effective Use of the Darkroom, Dental Clinics of North America, July, 1961, p. 363.

SUGGESTED READINGS

ADELSON, J. J.:   Handicapped and Problem Patient—Radiodontic Examination and Treatment, Dent. Radiog. & Photog., *34*, 27, #2, 1961.
BARBER, T. K.:   Roentgenographic Evaluation of Growth and Development, Am. Dent. A. J., *67*, 329, September, 1963.
COHEN, B. and STANFORD, R. W.:   Review of the Dangers of Radiation in Dentistry, Internat. D. J., *10*, 368, September, 1960.
MANSON-HING, L. R.:   Vision and Oral Roentgenology, Oral Surg., Oral Med., & Oral Path., *15*, 173, February, 1962.
MANSON-HING, L. R. and FINN, S. B.:   Roentgenography, in Finn, S. B.: *Clinical Pedodontics*, 2nd ed. Philadelphia, Saunders, 1962, pp. 104–122.
ORBAN, T. R. and ORBAN, B. J.:   Three Dimensional Roentgenographic Interpretation in Periodontal Diagnosis, J. Periodont, *31*, 275, September, 1960.
PRITCHARD, JOHN: Role of Roentgenogram in the Diagnosis and Prognosis of Periodontal Disease, Oral Surg., Oral Med., & Oral Path., *14*, 182, February, 1961.
RAPER, H. R.:   Uses of Bite-wing Radiographs, Dent. Surv., *30*, 763, June, 1954.
RICHARDS, A. G.:   Dental X-Ray Equipment of the Future, Oral Surg., Oral Med., & Oral Path., *13*, 194, February, 1960.
RICHARDS, A. G.:   How Hazardous is Dental Roentgenography? Oral Surg., Oral Med., & Oral Path., *14*, 40, January, 1961. (Contains comprehensive Bibliography.)
RICHARDS, A. G.:   Shielding Requirements for Dental Installations, Am. Dent. A. J., *64*, 788, June, 1962.
RICHARDS, A. G.:   Sources of X-Radiation which Expose the Dentist, Dent. Radiog. & Photog., *37*, 51, #3, 1964.
SWEET, A. P. S.:   Radiodontic Pitfalls, Dent. Radiog. & Photog., *33*, 27, #2, 1960.
TROUT, E. D., KELLEY, J. P., and LUCAS, A. C.:   Conventional Building Materials as Protective Barriers in Dental Roentgenographic Installations, Oral Surg., Oral Med., & Oral Path., *15*, 1211, October, 1962.
WUEHRMANN, A. H.:   Responsibility of the Dental Profession in Reducing Exposure to Ionizing Radiation, Oral Surg., Oral Med., & Oral Path., *14*, 304, March, 1961.

Extraoral Radiography

DONALDSON, R. G.:   Lateral-Jaw Radiography, Dent. Radiog. & Photog., *35*, 58, #3, 1962.

ENNIS, L. M. and BERRY, H. M.:   *Dental Roentgenology*, 5th ed. Philadelphia, Lea & Febiger, 1959, pp. 117–135.

Eastman Kodak Company, X-ray Division: X-rays in Dentistry, pp. 53–63.

MANSON-HING, L. R.:   Utilization of Extraoral Roentgenographic Techniques in General Dental Practice, Dental Clinics of North America, July, 1961, p. 437.

McCALL, J. O. and WALD, S. S.:   *Clinical Dental Roentgenology*, 4th ed. Philadelphia, Saunders, 1957, pp. 54–80.

ROBINSON, M.:   Simplified Method for Office Roentgenograms of the Temperomandibular Joint, J. Oral Surg., Anes., & Hosp. Dent. Serv., *20*, 217, May, 1962.

SCHIER, M. B. A.:   Temperomandibular Joint Roentgenography: Controlled Erect Techniques, Am. Dent. A. J., *65*, 456, October, 1962.

STAFNE, E. C.:   *Oral Roentgenographic Diagnosis*, 2nd ed. Philadelphia, Saunders, 1963, pp. 386–389.

UPDEGRAVE, W. J.:   Practical Evaluation of Techniques and Interpretation in the Roentgenographic Examination of Temperomandibular Joints, Dental Clinics of North America, July, 1961, p. 421.

WUEHRMANN, A. H. and CHILCOAT, A. A.:   Extraoral Techniques, Oral Surg., Oral Med., & Oral Path., *12*, 1450, December, 1959.

Panoramic Radiography

KRASKE, L. M. and MAZZARELLA, M. A.:   Evaluation of a Panoramic Dental X-ray Machine, Dent. Prog., *1*, 171, April, 1961.

KUMPULA, J. W.:   Present Status of Panoramic Roentgenography, Am. Dent. A. J., *63*, 194, August, 1961.

MITCHELL, L. D.:   Panoramic Roentgenography, A Clinical Evaluation, Am. Dent. A. J., *66*, 772, June, 1963.

PAATERO, Y. V.:   Pantomography and Orthopantomography, Oral Surg., Oral Med., & Oral Path., *14*, 947, August, 1961.

UPDEGRAVE, W. J.:   Panoramic Dental Radiography, Dent. Radiog. & Photog., *36*, 75, #4, 1963.

Chapter 24

CHARTING

PERIODONTAL and dental chartings prepared completely or in part by the dental hygienist contribute significantly by providing the dentist with information essential to diagnosis and treatment planning for the care of the patient. The purpose of each type of charting is defined by its title: the dental charting includes diagrammatic representation of existing conditions of the teeth, whereas the periodontal charting indicates clinically determinable features of the periodontium. A separate type of chart form is designed which provides for recording the special features of each.

The dental hygienist does not diagnose; in charting, a picture of observations made during inspection is recorded. At no time would the charting be described specifically to the patient. In certain dental offices the dentist requires the dental hygienist to interpret aspects of the oral diagnosis to the patient. This is used as preliminary instruction for the patient in explaining the treatment plan and office procedures during treatment.

I. PURPOSES FOR CHARTING

Charting of the oral cavity has specific objectives. An accurate, detailed and carefully recorded charting is essential to dental and dental hygiene care as listed below.

A. Provides a graphic representation of the over-all dental or periodontal existing conditions.

B. Contributes to the prevention of oral diseases by early recognition of deviations from normal and calling such deviations to the attention of the dentist.

C. Assists the dentist in making the diagnosis and treatment plan.

D. Provides information for continuing records of the patient's dental and periodontal conditions which can be used for evaluating the response to treatment over a period of time and at recall appointments.

E. Defines areas of instruction needing emphasis if the patient is to understand his oral health problems and carry out personal daily routines which will aid in maintaining oral health.

F. Impresses the patient with the significance of a complete, exacting routine while studying his oral health.

G. Establishes a permanent record to protect the dental practice in case of misunderstandings or legal procedures concerning patient grievances.

H. Aids as a reference for the identification of a patient in the case of an emergency or accident.

II. **PRINCIPLES FOR CHARTING**

The dental hygienist must maintain a sincere sense of responsibility to the patient and an earnest desire to be of greatest possible assistance to the dentist. Neatness in the marking of symbols, drawings and labels goes hand in hand with the accuracy of the inspection itself. The principles listed below apply to both dental and periodontal charting.

A. **Preparation of Instruments**

Sanitize pencils or pen to be used by vigorously rubbing with gauze moistened in a chemical disinfectant.[1] Particular care must be exercised to keep sterile dental instruments apart from other equipment which cannot be sterilized. Transmission of oral microorganisms to chart forms, pencils, pens, erasers or radiographs presents a real problem in the maintenance of a clinically clean environment. Frequent handwashing is necessary.

B. **Radiographs:** bite-wing or periapical survey.

Radiographs should be prepared in advance of the charting in order to facilitate coordination between the clinical and radiographic inspections. The completely processed and dried radiograph provides greater assurance of a thorough analysis.

C. **Chart Form**

The wide variety of chart forms used by practicing dentists and dental clinic personnel, as well as the many requirements for and methods of recording on these chart forms, make any attempt to outline a specific universal procedure impractical. Characteristics of an adequate chart form are suggested below.

1. Contains space to show sufficient detail without requiring useless information.
2. Shows roots and all surfaces of the teeth clearly in a relationship convenient to recording necessary features.
3. Provides for recording information in a manner that may be interpreted readily by all who will use it.
4. Includes sufficient space for labeling clearly.

D. **Technique**

1. Adequate visibility and accessibility of field of inspection.
   a. Maintain correct position of patient and operator.
   b. Use maximum illumination.
      (1) Direct or reflected light.
      (2) Transillumination.
   c. Obtain necessary retraction.
   d. Maintain a dry field.
2. Sequence
   The use of a set routine is a prerequisite to accomplishing a complete and accurate charting. This is true not only for the tooth surface-to-surface pattern, but also for the parts of the charting itself. It is suggested that to chart all of one kind of item for the entire mouth, rather than completely charting one tooth, helps in obtaining accuracy since only one train of thought is required at a time. For example in the dental charting, record

all of the restorations and then start again at the first tooth inspected and chart all of the deviations from normal rather than chart all restorations and deviations for each tooth separately.

DENTAL CHARTING

Dental charting includes recording of the existing restorations and clinically and radiographically observable deviations from the normal appearance of the teeth. In certain dental practices the dental hygienist is responsible for completing the entire charting which is checked afterwards by the dentist. In other situations the dental hygienist charts only the existing restorations for the new patient and the dentist dictates the findings of the inspection for dental caries and other irregularities.

Charting of dental defects for public health or school health surveys is frequently a responsibility of the dental hygienist in private dental practice as well as the dental hygienist employed by school or health agencies. By such participation the dental hygienist in private practice is afforded the opportunity to contribute to the health of the entire community. Group methods used for a public health dental survey are adaptations of those used for the individual patient. The most frequently used type of survey is concerned only with the general status of the oral cavity, such as a dental caries survey to determine total decayed, missing and filled teeth.[2] This is in contrast to the charting made in private dental practice where the condition of each surface of each tooth is identified and recorded.

Essential to the preparation of a complete charting of teeth are an understanding of the terminology and clinical appearance of dental caries and knowledge of methods of inspection and recording.

I. PREPARATION OF THE TEETH FOR INSPECTION

    A. Oral prophylaxis usually precedes charting.
    B. Purposes for completing oral prophylaxis before charting
        1. Food debris and materia alba near cervical third of teeth and interproximally may mask or prevent detection of defects.
        2. Explorer can catch on dental deposits and complicate the detection of dental caries.

II. TECHNIQUE FOR DENTAL CHARTING

Chart forms, sequence and method of recording are adapted to the objectives and requirements of the supervising dentist. The teeth are dried before accurate observations can be made.

    A. **Radiographs:** the bite-wing radiographic survey is generally considered most useful for the detection of proximal dental caries and deficient or overhanging restorations. The right-angle view of the crowns provides the most accurate reproduction of the shape and size of the tooth.

    B. **Instruments**
        1. Sharp explorers: gentle manipulation to permit maximum tactile discrimination. The technique for use is described on page 79.

2. Clear, unscratched mouth mirror.
3. Dental floss (limited use in detection of irregularities of contact areas).

C. Types of Chart Forms

1. Anatomic: drawings of the teeth with surface characteristics and roots represented in their natural relative sizes.
2. Geometric: diagrammatic representation for each tooth divided to provide area for each surface; frequently does not include the roots. Example: 2 circles, inner circle representing occlusal and outer circle the rest of the crown.[3]

D. Suggested Sequence for Charting

1. Clinical visual and exploratory inspection
   a. Mark all missing teeth and identify closed spaces and partially erupted teeth.
   b. Mark all existing restorations (operative and prosthetic), making no attempt on the first round to identify any defects.
   c. Mark all deviations from normal after drying each tooth with compressed air and exploring each surface carefully.
2. Radiographic examination at viewbox
   a. Identify by label or symbol all teeth which are observable in radiographs which had not been evident in the mouth, such as impacted or congenitally missing.
   b. Mark existing restorations such as endodontic therapy and overhanging margins of restorations.
   c. Mark all deviations from the normal.

III. TERMINOLOGY USED IN DESCRIBING DENTAL CARIES

A. Cavity Nomenclature: carious lesions are named by the surface or surfaces involved.

1. *Simple Cavity:* involves one tooth surface (example: occlusal cavity).
2. *Compound or Complex Cavity:* involves more than one tooth surface (examples: mesio-occlusal cavity or disto-occlusal-lingual cavity).

B. G. V. Black's Classification of Cavities[4]

Class I.   Cavities in pits or fissures.
  a. Occlusal surfaces of bicuspids and molars.
  b. Occlusal two-thirds of buccal surfaces of molars.
  c. Lingual surfaces of maxillary incisors.
  d. Lingual surfaces of maxillary molars.
Class II. Cavities in proximal surfaces of molars and bicuspids.
Class III. Cavities in proximal surfaces of incisors and cuspids which do not involve the removal or restoration of the incisal angle.
Class IV. Cavities in proximal surfaces of incisors and cuspids which do require the removal and restoration of the incisal angle.
Class V.   Cavities in the gingival one-third (not pit cavities) of facial or lingual surfaces of teeth.

C. **Types of Dental Caries**
  1. Description by location related to etiology
    a. Pit and fissure cavities (Class I)
      (1) Cavity begins in minute fault of the enamel.
      (2) Location of pits
        (a) Where 3 or more lobes of the teeth join: imperfect closure of enamel plates (example: occlusal of bicuspid or molar).
        (b) At the endings of grooves (example: buccal of mandibular molar).
      (3) Areas are habitually clean except as the pit or fissure affords place for lodgment and fermentation of debris.
    b. Smooth surface cavities (Classes II, III, IV, V)
      (1) Cavities formed by dental caries beginning in smooth surfaces that are without pits, fissures or faults. May occur in the enamel or cementum (root caries).
      (2) Areas are habitually unclean because of their position.
        (a) Inaccessible to self-cleansing mechanisms.
        (b) Proximity to surfaces of adjacent teeth or prosthetic appliances.
  2. Description by occurrence
    a. Primary (initial or incipient): on surface which previously has not been affected.
    b. Secondary: on surface which previously has been affected and has been restored.
    c. Recurrent (generally referred to as secondary): on tooth surface adjacent to a restoration when the lesion is believed to be a continuation of the previous carious lesion.
    d. Rampant: widespread formation of chalky areas and incipient cavities in numerous teeth over a comparatively short time lapse. Most characteristically found in teen-age patients.

D. **Characteristic Route of Attack of Dental Caries**
  1. Starts in pits, fissures or smooth surfaces which are not self-cleansing.
  2. Follows general direction of enamel rods.
  3. Spreads at dentino-enamel junction.
  4. Continues along dentinal tubules.

E. **Clinical Detection of Dental Caries: Characteristic Changes in Tooth Structure Caused by Dental Caries**
  1. Visual inspection of color and translucency of tooth structure.
    a. Discoloration: brought about by ingress of foreign matter.
      (1) Chalky white areas of decalcification.
      (2) Grayish-white discoloration of marginal ridges due to dental caries on proximal surface.
      (3) Grayish-white color spreading out from margins of restorations due to lesions of secondary dental caries.
      (4) In relation to amalgam restoration: dental caries appears translucent in outer portion and white and opaque adjacent to the amalgam.
      (5) Open carious lesion may vary in color from yellowish-brown to dark brown (example: Class V).

(6) Less discoloration is present when dental caries progresses rapidly than when it progresses slowly.

b. Loss of translucency
  (1) Dull, flat white, opaque areas under direct light.
  (2) Dark shadow on proximal surfaces shown by transillumination: especially useful for anterior teeth and unrestored posterior teeth.

2. Exploratory inspection for hardness, roughness and continuity of tooth surfaces.
  a. Loss of hardness of tooth substance.
    (1) Roughness and/or indentation of enamel.
    (2) Developmental pit or fissure: explorer may "catch" but when dental caries is present there will be evidence of softening of tooth structure.
  b. Cavitation associated with nonself-cleansing areas where debris collects.
  c. Fraying of dental floss passing over proximal dental caries may mean one of several defects.
    (1) Calculus.
    (2) Defective margin of a restoration.
    (3) Sharp cavity margin.

PERIODONTAL CHARTING

Periodontal charting includes recording the position of the margin of the free gingiva, the depth of periodontal pockets as measured with a periodontal probe, and other factors which influence the periodontal condition of each tooth. As with the dental charting, the dental hygienist may complete the entire charting which is later checked by the dentist, or she may be required to make basic notations and then assist the dentist in the final steps.

Adaptations of periodontal charting are used for public health surveys of groups to determine characteristic patterns of periodontal diseases particularly the relative prevalence and severity. The P-M-A (papillary, marginal and attached) Index has been used to define gingival involvement.[5] Russell's Index defines by a scale each tooth according to the classic signs of destructive periodontal disease, inflammation, pocket formation and loss of function, and an average score is made for the number of teeth present in the mouth.[6] Such surveys are in contrast to a periodontal charting in private dental practice where the condition of the periodontium around each tooth is studied and recorded in detail.

Preparation of the periodontal charting requires knowledge of the general clinical features of periodontal conditions. The charting is prepared by comparing existing conditions with the characteristics of the normal supporting structures of the teeth. The characteristics of the normal gingiva have been described on pages 86–87.

I. TERMINOLOGY USED IN DESCRIBING PERIODONTAL CONDITIONS

A. **Pocket:** gingival sulcus pathologically deepened by periodontal disease.

B. **Gingival Enlargement:** increase in size of the gingiva.

    1. Localized: involving gingiva in relation to a single tooth or group of teeth.

    2. Generalized: involving the gingiva throughout the mouth.

    3. Marginal: involving only the margin of the free gingiva.

    4. Diffuse: involving the margin of the free gingiva and the attached gingiva.

C. **Gingival Recession:** progressive exposure of root surface by an apical shift of the gingiva following loss of alveolar crest and corresponding part of the periodontal ligament (membrane).

D. **Festoon** (McCall's Festoon): enlargement of the marginal gingiva with the formation of "life-saver"-like gingival prominence in relation to the tooth surface.

E. **Cleft** (Stillman's Cleft): apostrophe-shaped indentations which extend from and into the gingival margin along the root surface, most frequently on the labial or buccal.

F. **Mobility:** freedom of motion of teeth affected by loss of alveolar bone and inflammation of the periodontal ligament (membrane).

G. **Bi- or Trifurcation Involvement:** a pathologic condition in which the periodontal structures are destroyed to such an extent as to denude the tooth surface in the region of the bifurcation of the mandibular molars and maxillary bicuspids or the trifurcation of the maxillary molars.

H. **Food Impaction:** the wedging of food against the periodontal tissues by functional forces during mastication.

II. TECHNIQUE FOR PERIODONTAL CHARTING

Chart form, sequence and method of charting are adapted to the objectives of the supervising dentist. The gingiva must be dried before accurate observations can be made since light reflected from glistening, moist gingiva obscures detail.

A. **Radiographs:** the bite-wing survey is useful for observing the level of the alveolar bone and proximal defects of the teeth which affect the condition of the periodontium. A complete periapical survey is needed, however, to gain an over-all perspective of the supporting structures, particularly in cases of severe periodontal involvement.

B. **Instruments**

    1. Periodontal probe: the technique for use is described on page 80.

    2. Sharp explorers.

    3. Clear unscratched mouth mirror.

    4. Dental floss.

C. **Types of Chart Forms and Method of Recording**

For examples of chart forms and symbols used for recording, the reader is referred to textbooks of periodontics.[7-11] Two general methods frequently used are described below.

1. Diagrams to include lingual, facial and occlusal aspects of each tooth: the roots are crossed with horizontal lines at milli-meter intervals to permit designation of position of the margin of the free gingiva and the line of the alveolar crest by a continuous line.[7,9,11]
2. Diagrams to include lingual, facial and occlusal aspects of each tooth not in contact with each other. To chart the periodontal pocket, short individual lines are drawn parallel to the long axis of the appropriate tooth surface and the number of millimeters depth is marked at the end of the line.[8]

D. Sequence for Charting

Only major factors to be observed and recorded are listed below. The clinical visual and exploratory inspections are made in conjunc-tion with the radiographic. Clinical and radiographic inspections are compared to confirm the findings of each except in the measure-ment of the periodontal pocket. The depth of the periodontal pocket is not detectable in the radiograph.

1. Mark missing teeth, teeth not in the line of occlusion, and prosthetic replacements.
2. Mark mobile teeth as determined by digital inspection.
3. Mark insufficient contact areas and areas of food impaction as suggested by the use of dental floss and appearance of the gingival tissue.
4. Mark other deviations of the teeth such as faults of fixed or removable dentures, overhanging restorations, and bi- or trifurcation involvements as determined by the use of explorers and radiographs.
5. Mark position and characteristics of the gingiva.
   a. Enlargement.
   b. Recession.
   c. Clefts and festoons.
6. Mark depth of periodontal pockets as determined by the use of the periodontal probe.

TECHNICAL HINTS

I. When bleeding of the gingiva obscures tooth surfaces, postpone the preparation of a dental charting. Provide instruction in toothbrush-ing and other personal oral care procedures to promote healing.

II. Avoid inserting an explorer into obvious carious lesions visible to the naked eye to prevent unnecessary discomfort to the patient.

FACTORS TO TEACH THE PATIENT

I. The need for thorough, complete, exacting routine for dental and perio-dontal inspection at regular intervals.

II. Necessity for radiographic examination to complete the inspection and charting.

III. Reasons for requiring the completion of the oral prophylaxis prior to inspection for charting of the teeth.

REFERENCES

1. NEFF, J. H. and ROSENTHAL, S. L.:   A Possible Means of Inadvertent Transmission of Infection to Dental Patients, J. Dent. Res., *36*, 932, December, 1957.
2. WARNER, E. M.:   Public Health, in Bunting, R. W.: *Oral Hygiene*, 3rd ed.   Philadelphia, Lea & Febiger, 1957, pp. 292–297.
3. BODECKER, C. F.:   The Modified Dental Caries Index, Am. Dent. A. J., *26*, 1453, September, 1939.
4. BLACKWELL, R. E.:   *G. V. Black's Operative Dentistry*, 9th ed., Vol. II.   South Milwaukee, Medico-Dental Publishing Company, 1955, pp. 1–4.
5. MASSLER, MAURY and SCHOUR, ISAAC: The P-M-A Index of Gingivitis, J. Dent. Res., *28*, 634, December, 1949.
6. RUSSELL, A. L.:   System of Classification and Scoring for Prevalence Surveys of Periodontal Disease, J. Dent. Res., *35*, 350, June, 1956.
7. GLICKMAN, IRVING: *Clinical Periodontology*, 2nd ed.   Philadelphia, Saunders, 1958, pp. 475–478.
8. GRANT, DANIEL, STERN, I. B., and EVERETT, F. G.:   *Orban's Periodontics*, 2nd ed. St. Louis, Mosby, 1963, pp. 237–239.
9. GOLDMAN, H. M., SCHLUGER, SAUL, COHEN, D. W., CHAIKEN, B. S., and FOX, Lewis: *Introduction to Periodontia*, 2nd ed. St. Louis, Mosby, 1962, pp. 121–124.
10. BEUBE, F. E.:   *Periodontology.* New York, Macmillan, 1953, pp. 365–366.
11. MILLER, S. C.:   *Textbook of Periodontia*, 3rd ed.   New York, Blakiston Division, McGraw-Hill, 1950, pp. 117–120.

SUGGESTED READINGS

ARNIM, S. S.:   Utilization of Biologic Principles in the Practice of Operative Dentistry.   I. Diagnosis of Carious Lesions, Am. Dent. A. J., *28*, 598, April, 1941.
BRAUER, J. C. *et al.*: *Dentistry for Children*, 5th ed.   New York, Blakiston Division, McGraw-Hill, 1964, pp. 363–380.
FINN, S. B.:   *Clinical Pedodontics*, 2nd ed. Philadelphia, Saunders, 1962, pp. 145–146.
GREENE, J. C. and VERMILLION, J. R.:   Oral Hygiene Index: A Method for Classifying Oral Hygiene Status, Am. Dent. A. J., *61*, 172, August, 1960.
GREENE, J. C. and VERMILLION, J. R.:   Simplified Oral Hygiene Index, Am. Dent. A. J., *68*, 7, January, 1964.
KERR, D. A., ASH, M. M., and MILLARD, H. D.:   *Oral Diagnosis*. St. Louis, Mosby, 1959, pp. 182–239.
MANDEL, I. D.:   Dental Caries, in Cohen, M. M.: *Pediatric Dentistry*, 2nd ed. St. Louis, Mosby, 1961, pp. 186–190.
MILLER, S. C.:   *Oral Diagnosis and Treatment*, 3rd ed. New York, Blakiston Division, McGraw-Hill, 1957, pp. 436–445.

PART V

Patient Instruction

Chapter 25

AREAS AND PRINCIPLES FOR PATIENT INSTRUCTION

DENTAL health education is the provision of oral health information to people in such a way that they apply it in everyday living.[1] Knowledge of dental health facts is not enough; benefits result from the ability to make practical application.

Personalized patient instruction contributes first to the knowledge, habits, and attitudes of the individual, and then to the community through the individual. Directed efforts to improve the level of understanding and appreciation of the individual contribute to the oral health of the community, and in turn to the community's image of the dental and dental hygiene professions.

The scope of areas for instruction covers a wide range of topics related to the patient's personal oral health, community and school health, specific public health measures, and the contributions of members of other health professions. Interpretation of current dental research findings to all is a direct responsibility. The topics listed below are suggestive of the variety of areas for instruction.

I. THE INDIVIDUAL PATIENT

A. **Understanding of Procedures in the Dental Office:** clarification of purposes; benefits from continuing care through recall appointments.

B. **Personal Preventive Measures,** particularly for dental caries and periodontal diseases.

1. Oral physical therapy (Chapters 26 and 27)
2. Diet and nutrition
3. Fluorides (Chapter 21)
4. Accident prevention: use of safety belts in automobiles; aid to children in understanding prevention of fractured teeth; mouth protectors for contact sports.

C. **Factors to Teach the Patient:** listed at the end of many chapters in this book.

II. **COMMUNITY**[2,3]

A. **Fluoridation**

1. Promotion in communities not currently receiving benefits.[4,5,6] During a concentrated effort, every private dental patient should receive information in spoken and printed form.
2. Clarification of benefits in communities with natural fluoride or controlled fluoridation.

B. **School Health Programs:** familiarity with dental health teaching in schools permits supplementary teaching to children and parents.

C. **Other Health Professions**

1. Teach oral health as a part of general health.
2. Coordination of community education efforts: promotion for all health programs.

D. **Individual Teaching**

1. For patients who are physicians, nurses, health educators, teachers, and others involved in community education.
   a. Provide up-to-date reports on current dental research.
   b. Special emphasis for students in teaching careers: help them identify their responsibility in teaching oral health.
2. For patients in businesses concerned with the sale of dental health products: advice concerning approved materials and agents.

E. **Dental and Dental Hygiene Association Community Projects**

1. National Children's Dental Health Week Activities: publicity and promotion.
2. Mouth protectors for contact sports: explanation.

III. **INFORMATION ABOUT CAREERS IN DENTAL HEALTH**

A. **Education:** maintain lists of schools and sources of information about the education of dentists, dental hygienists, dental assistants, and dental laboratory technicians.

B. **Initiate Conversation about Potential Careers** to young people: provide leaflets which describe the different areas.

PRINCIPLES FOR INSTRUCTION

Since chairside discussion between patient and professional provides the most effective situation for dental health instruction, each visit to the dental office should be a learning experience for the patient. When he is seated in the dental chair, the patient's attention is focused on his oral condition and on the care he will receive. He will be more receptive to professional recommendations if time is allowed for unhurried discussion of his oral health problems and the operator demonstrates considerate attention to these problems.

I. **DEFINITIONS**

A. **Education:** the process by which the learner acquires knowledge, understanding and new modes of behavior.

B. **Learning:** a sustained change in an individual's behavior as a result of his previous and present experiences.

C. **Teaching:** the communication of knowledge; effective communication depends upon the teacher's skillful utilization of the "Principles of Learning," listed below.

D. **Instruction:** the performance or act of teaching.

E. **Motivation:** a stimulation of behavior that is directed toward fulfillment of a consciously or an unconsciously recognized goal. *Motives* initiate, direct and sustain the individual's behavior.

II. PRINCIPLES OF LEARNING[7]

The Principles of Learning guide the professional person as objectives are formulated, methods are adapted, and outcomes of oral health instruction for each patient are evaluated.

A. Learning takes place more effectively when the individual is physiologically and psychologically ready to learn.
B. Individual differences must be considered if effective learning is to take place.
C. Motivation is essential for learning.
D. Interpersonal relationships are important in motivation and in determining the kinds of social, emotional and intellectual behavior which emerge from the learning situation.
E. What the individual learns in any given situation depends upon what he recognizes and understands.
F. Transfer of learning is facilitated by recognition of similarities and dissimilarities between past experiences and the present situation.
G. An individual learns what he actually uses.
H. Learning takes place more effectively in situations where the individual derives feelings of satisfaction.
I. Evaluation of the results of instruction is essential to determine whether or not learning is taking place.

III. MOTIVATION FOR ORAL HEALTH PRACTICES

An individual is motivated to practice behavior that leads to achievement of goals which he values. The patient's degree of acceptance of the values of oral health and his recognition of the serious consequences of neglect will determine in large measure the extent to which he is motivated to follow professional recommendations.

Dental health instruction can be effective if the patient considers his oral health as a valuable asset or goal. Often the patient needs to have the values of oral health identified for him. The general goals suggested below may be emphasized in order of their importance to the individual, and more specific goals may be identified on the bases of the patient's age, his vocational or socio-economic status, or even casual remarks.

A. General Goals for Maintenance of Oral Health

1. Oral health promotes:
   a. Comfortable service of the masticatory apparatus throughout life.

      b. General health and strength because all nutrients pass through the oral cavity.

      c. Social and peer acceptance as a result of a pleasant smile, inoffensive breath odor, retention of natural facial contours, and maintenance of clear speech with unhindered enunciation.

  2. Oral health prevents:

      a. Unnecessary pain or uncomfortable dental procedures (often more important than esthetics).

      b. Loss of time and money, since it reduces the necessity for professional care appointments.

B. Specific Goals for Maintenance of Oral Health: Examples

  1. *Child's goals:* care for own teeth, thus assert independence; recognize feeling, taste, comfort of clean, healthy mouth.

  2. *Adolescent's goals:* preserve teeth, especially related to careers in military, athletics, movies, television.

  3. *Parent's goals:* improve child's health, appearance, social standing, self-confidence; provide child with opportunity for oral health that parent missed in own youth.

IV. PREPARATION FOR INSTRUCTION

Communication is accomplished on both the conscious and the subconscious levels. The patient consciously receives verbal instruction; subconsciously, he perceives the professional's personality, conviction, and sincerity. The latter factors often determine whether or not the patient accepts the operator's recommendations. Effective communication is based on intelligent preparation of the operator, the patient, and the environment.

A. Preparation of the Operator

  1. Set a good example: maintain general and oral health that demonstrate goals to be valued by the patient.

  2. Develop a positive approach.

      a. Speak firmly and clearly; avoid hesitancy in response.

      b. Use correct grammar and terminology that is meaningful to the patient.

      c. Demonstrate enthusiasm and optimism with regard to the patient's oral health.

B. Preparation of the Patient

  1. Show courtesy to the patient at all times.

  2. Establish friendly professional rapport: guide discussion to focus attention on the patient's oral health; avoid excessive irrelevant conversation.

C. Preparation of the Environment

  1. Before or after operative procedures:

      a. Seat patient in erect position, turn off dental light, and move instruments and equipment out of the way.

      b. Sit or stand so discussion can be conducted at eye level.

2. During operative procedures: continue discussion of patient's oral health but do not ask questions that require complex responses.

V. **METHODS OF INSTRUCTION**

Dental health instruction presented simply and concisely by the methods outlined below will permit efficient use of appointment time and should accomplish the desired results.

A. *Identify* the patient's attitudes, goals and motives for oral health practices.

B. *Explain* and show the patient *what* undesirable conditions exist: give the patient a mirror and use visual aids to clarify explanations.

C. *Explain why* improvement is necessary: emphasize the positive outcomes of improved habits but mention the potential results of neglect and reassure the patient that his oral health can be improved.

D. *Explain* and demonstrate *how* he may attain and maintain oral health: demonstrate techniques exactly as the patient is to practice them and describe the effects of these techniques.

E. *Evaluate* the patient's degree of *perception:* ask him to restate instructions or to demonstrate procedures.

F. *Repeat* instructions or *redemonstrate* procedures to clarify misunderstandings and to reinforce the patient's perception; compliment him for successful endeavors.

G. *Reevaluate* and continue instruction until the patient exhibits satisfactory understanding and a reasonable degree of proficiency in performance of new techniques.

REFERENCES

1. STRIFFLER, D. F.: Dental Health Education; Some Essentials for a State Dental Association's Program, Mich. S. Dent. A. J., *43*, 323, December, 1961.
2. HILL, T. J.: Obligation of the Dentist to His Community, Am. Dent. A. J., *60*, 327, March, 1960.
3. GALAGAN, D. J.: Community Projects for Better Dental Health, Am. Dent. A. J., *66*, 322, March, 1963.
4. McNEIL, D. R.: Time to Walk Boldly, Am. Dent. A. J., *63*, 333, September, 1961.
5. Fluoridation, Am. Dent. A. J., *65*, 578–717, November, 1962 (entire issue).
6. MYERS, S. E.: Promotion of Fluoridation, Dent. Assistant, *30*, 23, July-August, 1961.
7. SAND, OLE: *Curriculum Study in Basic Nursing Education.* New York, Putnam's, 1955, pp. 53–60.

SUGGESTED READINGS

American Dental Association, Bureau of Economic Research and Statistics: A Motivational Study of Dental Care, Am. Dent. A. J., *56*, 435, March, 1958; 566, April, 1958; 745, May, 1958; 911, June, 1958.
DUNNING, J. M.: *Principles of Dental Public Health.* Cambridge, Harvard University Press, 1962, Ch. 15.
FESTINGER, LEON: Cognitive Dissonance, Scien. Amer., *207*, 93, October, 1962.
IRWIN, L. W., CORNACCHIA, H. J. and STATON, W. M.: *Health in Elementary Schools.* St. Louis, Mosby, 1962, Ch. 8.
JAN, H. H.: General Semantic Orientation in Dentist-Patient Relations, Am. Dent. A. J., *68*, 424, March, 1964.

KEGELES, S. S.:　An Interpretation of Some Behavioral Principles in Relation to Acceptance of Dental Care, in Proceedings of 1959 Biennial Conference of State and Territorial Dental Directors with Public Health Service and Children's Bureau. Wash. D. C., Government Printing Office, *Public Health Service Pub.* #698, 1959, pages 21–30.

KEGELES, S. S.:　Some Motives for Seeking Preventive Dental Care, Am. Dent. A. J., *67*, 90, July, 1963.

LEAHY, K. M. and BELL, A. T.:　*Teaching Methods in Public Health Nursing.*　Philadelphia, Saunders, 1952, Chs. 4, 5, 6, and 11.

STOLL, F. A.:　*Dental Health Education*, 2nd ed. Philadelphia, Lea and Febiger, 1960, Chs. 10, 13, 14 and Appendix.

WARNER, E. M.:　Guidelines to Dental Health Programs for Children, J. School Health, *31*, 193, June, 1961.

YOUNG, M. A. C.:　Dental Health Education—Whither? Am Dent. A. J., *66*, 821, June, 1963.

Chapter 26

ORAL PHYSICAL THERAPY: TOOTHBRUSHES AND TOOTHBRUSHING

ORAL PHYSICAL THERAPY: BASIC PRINCIPLES

Oral Physical Therapy consists of methods by which the patient cleanses and massages his oral tissues to maintain oral health. All oral physical therapy procedures are artificial, as compared to natural mechanisms (see page 104).

Natural cleansing of oral structures may occur when an individual masticates hard-textured foods and foods that stimulate salivary flow. However, optimum function of the tongue, lips, saliva, and normal anatomic tooth form and alignment usually cannot remove debris that adheres to retentive areas of the dentition, particularly the pits, grooves, and cervical and approximal surfaces, and in the interdental areas. Most individuals must supplement natural self-cleansing mechanisms with toothbrushes and other devices.

Natural periodontal stimulation results as crisp, hard foods are chewed. As the teeth are occluded, muscular force is applied to crush foreign material held between occlusal or incisal surfaces. Masticatory force depresses periodontal ligament fibers which in turn compress adjacent blood and lymph vessels. Waste products of tissue metabolism are forced out of the compressed capillaries, and as pressure is relaxed, fresh blood and lymph enter the vessels. Capillary stimulation proportionately increases circulation and elimination of waste products from the deeper vessels.[1]

Frequently, as a result of masticatory forces and friction, stratified squamous epithelium of the gingiva undergoes a protective physiological process called *keratinization*. Keratinization is recognized by the layman as cornification, or callousing of skin that has been subjected to friction. Stratified squamous epithelium is composed of many layers of cells. The bottom layer of uniform columnar cells rests on a basement membrane, and each cell extends to underlying connective tissue. Mitotic cell replacement forces older cells toward the outer surface away from the vascular supply, where the cells become less regular in shape. As the outermost layers are reached, cells become flattened, lose their nuclei and die. The protein material of the cell is transformed into *keratin*, and the keratinized remnants of the cell are hard and scaly. Some surface cells, called parakeratotic cells, retain small pyknotic nuclei and are incompletely keratinized. In either case, these calloused layers of epithelium are more resistant to trauma and inflammation than nonkeratinized epithelium.[2]

Supplementary artificial stimulation of the periodontal tissues, particularly the free gingiva, is required when the diet is predominantly soft and when tissues show evidence of breakdown or irritation from local factors. *Massage* is a kneading pressure systematically applied to the gingiva by the fingers,

(271)

toothbrush, or an instrument designed specifically for this purpose. Gingival massage will increase elimination of waste products and circulatory flow in both peripheral and deeper vessels. The amount of keratinization of the gingival epithelium is proportional to the degree, frequency, and method of massage, and to the patient's characteristic physiological responses.

Hundreds of devices have been developed and utilized for the care of the teeth and oral soft tissues. As commercial aspects have become apparent, manufacturers have intensified the development and advertisement of products for public use. Professional recommendations are based on the scientific results of current dental research, and each patient receives oral physical therapy instruction that is in accord with the dentist's beliefs and objectives for his practice.

An informed individual in modern society will agree with members of the dental profession that oral physical therapy measures should be practiced routinely. However, there is an evident gap between knowledge and practice of oral health habits. This barrier may be overcome to some extent if oral physical therapy instruction is planned on the bases of the patient's attitudes toward oral health and on his past practices as reflected by his present oral conditions. An individual's attitudes and values are determined by methods outlined in Chapter 25, pages 267 to 268, and his oral conditions are identified by careful inspection, pages 81 to 85.

ORAL PHYSICAL THERAPY: OBJECTIVES

The fundamental objectives for oral physical therapy are to *cleanse* the oral cavity, particularly the teeth, and to *massage* the gingiva. These objectives apply from either a preventive or a treatment aspect, depending on the status of the patient's oral health.

For the patient undergoing definitive care for periodontal disease, personal oral physical therapy becomes first an essential part of the treatment program, and then an equally essential part of the maintenance phase of care. For other patients, adequate habits of personal oral care contribute to the prevention of oral disease. In either case, the patient becomes an active participant in obtaining and maintaining his own oral health, which is in itself an important objective.

I. OBJECTIVES FOR CLEANSING THE TEETH

Removal of Debris, Materia Alba, and Dental Plaque Reduces the Number of Microorganisms on and About the Teeth. These two objectives contribute to the related objectives listed below. The time factor is of particular importance, since cleansing the teeth immediately following eating provides the greatest benefits.

A. **Aids in the Prevention of Calculus Formation** by removing the components of calculus prior to calcification (see page 126).

B. **Reduces Irritation to the Gingiva:** mechanical irritation from deposits and debris, and chemical irritation from breakdown products of bacterial metabolism.

C. **May Aid in Dental Caries Prevention** when food debris (fermentable carbohydrates) and microorganisms are removed promptly after eating (see pages 113–115).

D. **Combats Halitosis** related to oral uncleanliness.

E. **Improves Appearance** by the removal of unsightly debris.

F. **Enhances the Feeling of Well-Being** and refreshes the taste.

II. OBJECTIVES FOR MASSAGING THE GINGIVA

Effective gingival massage by oral physical therapy to supplement natural mechanisms contributes to oral health in the variety of interrelated effects listed below.

A. **Promotes Keratinization of the Gingiva** which renders it more resistant to infection, inflammation, trauma, and mechanical and bacterial irritation.

B. **Stimulates Blood and Lymph Circulation.**

C. **Improves and/or Maintains Gingival Tone** which contributes to lowered gingival sensitivity to pressure or thermal changes.

D. **Reduces Tendency for Gingival Hemorrhage.**

E. **Contributes to Oral Comfort,** particularly during mastication.

F. **Aids in Maintaining the Normal Characteristics of the Gingiva:** color, size, contour, consistency, surface texture, and position (see page 87).

G. **Prevents Deposit Accumulation** in the submarginal areas since tissue tone and normal characteristics minimize retentive areas, and pressure from massage may force particles of debris out of the gingival sulcus.

Knowledge and understanding of the objectives for oral physical therapy become an essential part of patient instruction. As the patient appreciates what can be accomplished by conscientious, careful, and appropriately-timed oral care, and recognizes the optimum conditions which may be attained, he can learn to evaluate his oral status.

The interpretation of the objectives by the patient depends to a large extent on his motivation. With certain patients the primary purposes for daily routine personal care will be the social aspects of appearance, comfort, particularly during mastication, a pleasant breath, and personal cleanliness in general. Other patients, particularly those threatened by periodontal disease involvement, will be motivated by a fear of losing their teeth. With others, the scientific aspects related to disease prevention will have significance.

Previous neglect or other factors may make it difficult or impossible for a patient to attain ideal conditions even when oral physical therapy measures are conscientiously carried out. One patient will require more emphasis on the cleansing aspects, another on the massaging, whereas a third may need to improve both cleansing and massage. When the patient attains optimum oral conditions for his mouth, he will be rewarded with a feeling of satisfaction that will reinforce his motivation to continue the recommended regimen.

TOOTHBRUSHES

Toothbrushes are the devices used most universally for oral physical therapy procedures in civilized society. The variety of toothbrushes available and the pressures of mass media advertising seriously handicap the consumer when he attempts to select a product best suited to his needs. Without professional counsel, the layman's selection is influenced by persuasive advertisements or displays, a salesperson's advice, or previous conditioning that causes him to buy the same type of product or the least expensive article in the store. Of the foregoing, persuasive advertisements appear to be particularly influential determinants in the consumer's final selection of a toothbrush.

Advertising that claims therapeutic benefits from the use of a product often misleads an individual and gives him a false sense of security in the belief that his oral health will be safeguarded. Beneficial results usually depend upon the individual's requirements and the manner in which a product is used rather than upon its cost, claimed superiority or potential usefulness. To combat misconceptions, each individual is counseled with regard to the many factors specifically involved in his personal oral care.

DEVELOPMENT OF MODERN TOOTHBRUSHES

Before the 17th century, man cleansed his teeth with implements or solutions improvised from his surroundings. A "chewstick," forerunner of the toothbrush, was a twig, chewed at one end to splay the fibers, and used to cleanse teeth and gingiva by drawing the splayed fibers along surfaces of the oral tissues.

In 1600 the ingenious Chinese provided the earliest known literary record of implements designed specifically for oral care procedures. Pierre Fauchard in his classic 1728 publication, *The Surgeon Dentist,* advocated wet sponges and specially prepared herb roots for oral hygienic measures. He indicated that toothbrushes were expensive novelties in the nature of textile mops.[3]

In 1780 an Englishman, William Addis, designed the first toothbrush that resembled modern articles. It consisted of a bone handle with natural bristles drawn into holes bored in the head and secured by wires. By 1840, England, France and Germany began to produce bristle toothbrushes. The first American toothbrush was patented by H. N. Wadsworth in 1857.[3]

Many new varieties of toothbrushes were developed about 1900 when celluloid was introduced and used to manufacture toothbrush handles. In 1919, the American Academy of Periodontology defined specifications for toothbrush design in an attempt to standardize professional recommendations for personal oral care.[4]

Nylon was used in toothbrush construction in 1938. The next year, World War II complications prohibited Chinese exports of hog bristles, and synthetic materials were substituted for natural bristles for the duration of the war. Since 1945, synthetic materials have been improved and manufacturers' specifications have been standardized. As a result, many modern toothbrushes are made exclusively of synthetic materials.[3]

Automatic toothbrushes have been developed over a period of years, but until 1960 the cost of these devices prohibited their widespread distribution. Since improved production methods have made these instruments available to the public, brushes with a variety of power sources and bristle actions have been marketed.

MANUAL TOOTHBRUSHES

According to Kauffman, a toothbrush is defined as follows:

"... an artificial hygienic device ... to brush the teeth, consisting usually of a handle and clusters of bristles so arranged as to exert the most beneficial cleansing action possible, under the conditions present in the mouth of the individual, without causing injury to the hard structures or adjacent soft tissues."[5]

The present criteria for the design of toothbrushes are based on specifications prepared by a committee of the American Academy of Periodontology in 1919.[4]

I. DESCRIPTION (Figure 64)

A. **Handle:** the part intended to be grasped by the hand when the brush is manipulated.

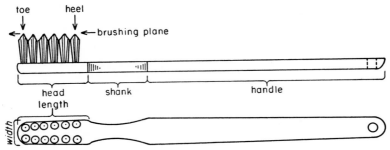

FIGURE 64.—Parts of the toothbrush. The brushing plane is the working end of the toothbrush. Toe end bristles are farthest from and heel end bristles are closest to the handle.

B. **Shank:** that portion which connects the handle and head of the brush.

C. **Head:** that portion which holds the bristles or filaments.

D. **Tufts:** clusters of natural bristles or synthetic filaments secured into the head of the brush.

E. **Brushing Plane:** the surface formed by the free ends of bristles or filaments.

II. HANDLES[5]

A. **Composition**
1. Materials: bone, wood, metal, rubber, celluloid and plastics.
2. *Recommended:* plastics which combine durability, imperviousness to moisture, pleasing appearance, low cost, and semiflexibility with sufficient rigidity for their purpose.

B. **Recommended Design**
1. Dimensions
   a. Adult: 4 to 5 inches long, $\frac{1}{2}$ inch wide, $\frac{3}{16}$ inch thick.
   b. Junior: about $\frac{1}{6}$ smaller than adult size.
   c. Child: about $\frac{1}{3}$ smaller than adult size.

2. Grasp: comfortable and reasonably rigid.
3. Shape: straight. A twist, curve, offset or angle with respect to the brushing plane or head tends to complicate manipulation, although gross deviations of less than 25° do not affect control appreciably.
4. Shank: constricted in width and aligned on handle axis.
5. Finish: smooth and strong.

III. HEADS

A. Composition

1. *Natural bristles*[6]
   a. Source: obtained from the backs of swine. China is the greatest producer and exporter of fine-quality bristles, but with trade prohibited and stockpiles depleted, home products may be used.
   b. Color: bronze and black bristles are superior in quality but not in esthetics. Bleaching, a routine process in preparation, tends to reduce durability.
   c. Stiffness: influenced by factors listed below.
      (1) Diameter of bristle: larger diameters are stiffer. Bristles taken from hogs in the winter or in cold climates are thicker; bristles are thicker near roots than at free ends.
      (2) Length of trim: shorter bristles are stiffer.
      (3) Inherent resiliency: varies with the breed of swine and the degree of absorbency after processing; bristles with retained natural oils absorb water, thus are more resilient.
2. *Nylon filaments*[7]
   a. Source: manufactured according to Federal specifications that govern temperature resistance, stable physical properties, composition, and diameter.
   b. Color: usually translucent and colorless, but can be supplied in opaque, white, black, or colors.
   c. Stiffness: generally, proportional to the square of the diameter and inversely proportional to the square of the length.[8]
      (1) Diameter: thicker filaments are stiffer; $0.010'' =$ soft; $0.012'' =$ medium; $0.014'' =$ stiff (hard); $0.016'' =$ extra stiff.
      (2) Length: shorter filaments are stiffer; a $\frac{1}{32}''$ decrease in length increases stiffness by as much as a $0.001''$ increase in diameter, but marked reduction in length impairs flexibility.[9]
3. Comparison of natural bristles and nylon filaments.[3,7,10]
   a. *Uniform stiffness:* the composition and diameter of nylon filaments can be controlled, which allows a greater uniformity of texture than that obtainable in natural products.
   b. *Resiliency:* nylon filaments retain resiliency longer than natural bristles which lose natural oils during use.
   c. *Durability:* nylon filaments apparently retain their tensile strength longer than natural bristles.[11]
   d. *Drying efficiency:* smooth finish and solid structure of nylon filaments permit easier cleaning than natural bristles which are hollow tubes and may harbor microorganisms.

e. *Cleansing effectiveness:* inconclusive evidence. Natural bristle tips splay during use, thus cover greater surface area, and may be more effective in cleansing action than the smoother nylon filaments.[12] However, little difference in polishing ability between natural bristles and nylon filaments of various diameters has been demonstrated.[13]

f. *Abrasive action:* conflicting evidence.

Neither natural bristles nor nylon filaments abrade tooth structure significantly when used without abrasive dentifrices.[14,15] One report indicated that nylon filaments may abrade enamel surfaces.[16] In another study, natural bristles caused twice as much abrasion of ivory and acrylic resin as nylon filaments.[8]

Bristle texture and resiliency may be of greater importance than composition. Soft nylon filaments of less than 0.009″ diameter abraded simulated dentin more than thicker filaments, presumably because soft bristles bent and matted, therefore covered a greater surface area than thicker filaments.[8,15]

g. *Effect on gingiva:* depends on gingival condition and the method and frequency with which the brush is used.[17,18,19,20]

B. **Recommended Design**

1. Brushing plane
   a. Trim: straight (Figure 65, A and F).
      (1) Flat plane formed by bristles of even trim can be adapted to the curvilinear alignment of teeth and their surrounding gingiva in limited space of oral cavity.[21]

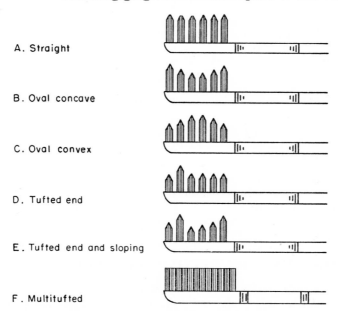

FIGURE 65.—Various trims of brushing planes of toothbrushes. *A.* and *F.* are straight trim, recommended as easiest to manipulate in all areas. *A.* is an example of a "tufted" and *F.* is an example of a "multitufted" brush. *B., C., D.* and *E.* represent typical varieties of unevenly trimmed tufted brushes. The longer tufts strike first and hardest, while the shorter tufts barely reach, or do not reach the surfaces of teeth and soft tissues.

(2) Uneven planes (Figure 65, B through E) are less efficient and may injure teeth and gingiva; short bristles fail to reach proximal areas; longer tufts may exert excessive pressure against facial and lingual surfaces.

b. Dimensions: recommendations are based on the size of the patient's oral cavity, presence of anatomic limitations for brush manipulation, and the ease with which the mouth can be opened. Dimensions suggested below are for average individuals.

(1) Adult: 1 to $1\frac{1}{4}''$ long and $\frac{5}{16}$ to $\frac{3}{8}''$ wide.[21]

(2) Junior: 1 to $1\frac{1}{8}''$ long and $\frac{5}{16}$ to $\frac{3}{8}''$ wide.

(3) Child: $\frac{7}{8}$ to $1''$ long and $\frac{1}{4}$ to $\frac{5}{16}''$ wide.

2. Number of tufts

a. Tufted design: 5 or 6 tufts long and 2 or 3 rows wide.

b. Multitufted design: 10 or 12 tufts long and 3 or 4 rows wide.

IV. THE PROFESSIONAL TOOTHBRUSH

The Council on Dental Therapeutics of the American Dental Association has specified desirable characteristics for toothbrush design.[21] While the Council recognizes that individual preference and manual dexterity may permit successful use of a wide variety of designs, toothbrushes are required to meet specifications for utility, efficiency and cleanliness. A professional toothbrush must:

1. Conform to individual requirements in size, shape and texture.
2. Be manipulated easily and efficiently.
3. Be cleaned and aerated readily.
4. Be impervious to moisture, durable and inexpensive.
5. Have prime functional properties of flexibility, elasticity and stiffness of the bristles; strength, rigidity and lightness of the handle.

A. **Handle:** straight and aligned on same plane as the head.

B. **Head**

1. Length: sufficient to cover approximate width of three adjacent teeth.
2. Width: sufficient inter-row spacing to permit full use of flexibility of bristles and promote cleaning, drying and exposure to air.[3]

C. **Bristles:** tufts and texture suited to the patient's individual requirements and preference. If a patient requires a specific bristle texture related to his oral condition, nylon filament stiffness is uniform, whereas natural bristle stiffness is not standardized.

V. BRISTLE TEXTURE RECOMMENDATIONS

When a patient accomplishes adequate cleansing and massage with his current toothbrushes, no change is necessary and he is encouraged to continue his successful procedures.

A. **Tufted, Hard Texture:** for a patient with normal, healthy gingiva, who brushes carefully and does not injure his gingival epithelium.

B. **Tufted, Medium Texture**
   1. Patient
      a. Adult who may abrade soft tissues with careless use of stiffer bristles.
      b. Child who needs to develop dexterity before stiffer bristles can be used safely.
   2. Cleansing
      a. Teeth out of normal alignment, crowded or overlapped.
      b. Tooth surfaces which are difficult to reach: buccal of maxillary third molar, lingual of mandibular third molar, distal of most posterior tooth, proximal of abutment tooth.
   3. Massaging
      a. Healthy normal gingiva with good tone and in normal position.
      b. Healthy interdental and marginal gingiva: where band of attached gingiva is narrow; where vestibular area is decreased, for example, buccal surfaces of mandibular second and third molars.
      c. Healing gingiva after sufficient epithelization: for example, after control of acute phase of necrotizing ulcerative gingivitis.

C. **Multitufted, Soft Texture**
   1. Patient
      a. Adult: who can accomplish adequate cleansing and massage with soft bristles; who cannot master recommended toothbrushing methods and may abrade soft tissues with stiffer bristles.
      b. Young child who evidences interest in brushing but has not developed sufficient coordination and manual dexterity to control the brush.
   2. Cleansing
      a. Cervical areas of teeth that are malaligned, surrounded by collared gingiva, with exposed root surfaces; or areas adjacent to orthodontic bands.
      b. Proximal surfaces of teeth: that are crowded or overlapped or that are abutments for fixed or removable partial dentures; with receded interdental gingiva.
      c. Teeth with attached orthodontic bands and wires or periodontal splints.
      d. Teeth after gingival surgery until tissue heals to allow application of stiffer bristles.
      e. Gingival surfaces of fixed partial dentures.
   3. Massaging
      a. Hemorrhagic, edematous or enlarged gingiva, until tissue heals to permit use of stiffer bristles.
      b. Hypersensitive gingiva after extensive instrumentation, until tissue heals and stiffer bristles can be used.
      c. Abraded gingiva injured by improper toothbrushing, until tissue heals and toothbrushing method is corrected.

VI. CARE AND SUPPLY OF TOOTHBRUSHES

A. Procedure for Cleaning the Toothbrush
New brushes are supplied in contamination-resistant containers.

Routine rinsing after use will maintain the toothbrush in a hygienic state, and thorough cleansing will decrease the time necessary for bristles to dry and regain their stiffness.

1. Hold head of brush under strong stream of cold water. Hot water softens bristles and reduces their resiliency.
2. Tap the handle against edge of wash basin to loosen remaining particles of dentifrice and debris.
3. Rinse head of brush under stream of cold water.

B. **Procedure for Drying and Storing the Toothbrush**

1. Tap the handle against edge of wash basin to remove excess water.
2. Hang brush with head upward in a rack separate from other brushes to prevent cross-contamination.
3. Do not store wet brush in closed container because this affords an ideal situation for growth of microorganisms.

C. **Supply**

1. Alternately use two, preferably three toothbrushes.
   a. Handle colors should allow differentiation between brushes of various members of a household.
   b. Economic savings result when several brushes are used and bristles are allowed to regain their resiliency between brushings.
   c. Replace worn brushes at spaced intervals so set contains at least one brush in peak condition for daily use.
2. Replace toothbrushes before bristles become frayed, lose resiliency, or become difficult to clean after use.
   a. Durability depends on the original quality of the bristles or filaments and the frequency and manner of their use.
   b. Frayed and broken bristles may puncture or abrade soft tissues.
   c. Soft, nonresilient bristles are less effective and may cause patient to use greater pressure which increases potential for soft tissue injury.

GENERAL PRINCIPLES FOR THE USE OF THE TOOTHBRUSH

The existing oral conditions and requirements of each individual must be considered before oral physical therapy measures are introduced. Many patients can maintain oral health by the correct use of any one of several procedures. The common factor to all successful toothbrushing methods is the systematic and thorough application of the toothbrush to cleanse the teeth and avoid injury of the soft tissues. Fundamentally, the principles listed below apply to all recommended techniques. Specific methods are described on pages 284 to 292.

I. GRASP AND CONTROL

A. **Grasp:** Hold the toothbrush handle firmly in the palm of the hand with fingers curved around the handle.
B. **Control:** Place the thumb against the shank and use wrist action to move the handle.

II. MANIPULATION OF BRUSHING PLANE

A. Cleansing

  1. Lingual and facial surfaces
     a. Place *sides* of bristles on teeth and adjacent gingiva so bristle tips do not lacerate or puncture soft tissues.
     b. Slowly draw bristles over lingual or facial surfaces with bristles flexed onto proximal surfaces.
  2. Cervical areas, submarginal and proximal surfaces
     a. Gently apply bristle tips to surface to be cleansed, with bristles at oblique angle to surface so tips do not lacerate or puncture soft tissues.
     b. Vibrate or rotate brush: move bristles with very short horizontal or circular strokes over surface to be cleansed.
  3. Occlusal surfaces: place bristle *tips* on occlusal surfaces and work tips into pits and fissures to remove debris.

B. Massaging

  1. To promote keratinization: place *sides* of bristles on attached gingiva, flex bristles against marginal and interdental gingiva, and slowly *draw bristles across* soft tissue toward occlusal plane.
  2. To promote circulation: place *sides* of bristles on gingiva, flex bristles against gingiva, and vibrate or rotate brush to provide intermittent pressure and relaxation; *hold free ends of bristles in position.*

III. GENERAL BRUSH PLACEMENT

Because of the curvature of the dental arches and the relative inaccessibility of certain tooth surfaces, particular attention should be given to the systematic placement of the toothbrush on all exposed tooth surfaces and surrounding gingiva. A routine order of brushing will prevent overbrushing or omission of particular areas.

A. Recommended Brushing Routine

Recommendations are based on knowledge of the patient's oral condition, the results of his previous personal oral care habits, his preferences, and his capability to perform suggested procedures. Areas that the patient has missed or brushed incompletely are brushed first to take advantage of the stiffness and peak efficiency of the bristles. The patient usually is alert and careful at the beginning of the toothbrushing routine, and if he brushes difficult areas first, he may establish desired habits more quickly because his attention is concentrated on new procedures.

  1. *Arch:* mandibular teeth first. Research has indicated that maxillary teeth are brushed more thoroughly.[22,23,24,25,26,27]
  2. *Surfaces:* lingual, facial, then occlusal. Most individuals brush labial surfaces of anterior teeth most thoroughly, then buccal surfaces of maxillary molars; many individuals fail to brush lingual surfaces.[25,26,27]
  3. *Side:* right for right-handed individuals, left for left-handed, although research has not indicated conclusively that these areas are more difficult.[24,25]

4. *Order:* lingual surfaces, right to left; facial surfaces, right to left; occlusal surfaces, right side, left side; order can be reversed if the patient finds it simpler to perform.

B. **Brush Placement for Systematic Coverage of Entire Arch** (Figure 66)

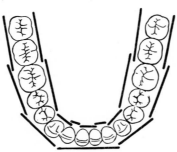

FIGURE 66.—Positions for bristle placement to provide complete coverage of all teeth. Each position overlaps the adjacent position. Short lines adjacent to lingual surfaces of anterior teeth indicate the width of the brushing plane, while longer lines elsewhere indicate the length of the toothbrush head.

The length of the brushing plane usually covers surfaces of three adjacent teeth, and the width covers approximately one tooth surface. The first brush placement allows toe-end bristles to extend past the most posterior tooth on one side of the arch. In succeeding positions, end bristles overlap previously brushed teeth to provide thorough coverage of the entire arch.

1. Posterior teeth: use full length of brushing plane; two positions are minimum when second and third molars present.
2. Anterior teeth
   a. Facial surfaces: use full length of brushing plane; three positions are minimum from cuspid-to-cuspid if teeth are in normal alignment.
   b. Lingual surfaces: use width of brushing plane; five to seven positions are minimum from bicuspid-to-bicuspid.

IV. **BRUSH PLACEMENT ADAPTATIONS FOR LIMITED ACCESSIBILITY**

Certain areas are difficult to brush no matter which method or toothbrush is used. Procedures suggested below involve brush placement adaptation when access is limited because of tooth position, gingival condition, anatomic form or oral anatomy.

A. **Hard-to-Reach Tooth Surfaces**

1. *Distal surfaces of most posterior teeth* (Figure 67).
   a. Distobuccal surface: insert brushing plane parallel to buccal surface with toe-end bristles extended past distal surface; then press handle against cheek and partially occlude teeth.
   b. Distolingual surface: insert brushing plane parallel to lingual surface with toe-end bristles extended past distal surface; then retract tongue with back of brush head and extend handle across incisal edges of opposite anterior teeth.

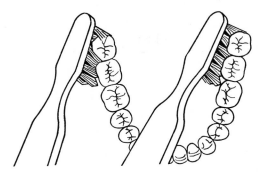

FIGURE 67.—Brush placement to cleanse distal surfaces of most-posteriorly-erupted teeth using Rolling Stroke or Modified Stillman's Method. Brush is held at oblique angle to distal surface so toe-end bristles cover surface to be cleansed.

2. *Proximal surfaces of teeth adjacent to edentulous areas.*
   a. Distal surfaces: see A. 1, above.
   b. Mesial surfaces: place brushing plane at right angle to facial surface of tooth and apply sides of toe-end bristles to mesial surface; or place brushing plane at oblique angle to mesial surface and retract cheek with handle to gain access.
3. *Exposed surfaces of malposed teeth:* place sides of bristles against free gingiva, then with short strokes, slowly shimmy bristles over cervical areas and proximal surfaces of teeth.
4. *Cervical areas and exposed root surfaces:* place sides of bristle tips just above margin of free gingiva, flex bristles onto tooth surface, and gently shimmy bristles over cervical areas onto exposed root surfaces.
5. *Occlusal surfaces of erupting teeth partially covered by soft tissue:* carefully work toe-end bristle tips into occlusal pits and grooves to loosen debris, but do not puncture soft tissue.

B. **Anatomic Limitations**
   1. *Taut cheek musculature*
      a. Insert brushing plane parallel to buccal surfaces of molars, then press handle against cheek and partially occlude teeth to bring mandible into lateral excursion.
      b. Use a junior-size toothbrush if necessary to gain access.
   2. *Taut lip muscles or short labial frenums:* retract lip with back surface of brush head or with fingers of free hand.
   3. *Narrow arch:* place width of brushing plane over cingulum of each anterior tooth and adjacent interdental areas.
   4. *Short lingual frenum:* use brush with shorter brushing plane (but not shorter trim), or cut off one or two heel rows of bristles until length of brushing plane can be adapted to lingual surfaces.
   5. *Macroglossia:* retract tongue with back of brush head to gain access to lingual surfaces of mandibular molars.
   6. *Hypersensitive gag reflex:* have patient raise head which relaxes muscle tension and places tongue in a more distal rest position.

V. AMOUNT OF BRUSHING

No correlation has been found between efficiency of results and the length of time expended to brush the teeth.[28] In a group of 7- to 12-year-old children, less than two minutes were used per brushing, and the second minute was used by most to brush labial surfaces of anterior teeth.[27] Seventy-five per cent of a group of 2- to 5-year-olds brushed for less than 20 seconds.[9] Fifty dental students, who should have been motivated to brush thoroughly, averaged 2.3 minutes per brushing with standard brushes in a controlled test.[28]

The lack of correlation between brushing time and efficiency may be due to two factors: first, an individual cannot judge the passage of time accurately while he concentrates on the performance of a manual skill; secondly, he brushes accessible areas for longer periods of time than he brushes hard-to-reach areas. Because timed procedures cannot assure thorough coverage, it is recommended that the patient count the number of strokes for each brush position. Suggestions below are minimum for a patient with normal or slightly subnormal oral conditions.[29]

A. **Six Strokes in Each Area:** to cleanse teeth and promote keratinization of gingiva.

B. **Count of Ten** (while brush is vibrated and bristle ends are held in position): to massage gingiva and loosen debris in interdental and cervical areas and on proximal surfaces.

VI. BRUSHING THE TONGUE

A. **Objectives:** removes debris and dead epithelial cells and thereby stimulates circulation and imparts a feeling of oral cleanliness and a temporary improvement of breath odor.

B. **Procedure**[30]
1. Extrude the tongue.
2. Hold brush handle at right angle to dorsal surface of tongue (as for labial surfaces of anterior teeth).
3. Direct bristle tips toward throat.
4. Place sides of bristle tips on surface of tongue, as posteriorly as possible, avoiding initiation of the gag reflex.
5. Exert very gentle pressure, and draw the brush forward and over the tip of the tongue. Avoid "scrubbing" the papillæ.
6. Repeat several times until debris is removed.

RECOMMENDED PROFESSIONAL TOOTHBRUSHING METHODS

When performed conscientiously, most toothbrushing methods can accomplish their dual objectives: cleansing and massage. Successful results without injury to the teeth or soft tissues are the criteria by which a method of toothbrushing is evaluated. If a patient's method is successful in all but a few areas, he is instructed to use a supplementary technique that will improve results in those areas.

Professional toothbrushing methods described in this section are recommended by most dental authorities and may be accomplished with the use of manual toothbrushes. These methods are compared on the bases of indications for use, techniques, advantages and disadvantages in Table 11.

I. **ROLLING STROKE METHOD**

The American Dental Association recommends this method for use by an individual with a normal, healthy mouth to cleanse the teeth and massage the gingiva.[31]

A. **Indications for Use**

1. Patient: child or adult with sufficient coordination and manual dexterity to manipulate brush.
2. Cleansing: teeth in normal or slightly deviant alignment.
3. Massaging
   a. Normal, healthy gingiva when interdental gingiva has not receded, to promote keratinization.
   b. Spongy, but not hemorrhagic gingiva; example: before oral surgery, to increase tone.

B. **Technique**[31]

1. Facial surfaces, all teeth; lingual surfaces, posterior teeth.
   a. *Place* brush (Figure 68A).
      (1) Direct bristles toward apices of teeth; upward for maxillary and downward for mandibular teeth.
      (2) Place sides of bristles on attached gingiva, slightly beyond free gingival groove, with brush head parallel to occlusal plane.

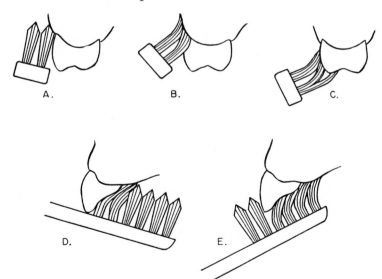

FIGURE 68.—Rolling stroke method of toothbrushing. *A.* Sides of ends of bristles placed against cervical areas of teeth and free gingiva. *B.* Brush turned to flex bristles against gingiva and onto interdental papilla. *C.* Brush drawn toward occlusal plane while brushing plane is swept across teeth. *D.* Brush placement for lingual surfaces of anterior teeth; handle held perpendicular to labial surfaces of adjacent teeth and heel end bristles flexed against cervical area of teeth and gingiva. *E.* Handle drawn forward and away from incisal edge to permit sides of bristle ends to contact lingual surfaces of teeth.

TABLE 11.—COMPARISON OF RECOMMENDED PROFESSIONAL TOOTHBRUSHING METHODS

Method	Indications for Use	Advantages	Disadvantages
ROLLING STROKE Bristles: toward apices and flexed onto gingiva, 45° angle. Stroke: long sweep over gingiva and teeth.	Patient—with sufficient coordination. Cleansing—normal dentition. Massaging—normal or slightly enlarged gingiva.	Simplest method to learn and use. Cleanses effectively. Stimulates periodontal circulation. Promotes keratinization.	Young child may have insufficient coordination. Careless technique may fail to cleanse cervical and proximal surfaces, and may lacerate gingiva. Quick strokes may be inadequate to cleanse proximal and cervical surfaces and interdental areas when gingiva is receded.
MODIFIED STILLMAN'S Bristles: toward apices and flexed onto gingiva, 45° angle. Stroke: vibrate to 10 count, then perform rolling stroke.	Patient—with sufficient coordination. Cleansing—normal dentition; interdental and cervical areas and proximal surfaces when gingiva slightly receded; exposed root surfaces; proximal surfaces of teeth next to edentulous areas. Massaging—hypersensitive, enlarged or slightly receded gingiva.	Easier than Charters' Method and can be learned by most who require supplementary gingival massage. Shimmying bristle action loosens soft deposits from cervical areas and proximal surfaces. Stimulates periodontal circulation more than Rolling Stroke.	Requires more time and effort than Rolling Stroke Method. Careless technique may injure soft tissues.
CHARTERS' Cleanse teeth first with Rolling Stroke or Modified Stillman's Method. Facial surfaces: Bristles: toward occlusal at 45° angle, flexed onto interdental gingival crests. Stroke: vibrate to 10 count. Lingual surfaces, posterior teeth: handle across opposite cuspid; toe-end bristles toward linguals and flexed interdentally. Lingual surfaces, anterior teeth: handle parallel with long axes of teeth; toe-end bristles toward linguals and flexed interdentally.	Patient—with high degree of manual dexterity and motivation. Cleansing—exposed proximal and root surfaces; malaligned teeth; gingival surfaces of fixed partial dentures and proximals of abutments; teeth after gingival surgery until tissue heals. Massaging—moderately or severely receded gingiva; healing gingiva after periodontal therapy or extensive instrumentation; gingiva underlying fixed partial dentures.	Most effective method for interdental gingival massage. Bristle position provides least potential for soft tissue injury.	Requires more skill and patience than other methods. May require substitution of Modified Stillman's Method for lingual surfaces. Since technique requires more time, patient may try to hurry and become careless.

(286)

    b. Press brush (Figure 68B).
        (1) Turn brushing plane toward teeth until head is at 45°
            angle to tooth surfaces.
        (2) Flex bristles onto interdental and marginal gingiva and
            press until tissue blanches.
    c. Roll brush (Figure 68C).
        (1) Slowly draw bristles across gingiva and tooth surfaces
            with a rolling motion toward occlusal plane.
        (2) Maintain pressure to flex bristles onto cervical areas and
            proximal surfaces of teeth.
    d. Repeat six times over each area covered by brushing plane.
    e. Continue to adjacent area; allow end tufts to overlap brushed
       area.
  2. Lingual surfaces, anterior teeth.
    a. Place brush (Figure 68D)
        (1) Position handle at right angle to long axes of teeth.
        (2) Place heel bristles on interdental gingiva so bristle tips
            extend apically beyond cervical areas of adjacent teeth.
    b. Press brush: flex bristles over interdental gingiva onto cer-
       vical areas of adjacent teeth (Figure 68D).
    c. Roll brush: slowly pull handle forward and away from incisal
       edges in an arcuate motion (Figure 68E).
    d. Repeat six times, then *continue* to next embrasure.
  3. Occlusal surfaces (see II. A. 3., page 281).

C. **Advantage:** the simplest professional method which provides ade-
    quate cleansing and stimulation for most individuals.

D. **Disadvantages**
  1. A young child with undeveloped muscular coordination may not
    be able to master brush placement and manipulation; however,
    it is advisable to present an adequate professional method as
    early as possible to avoid the formation of undesirable habits.
  2. Careless bristle placement may lacerate soft tissues; bristle tips
    will puncture gingiva if pressed against it.
  3. If the rolling stroke is accomplished quickly, the bristles are not
    flexed onto debris-retentive areas: cervical areas apical to
    heights of contour; root surfaces and concave proximal sur-
    faces exposed by receded or blunted gingiva; receded inter-
    dental gingiva.

II. MODIFIED STILLMAN'S METHOD

    Stillman's Method originally was intended to massage the gingiva
rather than to cleanse the teeth. The modification of this method in-
corporates the rolling stroke which cleanses the facial, lingual and
cervical surfaces of the teeth, and the interdental gingiva.

A. **Indications for Use**
  1. Patient: adult with sufficient motivation and manual dexterity
    to vibrate the brush, yet maintain bristle tip position and
    avoid tissue injury.

2. Cleansing
   a. Concave proximal surfaces, cervical surfaces below heights of contour, and root surfaces exposed by blunted or receded gingiva.
   b. Proximal surfaces of teeth adjacent to edentulous areas.
3. Massaging
   a. Hypersensitive, spongy or swollen gingiva, to restore tone.
   b. Interdental gingiva that has receded slightly below contact areas of adjacent teeth.

B. **Technique**[32]

1. Facial surfaces, all teeth; lingual surfaces, posterior teeth.
   a. Place brush.
      (1) Direct bristles toward apices of teeth; upward for maxillary and downward for mandibular teeth.
      (2) Place sides of bristles on attached gingiva, but not beyond mucogingival junction, with brush head parallel to occlusal plane.
   b. Press brush (Figure 69A).

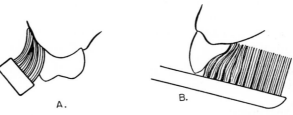

A.　　　　　　　　　　B.

FIGURE 69.—Modified Stillman's Method of toothbrushing. *A.* Sides of ends of bristles flexed against cervical areas of teeth and gingiva. *B.* Heel-end bristles flexed against lingual surface of anterior teeth and gingiva; handle extends at right angle to labial surfaces of adjacent teeth.

      (1) Turn brushing plane toward teeth until head is at 45° angle to tooth and gingival surfaces.
      (2) Flex bristles over interdental and marginal gingiva; press until tissue blanches.
   c. Vibrate brush.
      (1) Maintain pressure and bristle flexion.
      (2) Vibrate brush handle back and forth in short strokes to a count of ten; hold bristle ends in position on gingiva.
   d. Roll brush (Figure 68 C).
      (1) Slowly roll bristles across gingiva and tooth surfaces toward occlusal plane.
      (2) Maintain pressure to flex bristles onto cervical and proximal surfaces of teeth.
   e. Repeat six times over each area.
   f. Continue to adjacent area; allow end tufts to overlap brushed area.
2. Lingual surfaces, anterior teeth.
   a. Place brush (Figure 69 B).
      (1) Position handle at right angle to long axes of teeth.

        (2) Place heel bristles on interdental gingiva so bristle tips extend beyond cervical areas of adjacent teeth.

    b. Press brush: flex bristles over marginal gingiva and proximal and cervical surfaces of teeth.

    c. Vibrate brush.

        (1) Maintain pressure and bristle flexion.

        (2) Vibrate brush handle from side-to-side in short strokes to a count of ten; hold bristle ends in position on gingiva.

    d. Roll brush: slowly pull handle forward and away from incisal edges in an arcuate motion (Figure 68 E).

    e. Repeat six times, then *continue* to next embrasure.

  3. Occlusal surfaces (see II. A. 3., page 281).

C. Advantages

1. Most patients who require supplementary massage can master these brush placements and vibratory movements.
2. As brush is vibrated, bristle ends move slightly over smooth tooth surfaces and loosen debris attached to retentive areas ordinarily missed with the rolling stroke.
3. Vibratory movements stimulate circulation of the deeper vessels of the periodontium and massage interdental gingiva to a greater extent than the rolling stroke.

D. Disadvantages

1. More time and effort are required than for the Rolling Stroke Method, and patient must be motivated to perform more complex technique.
2. Method requires muscular coordination and manual dexterity to avoid injury to gingiva as brush is vibrated.

III. CHARTERS' METHOD

Charters' Method frequently is employed in the maintenance phase of periodontal therapy. It provides the greatest measure of gingival massage when correctly used by the patient.

A. Indications for Use[33]

1. Patient: who requires supplementary interdental gingival massage and who possesses sufficient patience, coordination and manual dexterity to perform the technique without injury to the soft tissues.
2. Cleansing
   a. Cervical and root surfaces and concave proximal tooth surfaces exposed by receded, blunted or hyperplastic gingiva.
   b. Retentive surfaces of malaligned teeth.
   c. Gingival surfaces of fixed partial dentures and proximal surfaces of abutment teeth.
   d. Teeth after periodontal surgery until tissue heals.
3. Massaging
   a. Moderately or severely receded gingiva, particularly interdental gingiva.

    b. Healing gingiva that has epithelized after: surgery, particularly where tissue tends to proliferate; conservative periodontal therapy, for example, after acute phase of necrotizing ulcerative gingivitis has subsided; extensive removal of submarginal calculus.

    c. Gingiva underlying fixed partial dentures and around abutment teeth.

B. Technique[34]

 1. Use Rolling Stroke or Modified Stillman's Method first to cleanse facial and lingual surfaces and to loosen food and debris impacted in proximal and cervical areas.

 2. Facial surfaces, all teeth.

   a. Place brush (Figure 70*A*).

    (1) Direct bristles toward occlusal plane, downward for maxillary and upward for mandibular teeth.

    (2) Place bristles at a 45° angle to occlusal plane with brush parallel to occlusal plane.

    (3) Bring edge of brushing plane to gingival margins; maintain the 45° angle between the occlusal plane and bristles.

   b. Press brush (Figure 70 B).

    (1) Flex sides of bristles over marginal and interdental gingiva until tissue blanches.

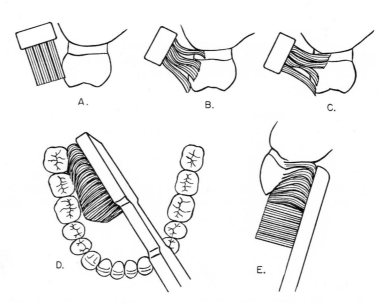

Figure 70.—Charters' Method of toothbrushing. Facial surfaces: *A.* Brush head parallel to occlusal plane; bristles directed occlusally and at a 45° angle to occlusal plane. *B.* Sides of bristles flexed over marginal and interdental gingiva and extended over proximal surfaces of teeth. *C.* Brush rotated to count of ten with sides of bristles flexed against soft tissues; *bristle tips do not move over soft tissues* during massage. *D.* Lingual surfaces, posterior teeth: brush handle extended across opposite cuspid; toe-end bristles flexed interproximally; sides of bristles flexed against marginal and interdental gingiva and proximal surfaces of teeth. *E.* Lingual surfaces, anterior teeth: brush handle held parallel to long axes of teeth; toe-end bristles flexed interproximally; sides of bristles against marginal and interdental gingiva and proximal surfaces of teeth.

(2) Allow some bristles to extend interproximally, flexed against crests of interdental gingiva and proximal surfaces of teeth.

    c. *Vibrate* brush (Figure 70 C).

      (1) Maintain pressure and bristle flexion.

      (2) Vibrate brush handle with slight rotary motion to a count of ten; hold bristles in position on soft tissue.

    d. Carefully *remove* brush and *repeat* 3 or 4 times in same area.

    e. *Continue* to adjacent area; allow end tufts to overlap brushed area.

3. Lingual surfaces, posterior teeth (Figure 70 D).

    a. *Place* brush.

      (1) Extend brush handle across incisal edge of opposite cuspid.

      (2) Direct bristles slightly apically and toward lingual surfaces of teeth.

      (3) Place toe-end bristles against interproximal embrasure.

    b. *Press* brush.

      (1) Flex sides of bristles onto marginal and interdental gingiva until tissue blanches.

      (2) Allow some bristles to extend interproximally, flexed against crests of interdental gingiva and proximal surfaces of teeth.

    c. *Vibrate* brush; hold bristles in position on soft tissue.

    d. *Repeat* 3 or 4 times in same area, then *continue* to adjacent interproximal embrasure.

4. Lingual surfaces, anterior teeth (Figure 70E).

    a. *Place* brush.

      (1) Insert brush handle parallel to long axes of teeth.

      (2) Direct bristles toward lingual surfaces of teeth.

      (3) Place side of toe-end bristles over interproximal embrasure.

    b. *Press* brush.

      (1) Gently press brush apically and toward lingual surfaces until bristles flex against marginal and interdental gingiva.

      (2) Allow some bristles to extend interproximally over crest of interdental gingiva and proximal surfaces of teeth.

    c. *Vibrate* brush; hold bristles in position on soft tissue.

    d. *Repeat* 3 or 4 times in same area, then *continue* to adjacent interproximal embrasure.

C. **Advantages**

1. Interdental gingival circulation is stimulated best by this method, since sides of bristles are extended over interdental crests and flexed onto the soft tissues.

2. There is less chance for soft tissue injury when bristles are directed occlusally and flexed over marginal and interdental gingiva, hence this is the method of choice for massage of hypersensitive gingiva.

D. **Disadvantages**

1. Performance of this technique requires a high degree of manual dexterity and much supervised practice to achieve desired results.

2. Brush placement on lingual surfaces of posterior teeth is difficult and the Modified Stillman's technique may be recommended in these areas; opposite direction of bristle placement may confuse the patient.
3. Charters' Method requires more time than other methods, and after the patient has learned the technique, he may try to hurry and become careless.

OTHER TOOTHBRUSHING METHODS

Toothbrushing methods described in this section are recommended less universally than those described in the preceding section. However, some of these methods may accomplish the desired cleansing or massage when used by a conscientious patient.

I. HIRSCHFELD'S METHOD

Hirschfeld's Method is similar to Charters' except that less pressure is applied and bristle action is used more effectively for cleansing than for massage.

A. Indications for Use
1. Patient: who lacks dexterity or ability to master Modified Stillman's or Charters' Method.
2. Cleansing: cervical and proximal surfaces of teeth and interdental tissues when gingiva is slightly receded.
3. Massaging: interdental and marginal gingiva.

B. Technique[29]
1. Facial surfaces: teeth are occluded and brush is placed as for Charters' Method; bristle tips are allowed to move slightly during vibration. Maxillary, then mandibular teeth are brushed before brush is moved to the next embrasure.
2. Lingual surfaces: toe-end bristles are placed and activated as in Charters' technique for lingual surfaces of anterior teeth.

C. Advantages: This method provides fairly effective interdental and marginal gingival massage and adequate cleansing of cervical areas of the teeth. With the teeth occluded, bristle flexion is stabilized somewhat by cheek pressure against the back of the brush head.

D. Disadvantages: Considerable dexterity is required to manipulate the brush on lingual surfaces; bristle placement on buccal surfaces of posterior teeth is difficult to visualize with the teeth occluded.

II. SCRUB BRUSH METHOD[35]

This method is used most often by very young children who apply bristles to occlusal surfaces of mandibular teeth and scrub vigorously as one would scrub a floor. If the circular scrubbing motions are applied with a soft-bristled brush, some debris may be removed and the soft tissues may not be injured. When bristle tips are drawn across soft tissues with sufficient force, abrasion may result. The lingual surfaces usually are not brushed by individuals who use this method.

III. FONES' METHOD

Fones' Method is similar to the Scrub Brush Method, except that it has been refined to include the facial and lingual surfaces in a systematic manner. This method may be recommended for very young children who evidence interest in toothbrushing but who cannot perform a more complex method.

A. Technique[36]

1. Facial surfaces: with the teeth occluded, place bristles against maxillary and mandibular teeth and quickly revolve brush head; draw bristles across teeth and against marginal gingiva of alternate arches.
2. Lingual surfaces: with mouth open, make small circular strokes on lingual surfaces of first one arch, then the other.
3. Occlusal surfaces: scrub the brushing plane over occlusal surfaces.

B. Disadvantages

1. Soft deposits impacted in interproximal areas are not removed.
2. May traumatize soft tissues, especially if a hard-textured brush is used.
3. May cause gingival recession or formation of McCall's festoons (collared gingiva, where marginal gingiva is blunted and forms collar around facial surface of tooth).
4. Deposits may be forced into gingival sulci.

IV. HORIZONTAL METHOD

A. Technique: place bristles at right angles to facial or lingual surfaces of teeth and gingiva, and forcefully draw bristles across surfaces with long horizontal strokes.

B. Disadvantages[37]

1. Proximal surfaces are not cleansed, and soft deposits are forced into interproximal areas.
2. Chronic use may cause gingival recession, particularly on labial surfaces of cuspids which are brushed vigorously and longer than other areas.
3. Chronic use with a dentifrice may cause root surface abrasion when marginal gingiva has receded.

V. VERTICAL (LEONARD'S) METHOD

A. Technique: with teeth occluded and anterior teeth held edge-to-edge, direct bristles at right angles to facial surfaces; use a slight rotary movement to draw bristles up and down over teeth.[38]

B. Disadvantages[39]

1. Proximal surfaces are not cleansed; cervical areas are not cleansed and deposits may be forced into gingival sulci.
2. Interdental and marginal gingiva are not massaged and may be traumatized by bristle tips.
3. Chronic use may cause gingival recession and formation of McCall's festoons.

VI. PHYSIOLOGIC (SMITH-BELL) METHOD[40,41]

A. **Technique:** use a very soft-textured brush; draw bristles over tooth surfaces and onto the gingiva in the same pathway that food travels (hence the name "Physiologic").

B. **Disadvantages**

1. Soft-bristled brush does not remove soft deposits from teeth nor massage gingiva effectively.
2. Careless performance of technique or use of stiffer brush will abrade soft tissues.

VII. BASS' METHOD[42]

This method requires the use of a toothbrush that has soft-textured nylon filaments with rounded ends, supplemented by the use of smooth, thin, unwaxed nylon dental floss to cleanse proximal surfaces of teeth.

A. **Technique:** with bristles directed apically at 45° angle to long axes of teeth, place bristle tips on gingival margins and submarginal surfaces of teeth, then vigorously apply bristles with short strokes.

B. **Advantage:** cervical areas of teeth below heights of contour and exposed root surfaces of teeth can be cleansed.

C. **Disadvantages**

1. Careless technique or use of stiffer-bristled brush can abrade gingiva and eventually cause gingival recession.
2. Use of abrasive dentifrice with this technique will abrade cementum.
3. Apical direction of bristles prevents effective massage of interdental gingiva.

AUTOMATIC TOOTHBRUSHES AND TOOTHBRUSHING

I. AUTOMATIC TOOTHBRUSHES

Automatic toothbrushes are the most recent innovations available on a wide-scale basis for oral physical therapy procedures. Differences between manual and automatic brushes lie in the mechanical action of the bristles and the size of the handles, which contain motors to activate the bristles. Motors are energized either by direct connection to a line current or by batteries in the handles. The head and shank are constructed as a unit that is detachable from the handle. Shorter brushing planes have been provided for automatic than for adult manual brushes, and soft-textured filaments have been used.

Principles for the care and supply of automatic brush units are the same as for manual brushes. If electricity is used as the energy source, the connecting cord should be inspected periodically to insure its safe condition.

The American Dental Association's Council on Dental Therapeutics has undertaken the study of automatic toothbrushes.[43]   Council specifications for these brushes are similar to those for manual brushes: durability, inexpensiveness, and design that promotes cleaning and aeration of the bristles. Basic criteria are related to the safe, unsupervised use of the brushes. They must be free from the hazards of electrical shock and they should be capable of cleansing the oral cavity effectively and efficiently without damage to the soft and hard tissues when used as directed.[44]

II. AUTOMATIC TOOTHBRUSHING

Consumer appeal of automatic brushes is based on bristle actions which are intended to perform the actual work of oral physical therapy while the user holds the brushing plane against the surface to be cleansed or massaged.   Various bristle actions include short horizontal strokes, arcuate strokes, rotary strokes, or combinations of these.

Instructions for the use of an automatic brush depend on its bristle action: a brushing plane that moves in short horizontal strokes or small circular strokes can be used to perform the Rolling Stroke, Modified Stillman's or Charters' Method; a brushing plane with an arcuate motion can be applied at the incisal or occlusal thirds of teeth, moved to the cervical areas, then returned to the original position.   Careless bristle placement and prolonged brushing in one area should be avoided, since the automatic bristle action is more rapid than that accomplished with manual brushes.

The Council has stated that automatic brushes may be especially useful for handicapped patients who cannot activate the manual brush effectively, or for patients whose handicaps require that their teeth be brushed by an attendant.[44] Regardless of the kind of toothbrush selected, successful results will depend primarily upon the conscientious method by which the device is used.

SUMMARY OF HARMFUL EFFECTS FROM IMPROPER TOOTHBRUSHING

Although the toothbrush has proven beneficial effects in the attainment and maintenance of oral health, carelessness in the use of this implement may produce harmful effects to the oral cavity.   According to Hirschfeld:

> "...injuries are induced mainly when the individual is uninstructed in proper brushing, lacks mechanical aptitude in the handling of the brush, or uses it when contraindicated; as well as when the brush is too old, or is improperly constructed."[45]

Since 1939 when Hirschfeld summarized the causes of toothbrush abrasion, dental scientists have corroborated his statements and added a significant finding: injurious effects of toothbrushing are magnified greatly when the brush is used with an abrasive dentifrice.[15,19]

Alterations of the gingiva and teeth listed in this section can be observed during the oral inspection. Since injury from improper use of the toothbrush is preventable, the operator needs to be alert to recognize traumatic effects in the early stages. Many times, inadequate habits of personal oral care can be corrected before permanent injury occurs.

As the patient demonstrates his toothbrushing method prior to oral physical therapy instruction, faulty habits of toothbrush manipulation often are apparent. After a relationship is established between improper toothbrushing and altered oral structures, the operator explains the condition, its etiology, and the necessary corrective procedures. The patient is instructed to follow professional recommendations carefully, because, as he attempts to use new methods, he may become overzealous and cause further injury.

I. ALTERATIONS IN THE GINGIVA

A. Acute Alterations[46]
1. Appearance
    a. Scuffed epithelial surface with denuded underlying connective tissue which results in a painful bruise.
    b. Punctuate lesions which appear as red, pinpoint spots.
    c. Diffuse redness and denuded attached gingiva.
2. Etiology
    a. Horizontal or vertical scrubbing toothbrushing method.
    b. Incorrect use of a new, hard-textured toothbrush.
    c. Overvigorous application of the toothbrush.
    d. Penetration of gingiva by bristle ends.
    e. Use of toothbrush with frayed, broken bristles.
    f. Application of bristles beyond attached gingiva.

B. Chronic Alterations[47]
1. Location
    a. Usually appear only on the facial gingiva, because of the vigor with which toothbrush is used.
    b. Frequently, inversely related to the right- or left-handedness of the patient.
    c. Areas most often involved are around cuspids or teeth in labio- or buccoversion.
2. Appearance
    a. Gingiva receded; cementum exposed.
    b. Large festoons (McCall's festoons): the interdental papillæ may remain at normal height and the tissue is usually pink and firm.
    c. Narrow grooves that extend from crest of free gingiva to the attached gingiva; tissue usually is pink and firm.
3. Etiology[46,47]
    a. Repeated use of a vigorous rotary, vertical, or horizontal toothbrushing method over a long period of time.
    b. Use of a long brisk stroke with excessive pressure, over a long period of time.
    c. Habitual prolonged brushing in one area.
    d. Excessive pressure applied with a worn, nonresilient brush.

C. Suggested Corrective Measures
1. Recommend substitution of a softer-bristled toothbrush until the acute phase of alteration subsides and normal tissue tone is restored.
2. Correct patient's toothbrushing method or recommend toothbrushing method better suited to his oral condition.
3. Recommend suitable method of gingival massage, including interdental massage, to improve gingival tone and to recontour the gingiva where possible.

II. **ABRASION OF THE TEETH**[48]

Harmful effects of the toothbrush on tooth structure are termed *abrasion*. Abrasion refers to loss of tooth substance produced by mechanical wear other than that produced by mastication.

A. **Location**

1. Primarily found on the facial surfaces, especially of cuspids and teeth in labio- or buccoversion.
2. Primarily found on the exposed cervical area of the root. The cementum is very thin near the cemento-enamel junction, and once the dentin is exposed, it abrades readily; on adjacent teeth, the cervical borders of the lesions are usually on the same plane.
3. Occasionally found on the cervical third of the anatomical crown.
4. Rarely found on the incisal or occlusal one-third.

B. **Appearance**

1. Wedge-shaped defect: horizontal V-shaped groove, bounded apically by the free gingiva and incisally or occlusally by the cervico-enamel junction.
2. Saucer-shaped defect: rounded concavity on the cervical one-third of the crown.
3. The concavities are usually smooth surfaced and shiny, in contrast to chalky, friable, pre-carious lesions.

C. **Etiology**

1. Generalized abrasion
   a. Chronic incorrect brushing with a very hard-textured tooth brush.
   b. Continued use of a dentifrice containing too harsh an abrasive.
   c. Vigorous horizontal or circular brushing.
2. Localized abrasion
   a. Vigorous or prolonged toothbrushing in one area.
   b. Bucco- or torsoversion of tooth or teeth: eminent surfaces often are over-brushed.

D. **Suggested Corrective Measures**

1. Recommend bristle texture suited to patient's strength and manual dexterity.
2. Suggest patient change to a less abrasive dentifrice (see pages 307–309).
3. Recommend method of toothbrushing better suited to patient's oral conditions.

III. **PREVENTION OF HARMFUL EFFECTS**

A. **Bristle Placement and Strokes**

1. Carefully place sides of bristles on, not above, attached gingiva; bristle tips may puncture gingiva if inserted at right angles.
2. Allow sides of bristles to transmit pressure and relaxation when brush is used to apply gingival massage; *hold bristle tips in position on soft tissues* as brush is vibrated.

3. Apply bristles carefully after extensive instrumentation, particularly when new toothbrush and/or new method are instituted.
4. Discard toothbrush when bristles start to splay.
5. Lift brushing plane off the teeth and gingiva between successive strokes so bristle tips are not drawn across soft tissues.
6. Use short vibratory movements on occlusal surfaces rather than long circular movements that extend bristle tips onto soft tissues.
7. Avoid overvigorous brushing on facial surfaces of cuspids and teeth in bucco- or torsoversion.
8. Hold lip away from teeth to gain accessibility and observe bristle placement in mirror to avoid accidental catch and pull by bristles on free margins of gingiva.

B. **Routine**

1. Use mirror to watch toothbrushing procedure to assure correct position of brushing plane and coverage of all surfaces.
2. Follow an orderly routine of brushing to avoid prolonged brushing in one area and insufficient brushing in other areas.
3. Concentrate on systematic brush placement and activation; do not become distracted or attempt to hurry.

C. **Untoward Results:** If sensitive areas persist for more than two days after initiation of a new toothbrushing method, consult the dentist or dental hygienist.

CONTRAINDICATIONS FOR TOOTHBRUSHING[49,50]

Although toothbrushing is of demonstrated benefit in the attainment and maintenance of oral health, certain oral conditions are not amenable to the mechanical action of the bristles. Open lesions present during the acute phase of periodontal or oral mucous membrane involvements can be irritated if bristles are drawn over the lesions.

Open lesions are hypersensitive and the patient usually will not brush teeth surrounded by these lesions unless he receives specific instructions. He needs to be encouraged to use a soft-textured brush to cleanse and massage these areas as soon as the epithelium is intact to promote complete epithelization. In all cases, the policy established by the dentist is followed when the patient is instructed in oral physical therapy measures for acute disturbances.

REFERENCES

1. MILLER, S. C.: *Textbook of Periodontia*, 3rd ed. New York, Blakiston Division, McGraw-Hill, 1950, pp. 320–322, 334–335.
2. WOLPE, P.: *Ueber Verhornungserscheinungen am Zahnfleischepithel, Deutsche Mschr. f. Zahnheilk, 45,* 1, 1927, cited by Glickman, I: *Clinical Periodontology*, 2nd ed. Philadelphia, Saunders, 1958, p. 21.
3. McCAULEY, H. B.: Toothbrushes, Toothbrush Materials and Design, Am Dent. A. J., *33,* 283, March 1, 1946.
4. American Academy of Periodontology, Committee Report: The Toothbrush and Methods of Cleaning the Teeth (Read Oct. 17, 1919), Dent. Items Interest, *42,* 193, March, 1920.
5. KAUFFMAN, J. H.: A Study of the Toothbrush, Dent. Cosmos, *66,* 300, March, 1924.
6. KAUFFMAN, J. H.: A Study of the Toothbrush. (IV.), Am. Dent. A. J., *26,* 32, January, 1939.
7. HINE, M. K.: The Toothbrush, Internat. Dent. J., *6,* 15, March, 1956.

8. HARRINGTON, J. H. and TERRY, I. A.:   Automatic and Hand Toothbrushing Abrasion Studies, Am Dent. A. J., *68*, 343, March, 1964.
9. KIMMELMAN, B. B. and TASSMAN, G. C.:   Research in Designs of Children's Toothbrushes, J. Dent. Child., *27*, 60, First Quarter, 1960.
10. WADE, A. B.:   A Clinical Assessment of the Relative Physical Properties of Nylon and Bristle Brushes, Brit. Dent. J., *94*, 260, May 19, 1953.
11. SWARTZ, M. L., PHILLIPS, R. W., and HINE, M. K.:   Effect of Certain Factors upon Toothbrush Bristle Stiffness, J. Periodont., *27*, 96, April, 1956.
12. HINE, M. K., WACHTL, CARL, and FOSDICK, L. S.:   Some Observations on the Cleansing Effect of Nylon and Bristle Tooth Brushes, J. Periodont., *25*, 183, July, 1954.
13. PHILLIPS, R. W. and SWARTZ, M. L.:   Effects of Diameter of Nylon Bristles on Enamel Surface, Am. Dent. A. J., *47*, 20, July, 1953.
14. MANLY, R. S. and BRUDEVOLD, FINN: Relative Abrasiveness of Natural and Synthetic Toothbrush Bristles on Cementum and Dentin, Am. Dent. A. J., *55*, 779, December, 1957.
15. PHANEUF, E. A., HARRINGTON, J. H., DALE, P. P., and SHKLAR, GERALD: Automatic Toothbrush: A New Reciprocating Action, Am. Dent. A. J., *65*, 12, July, 1962.
16. KRUSIC, VALTER: An Investigation of Toothbrushes and Toothpastes in Yugoslavia, *Zobozdrov Vest*, *10*, 239, October-December, 1955, (Abstracted in D. Abstr., *1*, 579, October, 1956).
17. STAHL, S. S., WACHTEL, N., DeCASTRO, C., and PELLETIER, G.:   The Effect of Toothbrushing on Keratinization of the Gingiva, J. Periodont., *24*, 20, January, 1953.
18. HINIKER, J. J. and FORSCHER, B. K.:   The Effect of Toothbrush Type on Gingival Health, J. Periodont., *25*, 40, January, 1954.
19. BEYELER, KARL, and MOOSER, MAX: Tooth Abrasions, Gingival Injuries and Daily Oral Hygiene, *Schweiz. Mschr. Zahnhk.*, *20*, 123, February, 1960, (Abstracted in D. Abstr., *6*, 51, January, 1961).
20. MAURICE, C. G. and WALLACE, D. A.:   Toothbrush Effectiveness: Relative Cleansing Ability of Four Toothbrushes of Different Design, III. Dent. J., *26*, 286, May, 1957.
21. American Dental Association Council, on Dental Therapeutics: *Accepted Dental Remedies*, 29th ed. Chicago, American Dental Association, 1964, pp. 175–176.
22. CHILTON, N. W., deDIO, ANTHONY, and ROTHNER, J. T.:   Comparison of the Clinical Effectiveness of an Electric and a Standard Toothbrush in Normal Individuals, Am. Dent. A. J., *64*, 777, June, 1962.
23. CROSS, W. G., FORREST, J. O., and WADE, B. A.:   A Comparative Study of Tooth Cleansing Using Conventional and Electrically Operated Toothbrushes, Brit. Dent. J., *113*, 19, July 3, 1962.
24. DERBYSHIRE, J. C. and MANKODI, S. M.:   Gingival Keratinization with Hand and Electric Toothbrushes: A Cytological Comparison, Am. Dent. A. J., *68*, 255, February, 1964.
25. ELLIOTT, J. R.:   A Comparison of the Effectiveness of a Standard and an Electric Toothbrush, J. Periodont., *34*, 375, July, 1963.
26. PARFITT, G. J.:   Cleansing the Subgingival Space, J. Periodont., *34*, 133, March, 1963.
27. LEFKOWITZ, WILLIAM and ROBINSON, H. B. G.:   Effectiveness of Automatic and Hand Brushes in Removing Dental Plaque and Debris, Am. Dent. A. J., *65*, 351, September, 1962.
28. QUIGLEY, G. A. and HEIN, J. W.:   Comparative Cleansing Efficiency of Manual and Power Brushing, Am. Dent. A. J., *65*, 26, July, 1962.
29. HIRSCHFELD, ISADOR: The Why and How of Toothbrushing, Am. Dent. A. J., *32*, 80, January, 1945.
30. GOLDMAN, H. M.:   *Periodontia*, 3rd ed. St. Louis, Mosby, 1953, p. 693.
31. American Dental Association: *Toothbrushing*. Chicago, American Dental Association, October, 1961. Pamphlet G6 200 M, 10–61. 6 pp.
32. STILLMAN, P. R.:   A Philosophy of the Treatment of Periodontal Disease, Dent. Digest, *38*, 315, September, 1932.
33. ROTH, HARRY, THALLER, JACK, and ALDERMAN, N. E.:   The Charters Method of Toothbrush Massage: A Valuable Supplement in Periodontal Therapy, J. Periodont., *27*, 309, October, 1956.
34. CHARTERS, W. J.:   Home Care of the Mouth. I. Proper Home Care of the Mouth, J. Periodont., *19*, 136, October, 1948.
35. COOLIDGE, E. D. and HINE, M. K.:   *Periodontia*, 3rd ed. Philadelphia, Lea & Febiger, 1958, pp. 414–415.
36. FONES, A. C.:   *Mouth Hygiene*, 4th ed. Philadelphia, Lea & Febiger, 1934, p. 300.
37. GOLDMAN, H. M., SCHLUGER, SAUL, FOX, LEWIS, and COHEN, D. W.:   *Periodontal Therapy*, 2nd. ed. St. Louis, Mosby, 1960, p. 46.
38. LEONARD, H. J.:   Conservative Treatment of Periodontoclasia, Am. Dent. A. J., *26*, 1308, August, 1939.

39. HIRSCHFELD, ISADOR: *The Toothbrush: Its Use and Abuse*. Brooklyn, Dent. Items Interest Pub. Co., 1939, pp. 369–371.
40. SMITH, T. S.: Anatomic and Physiologic Conditions Governing the Use of the Toothbrush, Am. Dent. A. J., *27*, 874, June, 1940.
41. BELL, D. G.: Teaching Home Care to the Patient, J. Periodont., *19*, 140, October, 1948.
42. BASS, C. C.: An Effective Method of Personal Oral Hygiene, II, Louisiana S. Med. Soc. J., *106*, 100, March, 1954.
43. American Dental Association, News of Dentistry: Other Actions—House of Delegates, 1963 Annual Meeting, Am. Dent. A. J., *67*, 709, November, 1963.
44. American Dental Association, Council on Dental Therapeutics: op. cit., p. 176.
45. HIRSCHFELD: op. cit., p. 181.
46. GLICKMAN, IRVING: *Clinical Periodontology*, 2nd ed. Philadelphia, Saunders, 1958, pp. 364–365.
47. HIRSCHFELD: op. cit., p. 262.
48. GLICKMAN: op. cit., pp. 471–472.
49. HIRSCHFELD, ISADOR: Gingival Massage, Am. Dent. A. J., *43*, 290, September, 1951.
50. SORRIN, SIDNEY, ed.: *Periodontia*. New York, Blakiston Division, McGraw-Hill, 1960, pp. 317–318.

SUGGESTED READINGS

American Dental Association, Council on Dental Therapeutics: Current Status of Electric Toothbrushes, Am. Dent. A. J., *69*, 404, September, 1964.
ASH, M. M., JR.: Manual Toothbrush and Use of Other Aids, Am. Dent. Hygienists' A. J., *38*, 78, Second Quarter, 1964.
BERTOLINI, ADRIANO and EMILIN, REGGIO: Experimental Research on the Effects of Mechanical Gingival Massage, *Paradontol.*, (Zurich) *9*, 114, Dec., 1955, (Abstracted in D. Abstr., *1*, 543, September, 1956).
BIRCH, R. H. and MUMFORD, J. M.: Electric Toothbrushing, Dent. Pract., *13*, 182, January, 1963.
BUEBE, F. E.: *Periodontology*. New York, Macmillan, 1953, pp. 220–242, 345–347.
BUNTING, R. W.: *Oral Hygiene*, 3rd ed. Philadelphia, Lea & Febiger, 1957, pp. 278–283.
COOLIDGE, E. D. and HINE, M. K.: *Periodontia*, 3rd ed. Philadelphia, Lea & Febiger, 1958, pp. 406–421.
COPENHAVER, W. M., ed. and JOHNSON, D. D.: *Bailey's Textbook of Histology*, 14th ed. Baltimore, Williams and Wilkins, 1958, Ch. IV., Epithelium.
CURTIS, G. H., McCALL, C. M., JR., and OVERAA, H. I.: A Clinical Study of the Effectiveness of the Roll and Charters' Methods of Brushing Teeth, J. Periodont., *28*, 277, October, 1957.
DUMMETT, C. O.: Prophylactic Periodontics, J. Periodont., *31*, 40, January, 1960.
GLICKMAN, IRVING: *Clinical Periodontology*, 2nd ed. Philadelphia, Saunders, 1958, pp. 364–365, 570–571, 929–946.
GOLDMAN, H. M., SCHLUGER, SAUL, FOX, LEWIS, and COHEN, D. W.: *Periodontal Therapy*, 2nd ed. St. Louis, Mosby, 1960, pp. 598–604.
GOLDMAN, H. M., et al.: *An Introduction to Periodontia*, 2nd ed. St. Louis, Mosby, 1962, pp. 324–343.
GRANT, DANIEL, STERN, I. B., and EVERETT, F. G.: *Orban's Periodontics*, 2nd ed. St. Louis, Mosby, 1963, pp. 25, 31, 105–106, 299–317, 326.
GREEN, ALBERT, ROSENSTEIN, S. N., PARKS, ALLEN, and KUTSCHER, A. H.: The Electric Toothbrush as an Adjunct in Maintaining Oral Hygiene in Handicapped Patients, J. Dent. Child., *29*, 169, Third Quarter, 1962.
GREENE, A. H.: A Study of the Characteristics of Stippling and Its Relation to Gingival Health, J. Periodont., *33*, 176, April, 1962.
HINE, M. K.: Use of the Toothbrush in Treatment of Periodontitis, Am. Dent. A. J., *41*, 158, July, 1950.
HIRSCHFELD, ISADOR: *The Toothbrush: Its Use and Abuse*. Brooklyn, Dent. Items Interest Pub. Co., 1939, pp. 180–329.
HOOVER, D. R. and ROBINSON, H. B. G.: Effect of Automatic and Hand Toothbrushing, Am. Dent. A. J., *65*, 361, September, 1962.
IWERSEN, A. E. and WERKING, D. H.: Hand and Automatic Toothbrushes: Effectiveness in Inhibiting Brown Pellicle, Am. Dent. A. J., *68*, 178, February, 1964.
KAPUR, KRISHAN and SHKLAR, GERALD: Effects of a Power Device for Oral Physiotherapy on the Mucosa of the Edentulous Ridge, J. Prosth. Dent., *12*, 762, July-August, 1962.
KELNER, MORRIS: The Use of an Electrically Powered Toothbrush in the Home Dental Care of Handicapped Children, Pennsylvania Dent. J., *28*, 3, November, 1961.
KOBYLANSKA, MARIA and NEYMAN, MARIA: Contamination, Disinfection and Preservation of Toothbrushes, *Czas. Stomat.*, *14*, 889, November, 1961, (Abstracted in D. Abstr., *7*, 530, September, 1962).

KRASSE, B. and BRILL, N.: Effect of Consistency of Diet on Bacteria in Gingival Pocket in Dogs, *Odont. Revy.*, *11*, 152, June, 1960, (Abstracted in D. Abstr., *6*, 175, March, 1961).

LOBENE, R. R.: The Effect of an Automatic Toothbrush on Gingival Health, J. Periodont., *35*, 137, March-April, 1964.

MELVILLE, T. H.: Bacteria on the Toothbrush, Brit. Dent. J., *111*, 90, August 1, 1961.

MERZEL, JOSE, VIEGAS, A. R., and MUNHOZ, C. O. G.: Contribution to the Study of Keratinization in Human Gingiva, J. Periodont., *34*, 127, March, 1963.

MILLER, S. C.: *Textbook of Periodontia*, 3rd ed. New York, Blakiston Division, McGraw-Hill, 1950, pp. 86–88, 320–342, 556–557.

ORBAN, BALINT: Clinical and Histologic Study of the Surface Characteristics of the Gingiva, Oral Surg., Oral Med. & Oral Path., *1*, 827, September, 1948.

ORBAN, BALINT: Hornification of the Gums, Am. Dent. A. J., *17*, 1977, November, 1930.

ROBINSON, H. B. G. and KITCHIN, P. C.: Effect of Massage with the Toothbrush on Keratinization of the Gingivae, Oral Surg., Oral Med. & Oral Path., *1*, 1042, November, 1948.

ROTH, HARRY: An Appraisal of the Motorized Toothbrush, J. Periodont., *34*, 517, November, 1963.

SANDERS, W. E. and ROBINSON, H. B. G.: Effect of Tooth Brushing on Deposition of Calculus, J. Periodont., *33*, 386, October, 1962.

SHICK, R. A. and ASH, M. M., JR.: Evaluation of the Vertical Method of Toothbrushing, J. Periodont., *32*, 346, October, 1961.

SLACK, G. L. and MARTIN, W. J.: Apples and Dental Health, Brit. Dent. J., *105*, 366, November 18, 1958.

SMITH, W. A. and ASH, M. M., JR.: A Clinical Evaluation of an Electric Toothbrush, J. Periodont., *35*, 127, March-April, 1964.

SOPARKAR, P. M. and QUIGLEY, G. A.: Power Versus Hand Brushing: Effect on Gingivitis, Am. Dent. A. J., *68*, 182, February, 1964.

SORRIN, SIDNEY, ed.; *The Practice of Periodontia*. New York, Blakiston Division, McGraw-Hill, 1960, pp. 12–14, 302–311, 318.

SORRIN, SIDNEY: The Use of the Toothbrush as a Preventive and Cure, Dent. Cosmos, *73*, 378, April, 1931.

STANMEYER, W. R.: A Measure of Tissue Response to Frequency of Toothbrushing, J. Periodont., *28*, 17, January, 1957.

STILLMAN, P. R.: Stimulation of the Gingiva, Am. Dent. A. J., *15*, 1077, June, 1928.

TERRY, I. A. and HARRINGTON, J. H.: Abrasion Tests on Acrylics, Am. Dent. A. J., *65*, 377, September, 1962.

TOTO, P. D.: The Clinical Usefulness of the Broxodent Automatic Action Toothbrush in Home and Institutional Oral Hygiene, Pub. Health Dent., *22*, 15, Spring, 1962.

VOLKER, J. F. and CALDWELL, R. C.: Prophylactic and Operative Techniques in Dental Caries Prevention, in FINN, S. B., ed.: *Clinical Pedodontics*, 2nd ed. Philadelphia, Saunders, 1962, pp. 682–685.

VOWELS, J. K.: Assessment of an Automatic Action Toothbrush (Broxodent) in Spastic Children, Brit. Dent. J., *115*, 327, October 15, 1963.

WILCOX, C. E. and EVERETT, F. G.: Friction on the Teeth and the Gingiva during Mastication, Am. Dent. A. J., *66*, 513, April, 1963.

Chapter 27

ORAL PHYSICAL THERAPY: SUPPLEMENTARY MEASURES

ALTHOUGH the toothbrush is the major instrument used for oral physical therapy procedures, various other implements and agents may be required for individuals with special needs and may be beneficial to all patients. Interdental areas and tooth surfaces that are inaccessible to bristle action of the toothbrush may be cleansed with dental floss, dental tape, mechanical devices by which streams of water can be directed through the interdental area, and various other devices. Enlarged or receded interdental and marginal gingiva may be massaged with instruments designed for this purpose. Dentifrices which provide slight abrasiveness are valuable aids in the removal of soft deposits and stains. Rinsing with lukewarm water dilutes retained fermentable carbohydrates and contributes to the removal of loosened debris.

A patient may need to use more than one supplementary aid described in this chapter, or he may require only a dentifrice and water rinse as supplements to an adequate toothbrushing method. The patient needs professional instruction in the use of all oral physical therapy devices that are recommended for him.

SUPPLEMENTARY AIDS TO CLEANSE PROXIMAL TOOTH SURFACES AND FIXED PARTIAL DENTURES

Areas of food impaction which appear to require restorative work are called to the dentist's attention, since the patient's routine use of temporary measures to relieve pressure and discomfort in these areas does not remove the cause of the symptoms. Permanent damage to the gingiva may result if proximal surfaces are contoured improperly or fail to contact adjacent teeth. When thorough toothbrushing is inadequate to cleanse the teeth, the patient is instructed to use supplementary devices after toothbrushing, to observe his performance in a mirror, and to rinse thoroughly with water afterward to assure the removal of loosened debris.

I. **DENTAL FLOSS AND DENTAL TAPE** (described on pages 186 to 188).

  A. **Indications for Use**

  1. Patient: who is interested and conscientious and who will follow instructions carefully to avoid injury to his soft tissues.
  2. Oral condition
     a. Proximal surfaces of: crowded or overlapped teeth; teeth surrounded by enlarged gingiva with deep gingival sulci, or by receded gingiva associated with exposed root surfaces.
     b. Gingival surfaces of fixed partial dentures and proximal surfaces of abutment teeth.

B. **Technique: Proximal Surfaces of Adjacent Teeth**

1. Prepare strand: use a 12-inch length; longer strands become contaminated and shorter cannot be grasped effectively.
2. Grasp about $\frac{1}{2}$ inch of strand and hold taut between thumbs and index fingers.
3. Position strand.
    a. Position at oblique angle against contact on facial aspect; place pad of index finger or thumb against contact area.
    b. Slowly tighten grasp and draw toward lingual through contact area. *Do not* use excessive pressure to snap through contact because the thin strand may lacerate crest of interdental papilla. (Figure 40, page 187).
    c. Draw strand against one proximal surface and gently work apically to the depth of the gingival sulcus; avoid laceration of marginal gingiva.
    d. Carefully return strand to contact area to remove debris from the sulcus, then draw strand $\frac{1}{2}$ inch facially or lingually to remove debris from interproximal area.
    e. Adapt unused area of strand to adjacent proximal surface and repeat 3 and 4, above.
    f. Remove strand from interproximal area: work occlusally or carefully pull from facial aspect until contact is cleared.
4. Polish proximal surfaces.
    a. Use dental tape which presents a wide, flat surface.
    b. Apply a small amount of dentifrice on facial aspect of contacts of one quadrant or arch at a time.
    c. Work dentifrice over proximal surfaces in the manner outlined in 3, above.

C. **Technique: Fixed Partial Denture and Abutments**

1. Prepare strand: use a 12-inch length.
    a. Fold one end to double thickness and press loop until it is reduced to smallest diameter.
    b. For very limited access where pontics are closely adapted: dip end of strand in molten wax and allow wax to harden; or use plastic floss threader.[1]
2. Position strand.
    a. Grasp double thickness of strand next to loop and thread loop between appliance and gingiva where access is greatest, usually adjacent to abutment tooth.
    b. Draw lingually until double thickness clears tissue and appliance, then grasp single thickness.
3. Remove soft deposits.
    a. Hold $\frac{1}{2}$-inch length of strand taut between thumbs and index fingers.
    b. Draw against proximal surface of abutment tooth and slowly work to depth of gingival sulcus, then back to gingival surface of appliance.
    c. Draw strand $\frac{1}{2}$ inch facially or lingually to remove debris from the area.
    d. Draw unused area against gingival surface of appliance, and with strand held taut against appliance, slowly work it over appliance to the other abutment.

    e. Draw strand ½ inch facially or lingually and repeat steps *a* through *c*, above, on proximal surface of other abutment.

    f. Draw another unused portion over the gingival surface of the appliance to the original position.

    g. Remove carefully from the embrasure: hold against junction between appliance and abutment and carefully draw strand through from the facial aspect.

4. Polish: apply dentifrice to facial aspect of abutments and appliance and work dentifrice over surfaces as in 3, above.

II. SOFT BALSA WOOD WEDGE

A. Indications for Use

1. Patient who will follow instructions carefully to avoid injury to interdental gingiva.
2. Oral conditions
    a. Exposed proximal surfaces when interdental papillae are receded and interproximal embrasures are constricted in width.
    b. Exposed concave proximal surfaces of teeth that are inaccessible to toothbrush bristles or dental tape.

B. Technique[2,3]

1. Soften wood: place pointed end in mouth and moisten with saliva.
2. Position wedge: apply base of wedge on slope of interdental papilla and insert into interdental embrasure until wedge fills the interdental area; avoid excessive pressure against crest of interdental gingiva.
3. Cleanse proximal surfaces: withdraw wedge slightly and replace 10 or 12 times.
4. Posterior teeth: break wedge in half and use pointed end from facial aspect.
5. Precautions
    a. Discard wedge after 2 or 3 embrasures are cleansed or when it has lost shape, before wood splays or splinters, to avoid injury to gingiva.
    b. Do not substitute flat, hardwood toothpick: shape not useful in interdental embrasures and wood may splinter.

C. Disadvantages

1. Careless use may injure interdental papillae: excessive pressure may cause further recession; use after wood is splayed may force splinters into soft tissues.
2. Wedge can be applied only from facial aspect.
3. Excessive pressure applied between adjacent teeth may force teeth apart.

III. HYDROTHERAPY (PRESSURE WASHING)[4]

A. Indications for Use

1. Receded interdental papillae, to cleanse interproximal area.
2. Following acute phase of gingival disease when epithelium is

denuded, or after gingival surgery until tissue heals, to remove debris and promote healing.

   3. Gingival surfaces of fixed partial dentures and proximal surfaces of abutment teeth to remove debris loosened with toothbrush or dental floss.
   4. Orthodontic appliances or periodontal splints, to cleanse interdental areas and proximal and cervical surfaces of teeth when use of toothbrush is inadequate or disturbs position of appliances.

B. **Description:** flow of lukewarm stream of water or physiologic saline solution directed to area of debris impaction by one of mechanical devices listed below.

   1. Pressure bottle with hand pump, with attached capillary tube.
   2. Commercially available device that can be attached to water faucet.[5]
   3. Water syringe (bulb holds water).
   4. Glass hypodermic syringe, 50 ml. capacity.

C. **Technique:** place tip of instrument next to interdental area and allow force of water or saline solution to remove debris.

IV. GAUZE STRIP[6]

A. **Indications for Use:** teeth which are spaced widely, or which border edentulous areas, to cleanse proximal surfaces inaccessible to toothbrush.

B. **Technique**

   1. Prepare strip: cut 1-inch gauze bandage into 6-inch length and fold down center.
   2. Position fold on cervical area of tooth, next to gingival crest and work back and forth several times; avoid excessive pressure of fold against soft tissue.

V. PIPE CLEANER[7]

A. **Indications for Use:** exposed bifurcation or trifurcation or proximal surfaces inaccessible to toothbrush bristle action.

B. **Technique**

   1. Carefully work end of cleaner through space between tooth and gingiva; avoid pressing wire end into soft tissue.
   2. Work about 1 inch of sides of cleaner back and forth against tooth surfaces several times, then withdraw from facial aspect.

SUPPLEMENTARY AIDS TO MASSAGE THE GINGIVA

When the gingiva is abnormal in contour, height, consistency or tone, the toothbrush usually cannot provide adequate massage. Supplementary devices for the application of artificial massage are selected on the basis of their proposed use, to massage either the interdental gingiva, or the facial and lingual gingiva. Massage can assist in the achievement of gingival

20

health when it is performed carefully according to instructions, and routinely after toothbrushing at least twice each day. Correct use of selected devices also will loosen debris from tooth surfaces inaccessible to toothbrush bristle action.

I. INTERDENTAL STIMULATORS

A. Composition and Design

1. Flexible rubber tip, conical or pyramidal in shape, attached to the end of a toothbrush or special handle.
2. Soft balsa wood or flexible plastic wedge, triangular in cross-section, and of toothpick length.

B. Indications for Use

1. Receded interdental papillae where space exists for insertion of device without injury to soft tissue, to stimulate circulation and promote keratinization.
2. Flattened or cratered interdental papillae, to recontour tissue.
3. After acute phase of gingival disease has subsided or when tissue has epithelized after surgery, to stimulate circulation, to promote keratinization and to aid in recontouring papillae.
4. Exposed bifurcations or trifurcations, to loosen debris and to promote circulation and keratinization of surrounding gingiva.
5. Unstimulated gingiva around abutment teeth for fixed or removable dentures, to promote circulation and keratinization.
6. Adjunct of choice
   a. *Recommended:* conical rubber tip used where interdental area permits access because it is least likely to cause injury to the soft tissues.
   b. Soft balsa wood or flexible plastic wedge: used where access is limited, and only as instructed to avoid injury to interdental papillae.

C. Technique: Conical Rubber Tip

1. Insert rubber tip from the facial aspect as far as possible into interdental area without excessive force or pressure.
2. Turn handle toward gingiva until side of cone rests on slope of interdental papilla (Figure 71A).
3. Slowly rotate handle with side of cone held in position on the soft tissue. Provide intermittent pressure against soft tissue and tooth surfaces (Figure 71B). Continue rotation to slow count of 10.

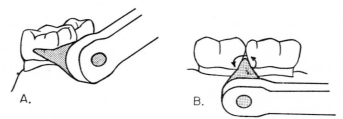

FIGURE 71.—Conical rubber tip interdental stimulator.
A. Side of cone in position on buccal slope of interdental tissue, causing slight compression.
B. Buccal view of conical rubber tip in position; arrows show direction of circular movement. Tip is not moved; massaging action results from slight pressure applied as handle is rotated.

4. Carefully remove tip and repeat procedure at next embrasure until all accessible areas are massaged.
5. Apply tip to lingual aspect where access permits.
6. *Exposed bifurcations and trifurcations:* apply tip to exposed root surfaces and underlying gingiva where access permits; rest side of cone on gingiva and direct tip obliquely toward occlusal plane.
7. *Gingiva surrounding abutment teeth or teeth adjacent to edentulous areas:* apply side of tip to gingiva at desired plane of contour; avoid excessive pressure on soft tissue.

D. **Technique: Soft Balsa Wood or Flexible Plastic Wedge:** see II, page 304.

II. GINGIVAL STIMULATORS

The side of the rubber tip stimulator may be used to massage marginal gingiva over facial and lingual surfaces of the teeth. However, when the margin of the free gingiva is enlarged or the gingival crest has receded excessively, the devices listed below may provide more effective stimulation.

A. **Digital Massage:** gentle intermittent pressure is applied by the thumb and forefinger (see page 194).

B. **Soft Rubber Cups**

1. Description: one to three soft rubber cups, similar in shape and size to those used by professionals to polish teeth, are attached to a handle. The rims of the cups form a "stimulating plane" similar to the brushing plane of the toothbrush.
2. Indications for use
   a. Grossly enlarged marginal gingiva, to reduce enlargement by pressure atrophy.
   b. Hypersensitive gingiva or epithelized gingiva following acute phase of gingival disease or surgery, to stimulate circulation and promote keratinization, and to cleanse exposed cervical areas of involved teeth.
3. Technique
   a. Place stimulating plane over enlarged tissue.
   b. Apply light pressure, then rotate handle to a count of 10 with the *cups held in position* on soft tissue.

DENTIFRICES

Dentifrices are pastes or powders that aid the toothbrush or dental tape in the removal of debris and stains from the teeth. Abrasive action of dentifrices is not required by every individual,[8] and in fact is contraindicated for a patient whose exposed root surfaces or nonkeratinized gingiva may be cut by abrasive particles. A patient may be advised to use a toothbrush moistened with water. If extrinsic stains accumulate after a period of two weeks, sodium bicarbonate may be recommended for a similar period and, if the mild abrasiveness of sodium bicarbonate is ineffective, the patient may use a commercial dentifrice periodically to remove the stain.[9]

The American Dental Association, Council on Dental Therapeutics studies and considers for classification the dentifrices that include biologically active ingredients for which therapeutic or prophylactic benefits are claimed, but does not consider dentifrices designated only to cleanse the teeth.[10]

All products evaluated by the Council are classified into one of four groups as follows:[11]

Group A: Products accepted by the Council and listed in *Accepted Dental Remedies*. These products may use the Seal of Acceptance as long as they conform to specifications of the Council.

Group B: Products for which reasonable evidence of usefulness and safety has been demonstrated and for which research is in progress. New evidence is reviewed each year, and a product may remain in this classification for three years.

Group C: Products for which there is inconclusive or limited evidence for accurate evaluation. Further study by qualified investigators is indicated.

Group D: Products which do not meet the Council's standards for acceptance.

Through its annual publication, *Accepted Dental Remedies*, and through periodic announcements in the *Journal of the American Dental Association*, the Council provides the profession with reliable information on the status of commercial dental products. Ingredients of commercial dentifrices are described in the section below.

I. CLEANSING DENTIFRICES

A. Indications for Use

1. Pleasant flavor encourages patient to brush his teeth.
2. Mild abrasiveness helps remove debris and stain and polishes teeth.
3. Toothpaste, rather than powder, is recommended for very small children because paste is easier to manipulate.

B. Basic Ingredients[12]

1. *Abrasive agent:* when drawn across tooth surfaces, aids in removal of soft debris and polishes surfaces.
   a. Proportion: comprises bulk of the dentifrice.
   b. Types currently used: calcium carbonates, phosphates, or sulfates; sodium metaphosphate, bicarbonate or chloride; magnesium carbonates or phosphates; hydrated aluminum oxide.[13,14,15]
   c. Criteria for selection: abrasive action that engages and removes soft deposits and stains that do not yield to chemical detergents, yet does not remove tooth structure with normal use. Properties of abrasive agents are described on pages 168–170.
2. *Surface-active detergent:* lowers surface tension, penetrates and loosens soft deposits, and emulsifies or suspends debris removed from tooth surfaces.
   a. Proportion: varies; claims for anti-cariogenic effects have been based on dentifrices' "foaming abilities," but claims are unsubstantiated.

    b. Types currently used: sodium lauryl sulfoacetate, sulfoco-laurate.[13]

    c. Criteria for selection: nontoxic, neutral in reaction, active in either acid or alkaline medium, stable, compatible with other dentifrice ingredients, no distinctive taste, and does not form precipitates in hard water or saliva.

  3. *Binding agents:* hold dry ingredients together in the form of a paste.

    a. Proportion: varies; adequate to maintain consistency of mixture.

    b. Types currently used
      (1) Liquids to retain moisture content: glycerin, propylene glycol, sorbitol.
      (2) Thickeners to prevent separation of liquid phase: starch, tragacanth, alginates, or cellulose derivatives.

    c. Criteria for selection: nontoxic and stable for storage of dentifrice.

    d. Objections: glycerin and propylene glycol dehydrate the mucous membrane and may cause irritation.[16]

  4. *Sweetening agent:* imparts a pleasant taste.

    a. Types currently used: saccharin, sucaryl.

    b. Criterion for selection: should be nonfermentable carbohydrate.

  5. *Flavoring agent:* a blend of essential oils imparts a pleasant, distinctive taste; flavoring agent should be nontoxic and stable for storage.

II. PROPHYLACTIC OR THERAPEUTIC DENTIFRICES

Prophylactic or therapeutic dentifrices are cleansing dentifrices that contain additional ingredients to prevent or reduce dental caries incidence, dental calculus accumulation, gingival disturbances, or hypersensitivity. The many variable factors which affect the processes listed above must be considered in the evaluation of beneficial effects obtained from the use of a dentifrice. Extensive, thorough laboratory and clinical studies are required to demonstrate the efficacy of any product before it can be accepted as safe and effective for public use. A prophylactic or therapeutic dentifrice may be recommended for patient use if the product has been classified in Group A or B by the American Dental Association, Council on Dental Therapeutics (see page 308).

Several approaches have been attempted with the use of dentifrices to prevent dental caries, including: modification of tooth enamel to make it less soluble in acids; neutralization of the acidity of the bacterial plaque; and control of the environment for cariogenic microorganisms or inactivation of their enzymes. To date, modification of the enamel surface has shown the more promising results.

A few of the many agents that have been added to dentifrices for the prevention of dental caries are described briefly below. Research related to the control of calculus formation is described on page 127, and dentifrices to reduce tooth sensitivity are described on page 211.

A. **Enamel Modifying Agents (Fluorides)**[15,17]

1. Action: fluoride ions combine with enamel surface to make it less soluble in acid. This method of incorporation of fluoride is superficial and cannot be construed as comparable to fluoridation of water, topical application of fluoride solution or ingestion of dietary fluorides (see pages 197–198).

2. Recommended prophylactic dentifrices: those currently classified as acceptable for unsupervised public use. Other fluoride dentifrices are under clinical study for classification.

B. **Antibiotic Agent** (Penicillin): purpose of use to inhibit or eliminate penicillin-sensitive organisms from the oral flora; ineffective since microorganisms restabilize and the flora returns to normal; also patient may become sensitized to penicillin and/or microorganisms may develop penicillin resistance.[18]

C. **Anti-enzyme Agents** (Foaming Detergents): aimed to destroy or block bacterial enzymes necessary for degradation of fermentable carbohydrates to acids. Example: sodium N-lauroyl sarcosinate: evidence of effectiveness not substantiated by sufficient data.[15,18]

D. **Environment-modifying Agents:** Examples: Urea and dibasic ammonium phosphate which were believed to prevent the breakdown of glucose by oral microorganisms, but clinical results have been controversial; chlorophyll, believed to inhibit acid production by oral microorganisms or destroy lactobacilli, but results have been inconclusive.[15,18]

RINSING AND MOUTHWASHES

To aid in the prevention of oral disease, rinsing must be accomplished many times each day, therefore the vehicle for this procedure should be readily available and inexpensive, and it should not irritate the tissues. Ordinary tap water meets these requirements. Commercial mouthwashes present a variety of flavors, colors and cosmetic properties; however, their major purpose is to remove debris from the oral cavity. The patient needs to be instructed with regard to the etiological factors of oral disease and halitosis. To combat misconceptions about claimed therapeutic benefits of commercial mouthwashes, he needs to know that these products impart a temporarily freshened breath odor and taste.

I. INDICATIONS FOR USE

A. After the ingestion of food or the use of an oral physical therapy device, rinsing mechanically loosens debris and microorganisms, removes these from the oral cavity, and temporarily refreshes the breath odor and taste.

B. After the ingestion of fermentable carbohydrates, the rinsing solution aids in the dissolution or dilution of retained sugar or acids formed from sugars.

C. When an individual is unable to brush his teeth after the ingestion of food, he may rinse or "swish" with water, although this procedure alone is less effective than when it is preceded by use of a toothbrush.

II. RINSING PROCEDURE

A. Take a mouthful of warm (body temperature) water, then close lips and occlude teeth.

B. With tongue and cheek action, force water through interdental areas with as much pressure as possible to loosen debris; then expectorate or swallow water and debris.

C. Repeat several times until loosened debris is removed.

III. ACCEPTED MOUTHWASHES[19]

A. Water.

B. Isotonic Sodium Chloride Solution ($\frac{1}{4}$ to $\frac{1}{3}$ teaspoonful salt added to 8 oz. glass water).

C. Mild Hypertonic Sodium Chloride Solution ($\frac{1}{2}$ teaspoonful salt added to 8 oz. glass water).

D. Sodium Bicarbonate Solution ($\frac{1}{2}$ teaspoonful soda added to $\frac{3}{4}$ glass water).

E. Sodium Chloride—Sodium Bicarbonate Solution (flavored).

1. Sodium chloride	2.0 Gm.	$\frac{1}{2}$ teaspoonful
2. Sodium bicarbonate	1.0 Gm.	$\frac{1}{4}$ teaspoonful
3. Amaranth solution	2.0 ml.	$\frac{1}{2}$ teaspoonful
4. Peppermint water to make	240.0 ml.	8 oz. glass

IV. PROPRIETARY MOUTHWASHES

A. General Classification[20]

Water and alcohol usually are the vehicles used in mouthwash preparation and each product is unique in its flavor, color and other properties. Similarities in formulation of proprietary mouthwashes allow general classification, but ingredients in a specific product may place it in two or more of the categories listed below.

1. *Cosmetic:* in addition to flavor and color, sometimes contain surface-active agents to assist in dissolution of essential oils and to aid in penetration of mucinous film that covers oral structures (example: denatured alcohol).

2. *Germicidal:* contain agents to remove or destroy oral microorganisms (examples: phenolic or quaternary ammonium compounds, essential oils). The Council on Dental Therapeutics considers these claims invalid because research has not demonstrated that clinical and laboratory results are comparable, that a nonspecific change in normal oral flora is beneficial, or that oral microorganisms, per se, are primary etiologic factors in oral disease.[19]

3. *Astringent:* contain agents to precipitate proteins from saliva and mucous secretions, shrink and protect inflamed mucous surfaces, and flocculate protein material so it can be flushed from the mouth (examples: zinc and aluminum salts). Frequent use of a concentrated astringent mouthwash may irritate the soft tissues or, because of the acidity of the solution, may gradually dissolve tooth structure.

4. *Buffered:* contain agents to raise the pH of saliva or mucinous deposits (example: alkaline compounds). This effect is transitory since saliva readily dilutes the buffer concentration.

5. *Deodorant:* contain agents to neutralize odors that arise in the oral cavity from microbial action on retained debris (example: chlorophyllin). As yet, no product has proved effective.

6. *Therapeutic* (medicated): contain agents to prevent the accumulation of dental calculus or the process of dental caries, or to relieve infection, pain or other symptoms of oral disease (examples: enzyme inhibitors, fluorides, antibiotics, antiseptics, effervescents). The Council has classified medicated mouthwashes for unsupervised use by the public in Group D, and has warned that use of these products to relieve symptoms of oral disease may delay the patient from seeking professional care needed to treat the disease. A product for use by the dentist is evaluated in terms of its effectiveness in adequate clinical tests to alleviate a specific condition.[19]

B. **Use**[19]

1. By the professional: cosmetic mouthwashes may be used as rinses or sprays to impart a pleasant taste after instrumentation; therapeutic mouthwashes may be prescribed by the dentist.

2. By the public: not recommended for routine use; see A, above. If a patient uses a mouthwash routinely, he should be instructed to follow the manufacturer's directions for dilution explicitly, and if breath odor persists, to consult a physician.

CARE OF FIXED OR REMOVABLE DENTAL APPLIANCES

Patients with orthodontic or prosthetic appliances may require one or several of the supplementary oral physical therapy measures outlined in this chapter. Because the addition of artificial structures within the oral cavity presents interference with the normal stimulation of gingival tissues and with cleansing of the teeth, these patients must be meticulous in their performance of oral physical therapy procedures.

I. CARE OF FIXED (CEMENTED) ORTHODONTIC APPLIANCE[21]

Because the appliance affords a high potential for food retention, the importance of thorough removal of debris immediately after ingestion of food cannot be overemphasized. The position of delicate wires and their attachments can be maintained if the patient brushes slowly and carefully, and avoids the use of toothpicks or other implements that could bend the wires.

A. **Recommended Toothbrush:** soft-textured multitufted, with small head or with short-trimmed center row of bristles.

B. **Recommended Toothbrushing Method**

1. Brush occlusal surfaces first to soften bristles.
2. Use Rolling Stroke Method (see page 285) to brush lingual surfaces and facial surfaces not covered by bands or wires.

3. Use Charters' or Modified Stillman's Method to brush surfaces covered by appliances (see pages 287 to 292).
   a. Carefully flex bristles onto proximal surfaces and cervical areas; avoid pressure against wires and attachments.
   b. With very light pressure, work bristle tips between wires and bands or tooth surfaces to loosen debris; avoid dislodgment or disturbance of wire position.

II. CARE OF COMPLETE DENTURES

A patient may believe that the necessity for careful hygienic measures has been removed with his natural teeth, but deposits and stains accumulate on surfaces of dental appliances and, if these accretions are not removed routinely, the soft tissues will become irritated. The importance of oral physical therapy procedures should be emphasized to the patient when he receives his dentures and at each appointment thereafter.

A. **Recommended Toothbrush:** a good-quality denture brush which has bristles of various lengths to permit adequate cleansing of the inner surface of the appliance.

B. **Cleansing Agents for Use in Conjunction with Denture Brush**[22]
   1. Castile soap.
   2. Sodium bicarbonate mixed with water to form paste.
   3. Precipitated calcium carbonate (chalk) mixed with water to form paste.
   4. Trisodium phosphate, $\frac{1}{4}$ teaspoonful dissolved in $\frac{1}{2}$ glass of water.
   5. *Do not use* kitchen cleansers or other harsh abrasives that may scratch the smooth surface of the appliance.

C. **Chemical Cleansing Agents**[22]
   Thorough mechanical cleansing with the denture brush or rinsing immediately after eating will prevent the formation of most stains and hard deposits on artificial appliances. Mild inorganic chemical cleansers can be used to assist in the removal of resistant stains and deposits from acrylic dentures. Appliances made of chromium-cobalt alloys corrode if allowed to remain in a solution containing chlorine.
   1. Mild white vinegar solution: not more than one tablespoonful per cup of water.
   2. Ammonia water solution.
      a. Formula: 2 ml. of 28 per cent ammonia water plus water to make 60 ml.
      b. Popular measure: scant teaspoonful of 28 per cent ammonia water in one cup water.
   3. Trisodium phosphate solution.
      a. Formula: 600 mg. trisodium phosphate plus water to make 60 ml.
      b. Popular measure: about $\frac{1}{3}$ teaspoonful trisodium phosphate in one cup water.

4. Sodium hypochlorite solution.
   a. Formula: 2 ml. of 5 per cent sodium hypochlorite solution plus water to make 60 ml.
   b. Popular measure: one teaspoonful 5 per cent sodium hypochlorite in one cup water.

D. Procedure for Cleansing Appliance

1. Firmly grasp appliance in palm of hand.
2. Protect from breakage if dropped
   a. Hold denture over sink half-filled with water which will cushion the impact.
   b. Place towel or wash cloth over surface of unplugged sink to cushion the impact.
3. Apply denture brush to all areas of appliance until debris is removed.
4. Rinse under moderate stream of warm (not hot) water.
5. For stains or deposits which resist mechanical removal
   a. Brush and rinse denture.
   b. Place denture in mild chemical solution for 1 to 2 hours. Denture can be stored in solution overnight if dentist has approved overnight removal of denture from the patient's mouth.

E. Procedure for Massaging Soft Tissues

1. Remove dentures and rinse the oral cavity thoroughly with warm water or saline solution.
2. Massage soft tissues by one of the methods suggested below.
   a. With thumb and forefinger, apply gentle pressure to the tissue that has been covered by the appliance. Repeat several times in each area.
   b. Cover the thumb and forefinger with soft terry cloth and massage the tissue as described in a, above.
   c. Use a toothbrush with soft-textured bristles. Direct bristle tips toward mucosa, then gently apply sides of bristles to tissue and use Modified Stillman's Method to massage (see pages 287 to 289). Avoid vigorous brushing or careless placement of bristles.

III. CARE OF REMOVABLE PARTIAL DENTURE OR SPACE MAINTAINER

The close adaptation of clasps or rests to teeth necessitates careful attention to the cleanliness of both the involved teeth and the appliance. Because soft tissues may receive continuous though slight pressure from appliances, supplementary stimulation is required to maintain healthy tissue tone.

A. Recommended Brushes

1. Toothbrush: suited to the patient's requirements (see page 278).
2. Clasp brush: bristles project from wire attached to handle; long bristles are close to the handle and are shorter-trimmed toward tip; tapered, cylindrical shape can be adapted to inner surfaces of clasps or precision attachments.
3. Denture brush: (see II, A, above) to cleanse smooth surfaces of appliance.

B. **Recommended Cleansing Agents:**   described under II, B, C
C. **Procedure for Cleansing Appliance**
   1. Firmly grasp appliance in palm of hand; use gentle pressure to maintain grip because excessive pressure may break fragile appliance.
   2. Protect from breakage if dropped.
   3. Carefully brush clasps and smooth surfaces to remove debris, then rinse appliance under gentle stream of warm (not hot) water.

REFERENCES

1. Zon Dental Bridge Cleaner, Johnson & Johnson Co.
2. GOLDMAN, H. M., SCHLUGER, SAUL, FOX, LEWIS, and COHEN, D. W.: *Periodontal Therapy*, 2nd ed. St. Louis, Mosby, 1960, pp. 606–607.
3. GRANT, DANIEL, STERN, I. B., and EVERETT, F. G.: *Orban's Periodontics*, 2nd ed. St. Louis, Mosby, 1963, pp. 320–321.
4. SORRIN, SIDNEY, ed.; *Periodontia*. New York, Blakiston Division, McGraw-Hill, 1960, pp. 314–316.
5. Water-Pik, Aqua-Tec Co.; Aquadent, Oral B Company.
6. GRANT, DANIEL, STERN, I. B. and EVERETT, F. G.: op. cit., pp. 317–318.
7. Ibid., pp. 319–320.
8. KITCHIN, P. C. and ROBINSON, H. B. G.: How Abrasive Need a Dentifrice Be? J. Dent. Res., *27*, 501, August, 1948.
9. American Dental Association, Council on Dental Therapeutics: *Accepted Dental Remedies*, 29th ed. Chicago, American Dental Association, 1964, p. 138.
10. American Dental Association, Council on Dental Therapeutics: New Policy on Dentifrices Announced by Council, Am. Dent. A. J., *35*, 522, October 1, 1947.
11. American Dental Association, Council on Dental Therapeutics: op. cit., p. viii.
12. GERSHON, S. D., POKRAS, H. H. and RIDER, T. H.: Dentifrices, in Sagarin, Edward: *Cosmetics Science and Technology*. New York, Interscience Pub., 1957, pp. 316–338.
13. HILL, T. J.: Therapeutic Dentifrices, in Ostrander, F. D.: Symposium on Practical Oral Therapeutics, Dental Clinics of North America. Philadelphia, Saunders, March, 1958, p. 179.
14. DOBBS, E. C.: *Pharmacology and Oral Therapeutics*, 12th ed. St. Louis, Mosby, 1961, pp. 514–515.
15. American Dental Association, Council on Dental Therapeutics: op. cit., pp. 138–140.
16. DOBBS: op. cit., pp. 74–75.
17. American Dental Association, Council on Dental Therapeutics: op. cit., pp. 134–135.
18. WALLACE, D. A.: Therapeutic Dentifrices: A Review of the Literature on Clinical Investigations, Dent. Prog., *2*, 242, July, 1962.
19. American Dental Association, Council on Dental Therapeutics: op. cit., pp. 140–141, 196.
20. GERSHON, POKRAS, and RIDER: op. cit., pp. 362–372.
21. WOODS, G. A.: Toothbrushing Procedure for Orthodontic Patients, Am. J. Orthodont., *41*, 370, May, 1955.
22. American Dental Association, Council on Dental Therapeutics: op. cit., pp. 173–174, 198.

SUGGESTED READINGS

ANTHONY, D. H. and GIBBONS, PAUL: The Nature and Behavior of Denture Cleansers, J. Prosth. Dent., *8*, 796, September-October, 1958.
BARTELSTONE, H. J., MANDEL, I. D., and CHILTON, N. W.: Critical Evaluation of Clinical Studies with Stannous Fluoride Dentifrices, N. Y. S. Dent. J., *28*, 147, April, 1962.
BASS, C. C.: The Optimum Characteristics of Dental Floss for Personal Oral Hygiene, Dent. Items Interest, *70*, 921, September, 1948.
BEUBE, F. E.: *Periodontology*, New York, Macmillan, 1953, pp. 226–227, 242–247.
BLAKE, G. C. and TROTT, J. R.: *Periodontology*. London, Butterworths, 1962, pp. 91–94.
BRUDEVOLD, F., CHILTON, N. W., and WELLOCK, W. D.: A Preliminary Comparison of a Dentifrice Containing Fluoride and Soluble Phosphate and Employing a Calcium-free Abrasive with Other Types of Fluoride Dentifrices. J. Oral Thera. and Pharm., *1*, 1, July, 1964.
CHARTERS, W. J.: Home Care of the Mouth. I. Proper Home Care of the Mouth, J. Periodont., *19*, 136, October, 1948.

COOLIDGE, E. D. and HINE, M. K.:   *Periodontology*, 3rd ed. Philadelphia, Lea & Febiger, 1958, pp. 128–129, 153, 421–427.

DOBBS, E. C.:   *Pharmacology and Oral Therapeutics*, 12th ed. St. Louis, Mosby, 1961, pp. 490–491, 504–511, 519–523, 546–547.

DUCKWORTH, R.:   Fluoride Dentifrices, Dent. Practitioner, *14*, 93, November, 1963.

DUDDING, N. J., DAHL, L. O., and MUHLER, J. C.:   Patient Reactions to Brushing Teeth with Water, Dentifrice or Salt and Soda, J. Periodont., *31*, 386, October, 1960.

EVERETT, F. G. and BETTMAN, M. M.:   Mouthrinsing, J. Periodont., *23*, 213, October, 1952.

EVERETT, F. G. and KUNKEL, P. W.:   Abrasion Through the Abuse of Dental Floss, J. Periodont., *24*, 186, July, 1953.

FOSDICK, L. S., McMILLAN, L., and BLACKWELL, R. Q.:   Some Observations of Tooth Enamel Surfaces, Arch. Oral Biol., *1*, 211, January, 1960.

GLICKMAN, IRVING: *Clinical Periodontology*, 2nd ed. Philadelphia, Saunders, 1958, pp. 571, 796, 938–941.

GOLDMAN, H. M., SCHLUGER, SAUL, FOX, LEWIS, and COHEN, D. W.:   *Periodontal Therapy*, 2nd ed. St. Louis, Mosby, 1960, pp. 605–608, 621–622.

HILL, T. J.:   Fluoride Dentifrices, Am. Dent. A. J., *59*, 1121, December, 1959.

KESEL, R. G.:   Methods of Prevention and Control of Dental Caries, Am. Dent. A. J., *52*, 455, April, 1956.

LeGRO, A. L.:   The Interproximal Spaces, Dent. Surv., *10*, 53, September, 1934.

MANLY, R. S.:   Factors Influencing Tests on the Abrasion of Dentine by Brushing with Dentifrices, J. Dent. Res., *23*, 59, January, 1944.

MUHLER, J. C.:   Effect of a Stannous-fluoride Dentifrice on Caries Reduction in Children During a Three-year Study Period, Am. Dent. A. J., *64*, 216, February, 1962.

SORRIN, SIDNEY, ed.:   *Periodontia*. New York, Blakiston Division, McGraw-Hill, 1960, pp. 311–316, 381–383.

SORRIN, SIDNEY and THALLER, J. L.:   The Interproximal Stimulator—An Adjunct in Periodontal Therapy, J. Periodont., *30*, 44, January, 1959.

THOMAS, B. O. A.:   Effective Interdental Stimulation, Am. Dent. A. J., *29*, 741, December, 1942.

VOLKER, J. F. and CALDWELL, R. C.:   Prophylactic and Operative Techniques in Dental Caries Prevention, in Finn, S. B.:   *Clinical Pedodontics*, 2nd ed. Philadelphia, Saunders, 1962, pp. 685–695.

Chapter 28

ORAL PHYSICAL THERAPY: PATIENT INSTRUCTION

PERSONALIZED oral physical therapy instruction transmits an attitude of concern for the patient's well-being that establishes confidence in the professional care received. Correct performance of oral physical therapy alone will not prevent oral disease, and instruction in these procedures is accompanied by appropriate recommendations of other measures required for maintenance of oral health. Procedures by which the professional communicates information and teaches the skills of oral physical therapy are described in this Chapter. These procedures cannot be regarded as rule-of-thumb practices, but they can serve as guides by which comprehensive instruction for each individual is planned.

Verbal instruction and demonstrations are geared to the patient's level of understanding and are kept as simple as possible within the limits of his requirements. It is difficult for a patient to see his own oral structures, and even more difficult for him to visualize an abnormality that is apparent to the experienced observation of a professional. Aids such as disclosing solution and the hand mirror can be used to assist the patient to evaluate his oral condition and to perform oral physical therapy techniques in the recommended manner. Pictures, models, and radiographs are used to illustrate normal and abnormal conditions of significance to the individual. Instructions printed in pamphlets or on office stationery and given to the patient for home use will reinforce spoken communication and visual demonstration.

A child learns to brush his teeth by observation and mimicry of members of his family. He may establish incorrect habits of oral physical therapy before he receives professional instruction, and he must learn to discard these habits when new procedures are introduced. If professional instruction is delayed or if a patient has failed to heed professional advice until habits are firmly established, additional instruction will be required to assist the individual to discard faulty practices and to use improved methods.

One period of instruction, demonstration and/or practice is insufficient to communicate all the dental health information needed by a patient or to allow him to master a new technique. Time and practice required for learning vary with the individual (see Chapter 25). Instructions are repeated until the patient demonstrates a reasonable degree of proficiency, then again after he has practiced at home so correct procedures can be reinforced and incorrect techniques altered. After a technique is mastered, the patient may become careless or forget important elements of the regimen. His oral condition may change over a period of time so that oral physical therapy procedures need to be directed, for example, toward prevention of dental calculus accumulation rather than control of dental caries. Each time the patient returns for dental and dental hygiene care his oral condition is re-evaluated and appropriate instructions are given.

PREPARATION FOR PATIENT INSTRUCTION

I. VISUAL AIDS

A. **Model of the Teeth** which can be used to demonstrate tooth-brushing methods, proper use of dental floss, interdental stimulators and/or other oral physical therapy measures.

B. **Study Model** of the patient's own teeth which may be used to individualize instruction to the fullest extent.

C. **Demonstration Toothbrushes**

   1. Purpose: to permit demonstration with the specific kind of brush recommended for the individual patient.

   2. Types

      a. Professional design of various sizes with natural and/or synthetic bristles.

      b. Denture brushes.

      c. Clasp brushes.

      d. Automatic toothbrushes of popular design.

D. **New Toothbrushes and Automatic Brush Inserts** for distribution to patients.

E. **Disclosing Solution:** liquid for office use and sample wafers for demonstration and distribution (see pages 191–192).

F. **Hand Mirror** for use by patient as he practices new techniques.

G. **Interdental Stimulators** for demonstration and distribution.

H. **Radiographs**

   1. Sample radiographs which show various conditions not visible clinically.

   2. Patient's radiographs may be used for instruction *only* if the dentist has made a previous diagnosis and the dental hygienist interprets the diagnosis to the patient.

I. **Viewbox** to provide adequate light for interpretation of radiographs.

J. **Printed Outline of Basic Instructions** for home use by patient.

II. SUGGESTED PROCEDURE TO PERSONALIZE INSTRUCTION

A. **Allow Sufficient Time.**

Plan sufficient time for explanation, demonstration and practice of oral physical therapy procedures. Instruction time and effort are invaluable investments, since the patient's motivation and ability to follow professional recommendations will result in longer service life of his dental restorations and in improved health of his soft tissues. The educated patient who appreciates his oral health is a good representative of the dental office.

   1. Begin instruction before the oral prophylaxis to allow consideration of the patient's present oral condition.

   2. Continue instruction throughout the appointment and review essential facts and techniques before the patient is dismissed.

3. Review information and practice techniques each time the patient returns for a series of appointments.
4. Provide special appointments to assist the patient to master a technique that is difficult for him and to correct misunderstandings or misconceptions.
5. Reevaluate the patient's oral condition and requirements at each recall appointment, and change the regimen when necessary.

B. **Establish Rapport** to gain the patient's confidence.

C. **Consider the Individual Patient**
1. Consider motivating factors of possible application to the patient's age, occupation, background and interests (see pages 267–268).
2. Consider the patient's manual dexterity.
   When a patient fails to demonstrate reasonable proficiency in the performance of a new technique, or fails to indicate interest or understanding of recommended procedures, he is reappointed for further instruction until his performance meets standards necessary for the maintenance phase of his dental care. The factors listed below may influence an individual's ability to follow recommendations.
   a. *Positive factors:* individuals whose occupations require manual or digital dexterity, such as machinists, typists, musicians, beauticians or key press operators, may master techniques more quickly because of transfer of digital skills.
   b. *Negative factors*
      (1) Age: children under eight years of age usually lack sufficient muscular coordination to control toothbrush manipulation; the onset of senility in older persons is accompanied by a loss of full muscular coordination.
      (2) Physical condition: for example, fatigue, debility, or extreme nervousness will tend to reduce the patient's ability to perform a digital skill.
3. Consider the patient's oral conditions, particularly those listed below which represent special problems that must be overcome through the use of appropriate oral physical therapy measures. When the patient is made aware of his "special condition" he may give more concerted attention to his entire regimen.
   a. Conditions that limit brush placement (see pages 83–85).
      (1) Oral cavity: limited opening and/or size.
      (2) Tongue: large and/or attached by short frenum.
      (3) Cheeks: thick and adapted closely to buccal surfaces of molars; taut musculature.
      (4) Teeth: malaligned, maloccluded, or missing.
   b. Conditions that predispose to deposit retention (see pages 103–109).
      (1) Saliva: viscous or slow rate of flow.
      (2) Teeth: malaligned, maloccluded, or missing.
      (3) Free gingiva and interdental papillae: enlarged or receded.
      (4) Oral habits: for example, mouth breathing.
      (5) Fixed or removable dental appliances.

    c. Dental calculus, soft deposits and stains: location, amount, tendency to form, and time interval since last oral prophylaxis.

    d. Conditions that may discourage the use of the toothbrush: denuded epithelium caused by faulty toothbrushing habits or active disease processes.

PROCEDURES FOR ORAL PHYSICAL THERAPY INSTRUCTION

I. PRINCIPLES

A. Demonstration

1. Provide the patient with a toothbrush for use in his own mouth.

    a. Give him a toothbrush of the recommended type when the dentist provides a new brush for each patient. Allow him to select from a variety of colors and to choose natural or synthetic bristles unless his oral condition requires a particular bristle texture (see pages 278–279).

    b. Provide a disinfected toothbrush that can be used at this appointment, and ask the patient to bring his own toothbrush next time if the dentist does not provide a new brush for each patient. When the patient brings his brush, check its condition and recommend purchase of a new brush if necessary.

2. Use patient's study models when available; if demonstration model is used and patient has edentulous areas, remove teeth from model so it corresponds to patient's condition.

3. Hold demonstration model so patient has direct view of brush placement, and hold demonstration brush handle as the patient must when he brushes his teeth.

4. Place and activate brush slowly and carefully so patient can follow demonstration; stress importance of thorough, careful technique.

5. Have patient observe his performance with use of mirror.

6. Allow patient to accomplish the recommended number of strokes correctly in each area before adjacent area is considered.

B. Instruction

1. State instructions simply and observe patient's facial expression as well as his performance for signs of confusion or misunderstanding.

2. Redemonstrate technique and repeat instructions to clarify problems; vary terminology or illustrations when necessary.

3. Correct patient's technique in a positive manner as errors arise during instruction; avoid direct criticism.

4. Encourage patient as he practices new technique; be liberal with compliments when they are deserved. Tell him to take extra time at first until he can perform the method successfully, and to continue to use thorough procedures when he gains proficiency.

5. Observe patient's approach to use of new device or method; caution him with regard to overvigorous procedures (see pages 295 to 298).

II. EVALUATE PATIENT'S PRESENT PROCEDURES

A. Give Patient a Toothbrush.
1. Explain merits of the recommended toothbrush (see page 278).
2. Explain the care and supply of toothbrushes (see pages 279–280).
3. Wet the patient's toothbrush under stream of water and give it to him.

B. Give Patient a Hand Mirror.

C. Ask Patient to Brush in His Accustomed Manner.
1. With certain patients it may seem appropriate to have a demonstration of the present method used. Generally, however, it is more effective to present the appropriate procedure for *this* patient in a positive manner.
2. When the patient is asked to brush first in his accustomed manner, observe his technique and compliment adequate methods. Note inadequacies, but reserve comment until recommended technique is demonstrated and reasons for the new method are explained.

D. Determine Whether Patient Uses Other Measures; for example, dental floss or toothpicks.

E. Show Patient Evidences of Faulty Techniques.
1. Show patient how to evaluate his state of oral cleanliness.
   a. Apply disclosing solution to his teeth or have him chew disclosing tablet; recommend daily home use of disclosing tablets.
   b. Ask him to feel tooth surfaces with tip of his tongue; note degree of smoothness or roughness.
   c. Ask him to note refreshed taste after he has brushed.
2. As patient observes in mirror, indicate retained deposits and stains and relate their presence to soft tissue abnormalities.
   a. Indicate disclosed deposits that were not removed when he brushed.
   b. Loosen materia alba to show its location and quantity.
   c. Loosen dental calculus deposit, then place it on patient's fingertip so he will feel its consistency and texture; compare submarginal deposit to splinter in skin.
3. Indicate areas of toothbrush abrasion (see page 297).
4. Indicate areas of soft tissue injury from use of other devices.

F. Select Oral Physical Therapy Measures to be Recommended: consider the patient's requirements and his demonstrated and potential ability to perform techniques.

III. DEMONSTRATE RECOMMENDED ORAL PHYSICAL THERAPY PROCEDURES.

A. Explain Objectives of Toothbrushing (see pages 272–273).
1. Relate objectives to patient's maintenance of oral health.
2. Relate his inadequate procedures to his oral condition.

B. Demonstrate the Recommended Toothbrushing Method.
1. Demonstrate the correct grasp of the toothbrush handle.

2. Demonstrate brush placement and activation on one group of tooth surfaces of the model.

3. With patient's brush, demonstrate bristle placement, pressure and activation on labial surfaces of his maxillary anterior teeth and gingiva while he observes in mirror.

4. Request patient to brush his teeth as demonstrated; observe his performance carefully and correct errors when necessary.

5. When patient achieves reasonable proficiency, repeat demonstration and practice on adjacent surfaces; continue until all tooth surfaces have been brushed.

6. Demonstrate adapted techniques for problem areas (see pages 282–283).

7. Review and stress the routine, number of strokes, and brush placement and activation.

C. **Explain and Demonstrate Supplementary Procedures.**

1. *Adjuncts for every patient*
   a. Brush the tongue (see page 284).
   b. Use a recommended dentifrice (see pages 307–309).
   c. Rinse thoroughly (see page 311).
   d. When the teeth cannot be brushed after ingestion of food, use a substitute measure: swish, or chew "nature's toothbrushes" at end of meal (fresh, raw fruits or vegetables).

2. *Procedures for selected patients*
   Aids to cleanse exposed root surfaces, proximal surfaces, cervical areas and fixed and removable appliances and their abutments, and aids to massage receded or enlarged gingiva and edentulous areas are described in Chapter 27. Instruction in the use of these aids is as important for selected patients as toothbrushing instruction. These devices are demonstrated and practiced.

D. **Evaluate Results of Recommended Procedures** (see II, E, 1.).

E. **Place Patient's Toothbrush in Original Container and Retain It for Future Use.**

IV. **CONTINUE INSTRUCTION THROUGHOUT APPOINTMENT.**

A. **Select "Teachable Moments"** when the patient is most receptive to instruction: for example, when he asks about his oral condition or expresses interest in professional procedures; when a parent asks about his child's oral condition; when operative procedures are performed in problem areas.

B. **Emphasize the Objectives of Oral Physical Therapy Procedures.**

1. Stress the patient's requirements and the value of thorough oral physical therapy measures to maintenance of his oral health.

2. Stress that debris is to be removed from the teeth with the toothbrush or with substitute measures when the toothbrush or other devices are not available immediately after the ingestion of food.

V. REVIEW AFTER INSTRUMENTATION IS COMPLETED:

A. **Redemonstrate Techniques:** Ask patient to practice use of toothbrush and other recommended devices in several areas, or if his soft tissues are hypersensitive, ask him to demonstrate on the model.

B. **Review the Recommended Regimen.**
1. Question the patient with regard to major points; for example, when teeth are to be brushed, how he will evaluate effectiveness of his regimen, how he will cleanse special problem areas.
2. Stress the importance of cleanliness and gingival stimulation to the more rapid attainment of oral health.

C. **Prepare Patient for Dismissal.**
1. Toothbrush
    a. Give him the toothbrush in its container if he is not reappointed for future instruction.
    b. Retain toothbrush in labeled container for use at next appointment and instruct him to purchase one to use at home.
2. Printed instructions: review material and indicate specific information he should consider; suggest he read material periodically.

VI. RECORD SUMMARY OF INSTRUCTION on patient's chart for future reference.

INSTRUCTION FOR CHILD UNDER 8 YEARS OF AGE

I. PREPARATION

A. **Perform Dental Hygiene Services First** to reduce apprehension; patient will be more receptive to instruction.

B. **Establish Rapport with Child** so he will respect suggestions for improved personal oral care habits.

II. INSTRUCT CHILD

A. **Principles for Demonstration and Instruction** (see page 320).
1. Use terminology child understands but avoid "talking down" to him.
2. Assist child to manipulate the brush when necessary to demonstrate correct position, but allow him to do as much as he can for himself.
3. Count strokes aloud; this helps him concentrate.

B. **Suggested Procedures for Oral Physical Therapy Instruction** (see page 318).

III. INSTRUCT PARENT

A. **Invite Parent into Operatory** and ask child to demonstrate the method he has practiced.

B. **Explain to Parent**

1. Objectives of thorough oral physical therapy procedures as related to child's requirements.
2. Merits of the recommended toothbrush.
3. Care and supply of toothbrushes.

C. **Explain to Parent and Child**

1. Parent will need to brush child's teeth at least once a day. Emphasize that parent's interest and supervision will assure thorough procedures.
2. Parent will be responsible for maintenance of child's oral cleanliness until child is 10 to 12 years old, and will retain partial responsibility for supervision of adolescent's oral care procedures.

D. **Demonstrate How Parent Can Evaluate Child's Oral Cleanliness.**

1. Give child a disclosing tablet to chew, then have him rinse.
2. Explain that stained debris can be removed with correct use of the toothbrush.
3. Show parent areas that are difficult for child to brush and which require special attention.

E. **Demonstrate a Method by Which Parent Can Brush Child's Teeth.**[1]

1. *Child's position:* child stands in front of operator with head tilted backward until full view of maxillary arch is achieved with child's mouth open; his head is cradled and supported by operator's left forearm.
2. *Retraction:* child's lips and cheeks are retracted with the operator's left thumb and fingers; his tongue is retracted with back surface of toothbrush head.
3. *Brush placement and activation:* labial surfaces of maxillary anterior teeth are brushed first to demonstrate bristle placement and activation, then other surfaces are brushed in recommended sequence.

F. **Request Parent to Practice Method with Child.**

1. Redemonstrate method of retraction that allows visibility, yet is comfortable for child.
2. Observe brush placement and activation, particularly on surfaces that are difficult to brush.
3. Allow parent to control child; avoid confusion that arises when two adults instruct child at same time.

G. **Review** necessity for parental supervision and assistance to assure thorough routine oral physical therapy procedures and reemphasize other preventive measures required for maintenance of the child's oral health.

FOLLOW-UP ORAL PHYSICAL THERAPY INSTRUCTION

I. GENERAL PROCEDURES

A. **Consult Patient's Record:**   note previous oral conditions and oral physical therapy recommendations.

B. **Inspect and Evaluate Oral Conditions:**   compare present to former conditions and record changes on patient's chart.
1. Give patient a hand mirror.
2. Apply disclosing solution to his teeth.
3. Show him conditions that have improved and areas that need more careful attention.

C. **Review Recommended Oral Physical Therapy Procedures.**
1. Give patient a moistened toothbrush.
2. Ask him if he was able to perform method at home; if he experienced difficulty, begin review with his problem.
3. Request patient to demonstrate complete procedure. Observe his technique carefully and compliment him when indicated. Correct his errors and attempt to relate faulty techniques to lack of improved cleanliness or tissue tone in specific areas.
4. Reapply disclosing solution and evaluate oral cleanliness while patient observes in hand mirror.

II. SPECIFIC PROCEDURES

A. **Patient Who Requires a Series of Appointments**
1. Allow sufficient time between appointments for sensitive tissues to heal and for the patient to practice recommended procedures.
2. Allow sufficient time at each appointment to review instruction and procedures.
3. If patient masters procedures, give him toothbrush to take home and remind him to review printed instructions often.
4. If patient fails to master procedures, keep toothbrush and reappoint him for further instruction. If he is unable to master techniques after further instruction, alter the method or substitue a less complex, but effective method by which he can cleanse his teeth and massage his gingiva without injurious effects.

B. **Recall Patient**
1. Consult the patient's oral inspection and oral physical therapy records; note changes that may require a new regimen.
2. Question the patient to determine his recall of previous instruction.
   a. If he is well-informed, compliment him and proceed as outlined in I, B and C, above.
   b. If he has forgotten essential elements of his regimen, proceed as with a new patient.

REFERENCE

1. STARKEY, P. E.:   Instructions to Parents for Brushing the Child's Teeth, J. Dent. Child., *28*, 42, First Quarter, 1961.

SUGGESTED READINGS

ARNIM, S. S.:   The Use of Disclosing Agents for Measuring Tooth Cleanliness, J. Periodont., *34*, 227, May, 1963.

ARNIM, S. S. and WILLIAMS, Q. E.:   How to Educate Patients in Oral Hygiene, Dent. Radiog. and Photog., *32*, 61, #4, 1959.

BASTIAN, E. H.:   Patient Education and Recall Systems, Austral. Dent. J., *8*, 31, February, 1963.

BEUBE, F. E.:   *Periodontology.* New York, MacMillan, 1953, pp. 230–233.

CUNNINGHAM, W. M.:   The Periodontal Patient, Dent. Practitioner, *12*, 365, June, 1962.

DERBYSHIRE, J. C.:   Methods of Achieving Effective Hygiene of the Mouth, in Grupe, H. E., ed.: *Symposium on Periodontal Therapy, Dental Clinics of North America.* Philadelphia, Saunders, March, 1964, pp. 231–244.

DE WEVER, J. E. and STRIFFLER, D. F.:   Exploratory Research in Tooth Brushing Instruction for Primary Schools, J. Dent. Res., *38*, 707, July-August, 1959.

GLICKMAN, IRVING: *Clinical Periodontology,* 2nd ed. Philadelphia, Saunders, 1958, pp. 931–932.

GOLDMAN, H. M., SCHLUGER, SAUL, FOX, LEWIS, and COHEN, D. W.:   *Periodontal Therapy,* 2nd ed. St. Louis, Mosby, 1960, p. 608.

GRANT, DANIEL, STERN, I. B., and EVERETT, F. G.:   *Orban's Periodontics,* 2nd ed. St. Louis, Mosby, 1963, pp. 302–304.

MANSON, J. D. and FORREST, J. O.:   A Method of Instruction in Oral Hygiene, Brit. Dent. J., *114*, 163, March 5, 1963.

SANDELL, P. J.:   Materials and Methods in Dental Health Education, Internat'l. Dent. J., *13*, 154, March, 1963.

SANDELL, P. J.:   Patient Education—A Practice Builder, Am. Dent. A. J., *64*, 14, January, 1962.

SORRIN, SIDNEY, ed.:   *The Practice of Periodontia.* New York, Blakiston Division, McGraw-Hill, 1960, pp. 318–321.

STARKEY, P. E.:   A Study of Four Methods of Presenting Dental Health Information to Parents, J. Dent. Child., *29*, 11, First Quarter, 1962.

SWENSON, H. M.:   Home Care Procedures in Oral Hygiene, Am. Dent. Hygienists' A. J., *37*, 82, Second Quarter, 1963.

WARNER, E. M.:   Patient Education for Dental Health, Am. Dent. Hygienists' A. J., *36*, 123, Third Quarter, 1962.

PART VI

Applied Techniques for Patients With Special Needs

INTRODUCTION

To understand each patient's general and/or oral health problems requires particular study. Actually each patient is a "special" patient and must be considered according to his individual needs. However, certain patients have problems peculiar to their age group and/or unusual health factors which may complicate the routine of care generally provided. These special patients require more skillful application of dental hygiene knowledge and ability to accomplish a comparably favorable result than for what might be called the "normal" patient.

Optimum oral health is frequently an important contributing factor in maintaining or restoring the patient's physical, emotional, vocational, economic, and social usefulness to the extent of his capabilities. *The dental hygienist's obligation is to see that no patient needs special rehabilitative dental services because of any condition which could have been prevented by dental hygiene care.*

To consider the patient as a whole requires attention to general physical and emotional problems as well as oral problems. Basic psychological needs for affection, belonging, independence, achievement, recognition and self-esteem frequently influence the outcome of treatment as well as the patient's whole attitude toward dental and dental hygiene care. With certain physical conditions, oral health has assumed less importance in the mind of the patient because other health problems have demanded so much attention. For some of these patients neglect has intensified the need for oral care.

The patients with special needs who will be considered in the chapters following include patients with oral and general systemic conditions. Variations with respect to age are brought out, and a chapter is devoted to a description of the aged.

SPECIAL ORAL PROBLEMS

In each specialty of dentistry, patients present problems which can be helped by the services performed by the dental hygienist. For example, patients with removable dentures require particular attention. The care of the denture has been described on page 182 and the instruction for the patient is on page 313. Patients with dentofacial handicaps who have missing teeth or congenital malformations, patients requiring surgery, and patients afflicted with habits conducive to the initiation of dental caries, all need special adaptations of the preventive care and instruction which the dental hygienist can afford.

SYSTEMIC DISEASES

Oral manifestations are evident in association with certain acute and chronic systemic diseases, particularly nutritional deficiences, endocrine disturbances, blood dyscrasias, and a number of chronic degenerative diseases. The presence of dental diseases may complicate and delay the rehabilitation of the patient with systemic illness. When an oral manifestation suggests the possibility of an undiagnosed systemic disease, dental personnel have the responsibility in the referral of the patient for medical examination.

As defined by the Commission on Chronic Illness,[1] chronic disease comprises all impairments or deviations from normal which have one or more of the following characteristics: are permanent, leave residual disability, are caused by nonreversible pathological alteration, require special training of the patient for rehabilitation, and may be expected to require a long period of supervision, observation, or care. According to the National Health Survey, 10 per cent of the population of the United States has one or more chronic conditions with some degree of activity limitation.[2] Approximately 50 per cent of the chronically ill are over 65 years of age, whereas only 5 per cent are under 15 years.[3,4] Arthritis, tuberculosis, diseases of the digestive system, cancer and other tumors, and the permanent results of accidents are primary causes of chronic disabilities. Other conditions include neuromuscular involvements such as cerebral palsy and muscular dystrophy, cardiovascular diseases, diabetes, epilepsy and mental illness.

Patients with chronic diseases may or may not be able to go to the dental office for appointments. Certain conditions, particularly during the advanced stages of a disease, require the patient to remain confined and in some instances, bedridden. Dental hygienists need to understand the special procedures for care in these instances.

The basic approach to chronic disease is prevention, and individual initiative is vital in prevention. The public, including dental personnel, must incorporate into their daily living fundamental health practices which contribute to optimum health and hence to the prevention of chronic disease.[5] Dental hygiene care improves the general health and influences the resistance to infection of the oral cavity. Through patient instruction, an important role in the prevention of chronic disease can be performed.

INTEGRATION OF APPLICATIONS TO SPECIAL NEEDS

It should be realized that a patient may have more than one special need. For example, the patient who requires dental hygiene care prior to oral surgery may have a blood disease. The pregnant patient may be diabetic. Here the use of the patient's medical history plays an important role in outlining the total needs of the patient.

The material included in Part VI is primarily for reference. There is an attempt to integrate learning in other areas of concentrated study in the dental, dental hygiene, medical, and social sciences. The dental hygienist is encouraged to supplement her knowledge and appreciation of the special needs of patients through the use of additional readings such as those suggested at the end of each chapter. Through application of understanding of the patient's needs, the dental hygienist may more skillfully direct her clinical techniques and patient instruction for complete *dental hygiene care.*

REFERENCES

1. Commission on Chronic Illness: Chronic Illness in the United States. I. *Prevention of Chronic Illness*. Cambridge, Harvard University Press, 1957, p. 320.
2. TRITHART, A. H.: Dental Care for the Aged, Chronically Ill, Institutionalized, and Home-bound, J. Am. Coll. Dent., *28*, 266, December, 1961.
3. LAWRENCE, P. S.: An Estimate of the Incidence of Chronic Disease, Pub. Health Rep., *63*, 69, January 16, 1948.
4. American Dental Association, Council on Dental Health: Role of Dentistry in Chronic Illness, Am. Dent. A. J., *48*, 687, June, 1954.
5. Commission on Chronic Illness: op. cit., p. 104.

SUGGESTED READINGS

BURKET, L. W.: Symposium on the Interrelationship of Oral and Systemic Disease, Foreword, Dental Clinics of North America. Philadelphia, Saunders, July, 1958, pp. 277–282.
Committee on Child Health, American Public Health Association: *Services for Children with Dentofacial Handicaps*. New York, American Public Health Association, Inc., 1955. 68 pp.
GALAGAN, D. J.: What the Dental Profession has to Offer in the Development of More Adequate Chronic Disease Programs, Am. J. Pub. Health, *46*, 450, April, 1956.
LAW, F. E.: Role of Dental Hygienist in the Care of the Chronically Ill, Am. Dent. Hygienists' A. J., *33*, 175, October, 1959.
SCHEELE, L. A.: Progress in Prevention of Chronic Illness, 1949–1956, J.A.M.A., *160*, 1114, March 31, 1956.
WALSH, J. P.: Correlation of Oral and General Diseases, Internat. Dent. J., *6*, 340, September, 1956.

Chapter 29

BEDRIDDEN AND HELPLESS PATIENTS

BEDRIDDEN PATIENTS

WITHIN recent years, efforts have been made through research and organized programming, to attend to the oral health needs of the chronically ill and handicapped. These patients represent all age groups. Many are confined to hospitals, institutions, nursing homes or private homes, which means that special adaptations for dental and dental hygiene care are required. Portable equipment is being developed and special training for dental personnel promoted. The reader is encouraged to study reports of research and program planning which have appeared in recent literature and which are listed as suggested readings at the close of this chapter.

Dental care for the chronically ill must be completed in a variety of surroundings. For the hospitalized, dental clinics frequently are available to provide care for inpatients. Those who are not hospitalized may be confined to their homes or may be able to be transported to the dental office in a wheel chair depending on the severity of the case and the extent of disability.

Dentists and dental hygienists in private practice have occasion to attend patients confined to their homes. Dental hygiene techniques lend themselves to care for the bedridden since the entire oral prophylaxis can be completed with manual instruments. Topical fluoride applications can be made by skillful adaptations for keeping the teeth dry. Instruction in personal oral care procedures has particular significance for the comfort as well as the health of the patient. Suggestions relative to planning and conducting a home visit are included in this chapter.

I. IMPORTANCE OF DENTAL HYGIENE CARE TO THE CHRONICALLY ILL (BEDRIDDEN) PATIENT

A. Aids in prevention of periodontal diseases which would require extensive treatment.

B. Assists in prevention of further complication of the patient's state of health by lessening dental care problems.

C. Contributes to the patient's comfort, mental ease, and general well-being.

D. Encourages adequate personal care procedures, whether performed by the patient or his attendant.

E. Contributes to general rehabilitation or habilitation of the patient.

II. PREPARATION FOR THE HOME VISIT

A. Understanding the Patient

1. Consider the characteristics associated with the particular chronic illness or disease.

2. Consider special problems related to age. (For example, for the gerodontic patient see pages 337–343.)

3. Review patient's medical history (by telephone if preliminary inspection visit is not practical) to determine unusual precautions which must be taken. Arrange with physician and dentist when premedication is indicated.

B. Instruments and Equipment

1. Sterile instruments, gauze wipes, cotton rolls and pellets, wood points and dappen dishes are wrapped in towels to make packages which will be convenient to open and use at the bedside.

2. Scalers for all possible adaptations should be included since the customary working positions may not be feasible.

3. Substances such as disclosing solution, postoperative antiseptic, polishing agent, and topical fluoride solution are carried in small, tightly closed bottles.

4. Coverall: a large plastic drape is of particular importance since in certain types of illness the patient's coordination during rinsing may be limited. Thoughtfulness in the care of bed linen is appreciated by the patient's attendant.

5. Emesis basin: for patient rinsing. Although a small basin undoubtedly would be available at the home, the kidney-shaped basin facilitates the rinsing process.

6. Lighting: adaptation of available possibilities.
    a. Headlight or reflector: dentist may have as part of his office equipment; with practice the dental hygienist can learn to use with ease.
    b. Photography spot light: might be available either from the dentist or from the patient's home; need a type with a narrow, concentrated beam.
    c. Gooseneck lamp: might be available in patient's home; need bulb of adequate wattage.

7. Miscellaneous facilities usually available at the home: arrangements must be planned (by telephone) in advance of appointment date.
    a. Large towels: for covering pillows.
    b. Types of pillows available which may be firm enough to assist in maintaining patient's head in reasonably stationary position.
    c. Hospital bed: can be adjusted most effectively for patient's position.
    d. Mouth wash: inquire as to whether the patient has a favorite kind and whether this would be available for use.

C. Appointment Time: Arrange during the patient's usual waking hours at as convenient a time as possible in relation to nursing care and mealtime schedule.

III. APPROACH TO PATIENT

Since a majority of patients who come to the dental office are active people with good general health, it is sometimes difficult for the dental hygienist to adjust to the relatively helpless, chronically ill person.

There may be a tendency to be oversolicitous which does not contribute to the development of a cooperative patient. Usually a direct approach with gentle firmness is most successful.

Establishment of rapport with the patient depends in part on whether the patient has requested and anticipated the appointment, or whether those caring for the patient have insisted on and arranged for the visit.

A. Psychological Characteristics of Patient

Frequently the well-adjusted chronically ill person may be more appreciative of the care provided than the patient who comes to the dental office, and may be well aware of the difficulties under which the dental hygienist is working. The cooperation obtained frequently depends on the patient's attitude toward his illness or disability.

A prolonged illness which may have been accompanied by suffering is not conducive to a healthy outlook on life. Monotonous confinement contributes to the development of characteristics such as those listed below.[1]

1. Difficulty in maintaining cheerful attitude.
2. Bored or dissatisfied with sameness of daily routine.
3. Easily depressed.
4. Discouragement about recovery leads to mental state which retards recovery.
5. Sensitive and easily offended.
6. Demanding; enjoy being waited on if used to having prompt attention to each request.
7. Indifferent to personal appearance and general rules of personal hygiene.

B. Suggestions for General Procedure

1. Regardless of inconvenience of arrangements, two appointments should be planned when extensive scaling is required.
   a. Patient may fatigue.
   b. Need for observing tissue response.
   c. Need to give encouragement in personal care procedures.
2. Request that visitors be asked to remain out of the room during the appointment to prevent distraction of patient.
3. Introduce each step slowly to be sure patient knows what is being carried out.
4. Do not make the patient feel rushed. When patient is inclined to want to talk extensively, listen as patiently as time permits. Socializing is one of the best ways to establish rapport.

IV. APPLIED DENTAL HYGIENE CARE

A. The Working Situation

Ingenuity is needed to arrange patient position, head stabilization, and proper lighting to maintain patient comfort and yet provide access for the operator.

1. Suggestions for patient positioning and head stabilization
   a. Patient in bed
      (1) Hospital bed: adjust to lift patient's head to desirable height.
      (2) Ordinary bed: use firm pillows to support patient.

  b. Patient in wheel chair
   (1) Tall back: may provide excellent headrest; back lowered
    to proper height.
   (2) Short back: although it is possible to back the chair
    against a wall and insert a pillow for the head, it may
    be better to have patient moved to a davenport or
    chair where a more stable headrest would be provided.
  c. Portable headrest may be attached to back of plain chair or
   wheel chair.
 2. Suggestions for lighting
  a. Turn off overhead lighting to reduce shadows in the mouth.
  b. Headlight: usually the most convenient and efficient form of
   lighting because of concentrated beam.
  c. Head reflector: reflect light from bed lamp attached to bed
   behind patient's head.
  d. Gooseneck or photographer's light: care must be taken not to
   direct light into patient's eyes.
 3. Instrument arrangement: on towel on table beside bed or chair.
 4. Operator position: standing beside bed. Resist urge to sit on
  the edge of the bed.

B. **Oral Prophylaxis:** Scaling and porte polishing are complicated by
 instability of head. Skill and patience are primary factors.

C. **Topical Application of Fluoride**
 1. Without the usual saliva ejector to aid in keeping the teeth dry,
  it may be well to perform the applications in four parts, one
  for each quadrant. Child's head may be held in steadier
  position.
 2. Use manual chip blower to dry the teeth (see page 81).

V. PATIENT INSTRUCTION

A. **Personal Oral Care:** Provide specific instruction for attendant of
 helpless or uncoordinated patient. Demonstrate in patient's
 mouth. An automatic toothbrush may prove valuable with
 certain cases (see page 295).

B. **Dietary Suggestions**
 1. Need for consultation with physician concerning prescribed diet.
  When important relationships of diet to oral health are suspected they should be reported to the dentist. He or the
  dental hygienist may discuss the patient's problem with the
  physician.
 2. Diet for dental caries prevention can be very important since
  the patient cannot go to dental office. Cariogenic foods should
  be avoided as snacks.
 3. Factors influencing suggestions for diet
  a. Patient's appetite may be poor, particularly if he is discouraged about the state of his health.
  b. Patient may be finicky in food selection which may have
   affected his general nutritional state or have resulted in
   excessive use of carbohydrate foods.
  c. Monotony of meals may have lessened his desire to eat.

THE HOSPITALIZED HELPLESS OR UNCONSCIOUS PATIENT

Personal oral care procedures for the hospitalized patient are accomplished by the attendant member of the nursing staff when the patient is unable to care for himself.   When a dental hygienist is employed in the hospital she will be called on to assist and advise.   Understanding the possible procedures is important to all dental hygienists if they are to appreciate ramifications of dental hygiene care for the many types of patients with special needs.

Skill is required to carry out routine methods of toothbrushing, rinsing and cleaning of removable dentures for the conscious patient who is able to cooperate.   Methods must be adapted when the patient's head cannot be elevated.   When the patient's illness or injury involves the oral cavity, the advice and recommendations of the attending oral surgeon are followed.

Maintenance of oral cleanliness for the acutely ill or unconscious patient requires special procedures because of the complete helplessness of the patient.   Objectives and methods described below have application for patients with other special needs, as for example, the patient with a fractured jaw (see page 373) or severe mental retardation (see page 396).

I. OBJECTIVES OF CARE

A. Prevent debris in the mouth from being aspirated and clogging air passages.
B. Minimize the possibility of oral infection.
C. Clean the mouth and provide comfort for the patient.

II. TOOTHBRUSH WITH SUCTION ATTACHMENT

Mouth cleaning may be accomplished by wiping the teeth and tissues and applying a lubricant to oral mucosa and lips, or by attempting to brush the teeth in a routine manner.   Removal of debris presents a problem by either method and rinsing is impossible because of the danger of aspiration of debris and water by the patient. The toothbrush with attached suction provides a more efficient and safe method for patient care.

A. **Description of the Brush**[2,3]
   1. Soft textured multitufted brush with hole drilled between the bristles in the middle of the head of the brush.
   2. Small plastic tubing inserted into hole; end adjusted slightly below level of brushing plane.
   3. Other end of tubing passed across back of brush handle and attached to handle by small rubber bands (Figure 72).
   4. Tubing is connected by an adapter to aspirator or suction outlet.

B. **Procedure for Use of Brush**
   The detailed procedure would be outlined for hospital personnel and included in the nursing procedures manual.[4]   An abbreviated outline of the basic steps is included here.
   1. Preparation of the patient.
      a. The patient may be aware of what is going on although not respond in his usual manner.
      b. Tell patient that he is going to have his teeth brushed.

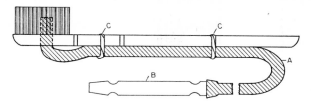

FIGURE 72.—Multitufted toothbrush with suction attachment for care of helpless patient. *A.* Plastic tubing. *B.* Adapter for attachment of tubing to aspirator or suction outlet. *C.* Rubber bands to attach tubing to toothbrush handle.

Plastic tube is inserted through a hole in the head of the brush and extended to a level slightly below the brushing plane.

  c. Turn patient on his side and place a pillow at his back for support.

  d. Place a face towel under patient's chin and over bedding.

 2. Attach toothbrush to suction outlet and lay brush on towel near patient's mouth.

 3. Place a rubber bite block on one side of the patient's mouth between the teeth. String tied to bite block is fastened to patient's gown with a safety pin.

 4. Pour mouthwash over brush; turn on suction.

 5. Gently retract lip and carefully apply Rolling Stroke toothbrushing procedures; apply suction over each tooth surface with particular care at each interproximal area. Moisten brush frequently.

 6. Move bite block to opposite side of mouth and continue brushing procedure.

 7. Place brush in cup of clear water to allow water to be sucked through and clear the tubing both during the procedure if there is clogging and after brushing to clean the tube.

 8. Remove bite block; wipe patient's lips with paper wipe and apply petroleum jelly.

 9. Wash brush and bite block; prepare materials for next use.

 10. One toothbrush usually is sufficient for the patient's stay in the hospital.

REFERENCES

1. Price, A. L.: *The Art, Science and Spirit of Nursing,* 2nd ed. Philadelphia, Saunders, 1959, pp. 752–753.
2. CAPPS, J. S.: New Device for Oral Hygiene, Am. J. Nursing, *58,* 1532, November, 1958.
3. TRONQUET, A. A.: Oral Hygiene for Hospital Patients, Am. Dent. A. J., *63,* 215, August, 1961.
4. University of Washington Hospital, Division of Nursing Services: How to Give Special Mouth Care to the Helpless and Unconscious Patient, March 6, 1959. (mimeographed)

SUGGESTED READINGS

AXELBAND, A. A.: Dental Treatment of Bedridden Patients at Home, Oral Hyg., *44,* 1197, September, 1954.
BALTZ, F. L.: How Can Local Dental Societies Cooperate with Nursing Homes in Development of Effective Dental Programs? Am. Dent. A. J., *64,* 162, February, 1962.
GALAGAN, D. J.: Development of Dental Health Care Programs for Persons with Chronic Illness, Am. Dent. A. J., *53,* 686, December, 1956.
GALAGAN, D. J.: Dental Care for the Chronically Ill and Aged: Emphasis on Rehabilitation. Introduction, Am. Dent. A. J., *64,* 155, February, 1962.

KLUMPP, T. G.:   Future Pattern of Medical Care of the Chronically Ill., Am. Dent. A. J., *58*, 67, February, 1959.

LAW, F. E.:   Dental Hygiene for the Chronically Ill and Aged, Am. Dent. Hygienists' A. J., *37*, 132, 3rd Quarter, 1963.

LOTZKAR, S. J.:   Dental Care for the Chronically Ill, Aged, and Homebound, Am. Dent. A. J., *67*, 71, July, 1963.

ST. MARIE, G. L.:   What Can the Dental Society Do? (Geriatric Care), Am. Dent. A. J., *64*, 157, February, 1962.

SHEARY, H. C.:   Role of the Dental Hygienist in Health Care of the Chronically Ill, Handicapped and Aged, Am. Dent. Hygienists' A. J., *37*, 135, 3rd Quarter, 1963.

SHELDON, M. P.:   Recent Developments Concerning Dental Care for the Chronically Ill and Aged, Am. Dent. A. J., *59*, 505, September, 1959.

SHELDON, M. P.:   Community Planning for the Dental Care of the Chronically Ill and Disabled, Dental Clinics of North America, July, 1960, p. 503.

ZUR, J. E.:   Role of State Dental Society and State Dental Division in Improving Dental Care of the Aged, Am. Dent. A. J., *62*, 384, April, 1961.

Chapter 30

GERODONTIC PATIENTS

PREVENTIVE measures for the aged through care and instruction assume greater importance since the number of people involved in this group is increasing steadily. In 1940 nearly 7 per cent of the population was over 65 years and it is expected that more than 14 per cent of the population will be over 65 in 1980 according to the United States Bureau of the Census. Dentists and dental hygienists are challenged by the need for helping the aging population to learn about personal care and seek professional care which will provide continuing oral comfort and function.

The biologic age is not synonymous with the chronologic age and hence signs of aging appear at different chronologic ages in different individuals. In reality aging begins at birth. Senescence, the process or condition of growing old, is a physiologic entity. Normal aging should not be confused with the effects of pathologic influences which accelerate the aging process.

Each age period brings changes in body metabolism, the activity of the cells, the endocrine balance and the mental processes. The knowledge and understanding of normal physical and emotional characteristics for each age level provide a guide for planning patient care and instruction.

I. GENERAL PHYSICAL CHARACTERISTICS

Changes with aging vary between individuals and between organs and tissues of the same individual. Major characteristics which may affect dental hygiene procedures have been included below.

A. **General Tissue Changes**
1. Dehydration.
2. Atrophy.
3. Diminished elasticity.
4. Decreased function including diminished reparative capacity.
5. Fibrosis.

B. **Basal Metabolism:** lowered.

C. **Skin:** thin, wrinkled, dry, loss of tone, pigmented spots, atrophy of sweat glands.

D. **Special Senses**
1. Sight: increased farsightedness, sensitivity to light, and night blindness.
2. Hearing: loss of sensitivity to high tones, gradual loss of hearing acuity.

E. **Muscular System:** loss of muscle tone, development of unsteadiness, tremor, lack of muscular strength.

F. **Cardiovascular System**
   1. Increase in blood pressure.
   2. Decreased circulation to tissues.

G. **Blood:** lowered red blood cell count and hemoglobin.

H. **Respiratory System:** shortness of breath.

I. **Digestive System**
   1. Degeneration of mucous membranes alters absorption of food elements.
   2. Gradual decrease in production of hydrochloric acid and other secretions necessary for digestion.
   3. Constipation; gas contained in stomach and intestine.

J. **Glandular Secretions:** diminished.

K. **Stress Reactions**
   1. Cannot tolerate extremes of heat and cold.
   2. Cannot tolerate muscular strain.
   3. Healing slower.
   4. Decreased resistance to infection.

II. ORAL CHARACTERISTICS

The same general tissue changes apply alike to oral tissues. Many older people may have lost some or all of their teeth as a result of dental caries or periodontal diseases.

A. **Lips:** dry, purse-string (related to dehydration within tissue).

B. **Mucous Membranes**
   1. Loss of elasticity.
   2. Diminished keratinization.
   3. Dryness.

C. **Tongue**
   1. Atrophy of papillæ resulting in smooth appearance.
   2. Taste bud degeneration; abnormal taste sensations.

D. **Salivary and Mucous Glands**
   1. Atrophy resulting in diminished secretion.
   2. Decrease in amount of ptyalin.

E. **Gingiva**
   1. Loss of stippling: shiny appearance.
   2. Diminished keratinization; lowered resistance to infection.
   3. Friable; easily injured.
   4. Recession.

F. **Teeth**
   1. Color: may be darker due to environment and changes in salivary secretion.
   2. Attrition: influenced by use: habits, dietary choices and occupational factors.

3. Pulp
    a. Narrowing of pulp chamber; formation of secondary dentin.
    b. Fibrotic changes.
    c. Formation of pulp calcifications (pulp stones or denticles).

G. **Epithelial Attachment:** migrates apically with continued eruption of tooth related to attrition.

H. **Periodontal Ligament** (Membrane): thickness varies with function more than age.

I. **Alveolar Bone**
    1. Reduction in height.
    2. Increased porousness or rarefaction (osteoporosis).
    3. Decreased vascularity.
    4. Reduction in metabolism and healing capacity.

III. PSYCHOLOGICAL CHARACTERISTICS

The list below should not be considered typical of all elderly patients since many are well-adjusted. These characteristics are suggested to help the dental hygienist better understand possible patient attitudes and actions.

A. **Insecurity**
    1. Related to reduced economic status, self-respect, and feeling of being needed due to inability to work.
    2. Influenced by rejection by family and desire for attention.
    3. Anxiety over health.

B. **Depression**
    1. Limited physical power; sensitivity about shortcomings of impaired vision, hearing, and lack of motor control.
    2. Changes in physical appearance.
    3. Loneliness: desire for attention.

C. **Inability to Adjust to Changes in Mode of Life;** tendency to develop fixed habits and ideas.

D. **Slowing of Voluntary Responses** and speed of association of thought.

E. **Difficulty in Perception** and timing sequential events.

F. **Tendency to Introspection;** narrowing of interests; living in the past.

G. **Slowing of Speed of Vocalization.**

IV. APPLIED TECHNIQUES FOR THE APPOINTMENT

In planning and conducting the appointment for the gerodontic patient, knowledge of the general physical, oral and psychological characteristics of the aging is applied. Suggested factors for consideration are listed in Table 12.

TABLE 12.—ADAPTATIONS IN CLINICAL TECHNIQUES FOR THE
GERODONTIC PATIENT

Appointment Factors	Characteristic of the Gerodontic Patient	Suggested Relation to Appointment Procedure
APPOINTMENT TIME	Tires more easily than younger patient. Shortness of breath. Inclined to be impatient.	Plan shorter appointments. Need more frequent recall to provide for shorter appointments. Appreciation of fact that he has made a real effort to get to the office.
	Cannot tolerate extremes of muscular strain; recovery from activity slow.	Prevent need for long appointments.
	Slower voluntary responses. Sensitivity about shortcomings of lack of motor control.	Do not rush him. Do not make him feel old by obviously assisting him into the dental chair.
	Lowered tolerance to extremes of heat and cold; less body cooling through perspiration.	Adjust room temperature.
	Impaired hearing.	Speak clearly and slowly, repeat names; provide written memorandum of details concerning appointment.
ORAL PROPHYLAXIS TECHNIQUES	Loss of elasticity of lips and oral mucosa.	Difficulty in retraction may provide patient discomfort.
	Slowing of voluntary responses. Cannot adjust to sudden muscular demands.	Do not demand quick response to request for change of position of head, rinsing.
	Increased susceptibility to irritations of the tissues. Friable tissues; epithelium tears easily. Tendency to develop canker sores, traumatic ulcers, or angular cheilosis under mild stress to tissues.	Need for unusual care during instrumentation or x-ray film placement to prevent irritation to soft tissues.
	Reduction in growth and repair processes. Decreased resistance to infection.	Provide as little trauma to gingiva as possible during instrumentation. Suggest postoperative care procedures for promoting healing.
	Inability to recover readily from stresses and strains; Unsteadiness; tendency to dizziness.	At completion of appointment straighten chair and let patient sit up for short time before dismissing; assist out of chair.
RADIOGRAPHY	Increased fibrosis of tissues.	Adjustment of exposure or processing time.

Attention to dental office arrangement which may provide physical barriers is important. The aged person's impaired vision, feebleness or lack of motor control must be considered. There is need for elimination of hazards such as small rugs which can slide on polished floors, corners of rugs which can be tripped over, and irregularities in floor levels.

V. PATIENT INSTRUCTION

Older individuals need to be as interested in their health and appearance as people of any age. Esthetic deterioration may create emotional unhappiness and when the aged feel insecure or unwanted they may lose their interest in personal oral care and diet. Motivation through expression of sincere interest on the part of dental personnel can be an influencing factor in helping the patient to better health.

In the younger age groups there are still many who believe it inevitable and normal to eventually lose the teeth. With older people who still have their teeth, there is a tendency to be very resistant about the loss of them. Certain people fear dentures because they associate them with "old" people. Patients with partial dentures will already have been impressed with the need for preservation of the remaining teeth. Here, in the desire to save the teeth, lies the appeal for preventive measures for both the teeth and their supporting structures, and good use should be made of this very real motivating force.

In patient instruction it is important not to try to change all lifelong habits since this may create frustration and unhappiness. Self-confidence, which has diminished because of lowering of physical capabilities and emotional satisfaction, must be built up. Major changes, required because previous habits are detrimental, must be brought about gradually if cooperation is to be expected. There is need for a more optimistic attitude about the degree of oral health which the elderly patient can be expected to achieve.

A. Personal Oral Care Procedures

Recommendations follow the same pattern as for other adult patients (see Chapters 26 and 27 and Table 11, page 286). Each procedure is related to the individual need. With the elderly patient the difference lies in the method of motivation and instruction. Suggestions for adaptation of instruction to physical and psychological characteristics are listed in Table 13.

B. Dietary Habits

Dietary and resulting nutritional deficiencies are common in older people. For example, characteristic changes such as burning tongue, angular cheilosis and atrophic glossitis may occur as a result of Vitamin B complex deficiencies. Unfortunately, many people believe that a diet rich in nutritive elements is important only for children.

1. *Factors contributing to dietary and nutritional deficiencies*
   a. Limited budget.
   b. Lives alone or eats alone.
   c. Does not eat regular meals; frequently uses nonnutritious snacks and foods for entertaining.
   d. Lacks interest in shopping for food or preparing it.

    e. Acuteness of senses lowered; may seek highly seasoned or sweetened foods.

    f. Childish likes and dislikes; unusual cravings.

    g. Tendency to follow food habits of lifetime; ignores newer knowledge of food preparation methods and dietary needs.

    h. Inadequate masticatory efficiency through tooth loss or inadequate dentures.

        (1) Adverse food selection may result from social embarrassment over inability to chew.

        (2) Adaptations in eating habits made to compensate for deficiency may interfere with adequate digestion and absorption of nutrients.[1]

    i. May follow dietary fads which provide only a very limited and unbalanced diet.

    j. Loss of appetite: may have physiologic, social, or economic causes.

    k. Lack of self-discipline; feeling that aging brings privilege to eat only preferred foods.

TABLE 13.—CHARACTERISTICS AFFECTING INSTRUCTION FOR THE GERODONTIC PATIENT

Characteristic of the Gerodontic Patient	*Suggested Relation to Appointment Procedure*
Tendency for introspection; desire for attention.	Patience needed in taking time to listen to complaints and accounts of past experiences.
Feelings of insecurity. Deprivation of physical capabilities. Mental weaknesses shown through touchy sensitiveness, exaggerated imaginary or real pains, or attitudes of suspicion.	Sympathetic understanding needed. Build up self-confidence.
Resistance to change; tendency to maintain fixed habits.	Should not attempt to change all life-long habits, only detrimental ones.
Vision impaired.	Provide eyeglasses while giving instruction.
Hearing impaired; loss of sensitivity to higher tones.	Speak distinctly in normal voice. Look at patient while speaking; many are lip readers (see page 423).
Slowing of voluntary responses. Slowing of speed of thought associations. Difficulty in timing sequential events; skills become separate movements as by a child. Least comfortable when must respond quickly to demanding sequential stimuli. Rate of learning changed, ability to learn not changed. Changes in speed of vocalization.	Make suggestions gradually, over series of appointments. Do not demand learning a completely new procedure; adapt procedure already used. Guide patient's demonstration of toothbrushing to prevent embarrassment. Do not expect perfection; go slow, anticipate difficulties, give cues, clues. Distinguish between slowness of learning and inability.
Memory shortened due mainly to lack of attention, lack of interest, or more selection of what patient wants to remember.	Use motivating factors carefully. Provide written instructions; spoken instructions may be forgotten or misunderstood.
Need for personal achievement.	Help patient gain sense of accomplishment; commend for any success, however minor.

2. *Dietary needs of the aged*

Adequate nutritional balance is one of the best safeguards for promoting health and efficiency at any age. Because of the factors mentioned above, elderly people frequently use a high carbohydrate diet and neglect other nutritional needs.

The first consideration in making recommendations for aging patients is that a well-balanced diet with limited fermentable carbohydrate for dental caries prevention is important as for any age. Caloric intake must be decreased because of lowered metabolic rate and activity. Protein, vitamins and minerals are particularly important for body function, repair and resistance to disease. Reviews of dietary and nutritional needs are available for study.[2-6] Recent research shows that fluoride in the diet of the elderly is beneficial in the prevention of osteoporosis and fractures of the bones.[7,8,9]

3. *Instruction in dietary habits*

A weekly dietary survey for evaluation of the patient's problems such as that used for a dental caries control study (see pages 356–361) could prove very helpful if handled tactfully. The dietary review would aid in calling deficiencies to the patient's attention.

Appeal to the patient is made through his own personal concern for the relationships of dietary deficiencies to appearance, lowered resistance to disease and premature aging, which may inspire the patient to improve his daily habits.

REFERENCES

1. O'ROURKE, J. T. and MINER, L. M. S.: *Oral Physiology.* St. Louis, Mosby, 1951, pp. 298–304.
2. BAVETTA, L. A. and NIMNI, M. E.: Nutritional Aspects, in Cowdry, E. V.: *Care of the Geriatric Patient,* 2nd ed. St. Louis, Mosby, 1963, pp. 288–316.
3. FISHER, W. T.: Prosthetics and Geriatric Nutrition, J. Pros. Dent., *5,* 481, July, 1955.
4. Detroit Dental Clinic Club, Complete Denture Section: Nutrition for the Denture Patient, J. Pros. Dent., *10,* 53, January-February, 1960.
5. MASSLER, MAURY: Tissue Changes During Aging, Oral Surg., Oral Med., & Oral Path., *9,* 1185, November, 1956.
6. O'ROURKE: op. cit., pp. 249–266.
7. Bone Density and Fluoride Ingestion, Nutrition Rev., *19,* 198, July, 1961.
8. BERNSTEIN, D. S., *et al.*: Use of Sodium Fluoride in Metabolic Bone Disease, J. Clin. Investig., *42,* 916, June, 1963.
9. LEONE, N. C.: Effects of the Absorption of Fluoride, Arch. Indust. Health, *21,* 324, April, 1960.

SUGGESTED READINGS

ALLEN, E. F.: Dental Aspects, in Cowdry, E. V.: *Care of the Geriatric Patient.* 2nd ed., St. Louis, Mosby, 1963, pp. 317–322.

American Dental Association, Council on Dental Health and Council on Legislation: American Dental Association Statement before the Subcommittee on Problems of the Aged and Aging, Am. Dent. A. J., *59,* 1003, November, 1959.

BERNARD, MARCELLE and HOGAN, W. J.: Geriatric Patient in the Office, Am. Dent. A. J., *63,* 670, November, 1961.

BILLS, E. D.: Counsel to the Aging Dental Patient, J. Pros. Dent., *9,* 881, September-October, 1959.

BIRREN, J. E.: Psychological Limitations that Occur with Age, Pub. Health Rep., *71,* 1173, December, 1956.

BROWN, A. F.: *Medical Nursing,* 3rd ed. Philadelphia, Saunders, 1957, pp. 60–87.

BURMAN, L. R.: Gerodontia, N. Y. J. Dent., *20,* 62, February, 1950.

DONAHUE, WILMA and STOLL, M. R.: Psychological Aspects, in Cowdry, E.V.: *Care of the Geriatric Patient*, 2nd ed., St. Louis, Mosby, 1963, pp. 37–62.

GLICKMAN, IRVING: Clinical Periodontology, 2nd ed. Philadelphia, Saunders, 1958, pp. 60–65.

HOMMA, KUMIKO and WILKINS, E. M.: Oral Health Education for the Gerodontic Patient, Am. Dent. Hygienists' A. J., *33*, 10, January, 1959.

JAMIESON, C. H.: Geriatrics and the Denture Patient, J. Prosthetic Dent., *8*, 8, January, 1958.

KRAJICEK, D. D.: Dental Treatment of the Elderly Patient, Am. Dent. A. J., *58*, 74, February, 1959.

KROGMAN, W. M.: Geriatric Research and Prosthodontics, J. Pros. Dent., *12*, 493, May-June, 1962.

MASSLER, Maury: Geriatrics and Gerodontics, N. Y. J. Dent., *26*, 54, February, 1956.

MOEN, B. D.: Statistics Relating to Dental Care for the Aged, J. Am. Coll. Dent., *29*, 94, June, 1962.

PRICE, A. L.: *The Art, Science and Spirit of Nursing*, 2nd ed. Philadelphia, Saunders, 1959, pp. 762–776.

RUTKIN, I. R. and LEEDS, M. H.: Dentistry for the Elderly, Am. Dent. A. J., *59*, 1248, December, 1959.

SCHWEIGER, J. W.: Prosthetic Considerations for the Aging, J. Pros. Dent., *9*, 555, July-August, 1959.

SEIFERT, I., LANGER, A., and MICHMANN, J.: Evaluation of Psychologic Factors in Geriatric Denture Patients, J. Pros. Dent., *12*, 516, May-June, 1962.

SILVERMAN, S. I.: Dental Care for the Aged: Role of Private Practitioner, Am. Dent. A. J., *64*, 165, February, 1962.

SILVERMAN, SOL: Geriatrics and Tissue Changes, Calif. S. Dent. A. J. and Nev. S. Dent. A. J., *33*, 194, May-June, 1957.

TAYLOR, R. G. and DOKU, H. C.: Dental Survey of Healthy Older Persons, Am. Dent. A. J., *67*, 62, July, 1963.

UHLER, I. V.: Oral-Facial-Speech Problems of the Aging: A Challenge to the Health Care Professions, J. Oral Surg., Anes., & Hosp. D. Serv., *19*, 380, September, 1961.

WATERBURY, C. H.: Dentist and Our Aging Population, Oral Hygiene, *47*, 52, July, 1957.

ZIEGLER, J. E.: Geriodontics, South. Calif. S. Dent. A. J., *24*, 29, September, 1956.

Chapter 31

DENTAL CARIES CONTROL PATIENTS

INTRODUCTION TO THE DENTAL CARIES CONTROL STUDY

PATIENTS who are subject to marked dental caries activity are a particular responsibility of the members of the dental profession. These patients* need special help in coping with the problem which, if left unattended, may well lead to extensive loss of teeth prematurely. To instigate a program of dental caries control requires thought, effort and patience on the part of the dentist and dental hygienist in determining the method of approach.

A dental caries control study may be described as a planned effort to analyze the patient's problem and initiate a program for dental caries prevention. This educational effort includes in part or whole, much of the same information that is provided for all patients. In the caries control study the instruction becomes more intensified as the patient is counseled to put into effect a specific program for diet and personal care.

Pertinent information is obtained through the oral inspection, dental and medical history, dental charting and a study of the diet made through use of a week-long diary kept by the patient. A dental caries activity test may be used as an indicator of the degree of susceptibility. Critical review of the information obtained leads to the definition of a specific plan for limitation of use of foods with high fermentable carbohydrate content in an attempt to curb the process of dental caries. Meticulous procedures for the patient's personal oral care are emphasized in their relation to the carbohydrates used in the diet. Through dental health instruction the patient comes to learn the purposes of each step in the study and to accept responsibility in carrying out his part of the program of action. Practical studies of this type have been described in the literature.[1-5]

The success of dental caries control measures is dependent upon the patient's clear understanding and appreciation of the procedures, as well as his ability and willingness to cooperate. In turn, the dental hygienist applies her knowledge of the physical and emotional problems at various age levels in her attempt to understand and motivate the patient.

I. OUTLINE OF THE PARTS OF THE STUDY

A. Preliminary Planning

1. Patient Selection.
2. Explanation of Procedures to Patient.

B. Obtaining and Summarizing the Data

1. Patient's Medical and Dental History.
2. Clinical Survey.
   a. Oral inspection.
   b. Dental charting.

*The word "patient" is used to mean patient *and* parent when patient is a child.

3. Complete Oral Radiographic Survey.
4. Dental Caries Activity Test.
5. Dietary Survey.
6. Analysis of Data.

C. **Clinical Procedures**
1. Oral Prophylaxis.
2. Topical Fluoride Application(s).
3. Restorative Dentistry.

D. **Instruction in Personal Oral Care Procedures**

E. **Dental Health Education Conference with Presentation of Program of Action**

F. **Evaluation of Progress**
1. Dental Caries Activity Test.
2. Follow-up Appointments.

G. **Case History Written Report**

II. **PATIENT SELECTION**

The study might be proposed at an initial appointment but more frequently at a recall appointment when the patient has shown real concern for the problem and has demonstrated a cooperative attitude. Interest in participation in a study can and should be developed in patients who need help in their dental caries problem.

A patient of any age who has high dental caries activity may benefit from the study. In proposing the need for the study, the probability of success is dependent on many factors including those listed below.

A. **Acceptance of Responsibility by Those Concerned**
1. The Dentist and Dental Hygienist: must sincerely want better oral health for the patient.
2. The Patient
   a. Young children: parents will bear weight of responsibility.
   b. Intermediate children: child will have certain responsibilities along with parents.
   c. Teen-agers: patient will have responsibility but must be able to obtain cooperation from parents.
   d. Adult: will take own responsibility.

B. **Patient's Prerequisites**
1. Interest in improving oral health.
2. Appreciation of services to be rendered.
3. Willingness to cooperate in keeping appointments.
4. Willingness to carry out required procedures conscientiously.

C. **Evaluation of the Patient**
Skill in recognizing the above mentioned prerequisites comes with experience in understanding people in general. It is difficult to determine in a brief meeting whether the enthusiasm evidenced at the beginning will carry on throughout a study. Probability of success will depend, in part, on the continued interest and enthusiasm of dental personnel as the patient is motivated in the course of the study.

III. **EXPLANATION OF PROCEDURES TO PATIENT**

The final outcome of the study frequently depends on the preliminary presentation. A well-informed patient is more cooperative and appreciative. At the outset at least the four factors listed below should be described and discussed.

A. Purposes and general objectives in terms of better oral health and the social and economic advantages.
B. Outline of the general procedures involved in the study.
C. Description of time involved and suggestions concerning the planning of the appointments.
D. Need for mutual cooperation.

IV. **PREPARATION FOR THE STUDY**

A. Study physical and emotional characteristics of the patient's age group.[6,7]
B. Plan approach to the patient according to the appraisal of his *individual* characteristics.
C. Outline objectives for the patient in terms of his basic oral health needs.
D. Plan how the patient (and parents) may be motivated.

APPOINTMENT PLANNING FOR THE DENTAL CARIES CONTROL STUDY

There is no standard or uniform procedure which can be applied for all patients. A number of factors will enter into the determination of the number and length of appointments, particularly the patient's capacity for learning. Overcrowded, hurried appointments with too much material presented at one time will make it difficult for the patient to absorb the information and follow instructions. A series of appointments permits time for review and to encourage the patient to ask questions.

Carefully planned appointments contribute much to the success of the study. When the entire series of appointments is outlined at the beginning, the time required is clear to the patient and misunderstandings are minimized.

A suggested plan for appointments is included here. At least 4 and preferably 5 appointments are recommended. Each phase of the study is described in succeeding sections of this chapter.

I. **FIRST APPOINTMENT WITH PATIENT**

A. Review objectives of study to enlist full cooperation.
B. Obtain or review the patient's medical history.
C. Obtain saliva sample.* Seal and label container.†

*Reliable patients can be instructed to collect their saliva samples at home immediately upon rising in the morning. The most accurate results are obtained from samples taken at that time since the oral flora is nearest to normal distribution. See section on Caries Activity Tests for instructions.

†Upon dismissal of patient at each appointment when a saliva sample has been obtained, attend promptly to laboratory procedures conducted in the dental office or to mailing of saliva sample to laboratory. Familiarity with the schedule of the laboratory is important in order that samples be mailed to reach the laboratory on a day when weekends or holidays do not interfere with interpretation of results after the required incubation period.

   D. Complete the oral inspection.

   E. Perform the oral prophylaxis.

   F. Make the topical fluoride application. (When a series of sodium fluoride applications is to be made, the successive applications are planned with the second, third and fourth appointments below.)

   G. Present preliminary toothbrushing instruction; avoid reference to relationship of fermentable carbohydrates in the diet.

   H. Introduce dietary survey which the patient will record for one week. Discuss directions carefully (see page 358).

   I. Following first appointment
     1. Reevaluate basic assumptions and redefine objectives for the patient.
     2. Review physical and emotional characteristics of the individual patient.[6,7]

II. SECOND APPOINTMENT

   A. Obtain saliva sample.

   B. Receive and review dietary survey with patient to complete any necessary details (see page 358).

   C. Continue personalized instruction in oral physical therapy, the cause of dental caries, and other information essential to the individual patient.

   D. Make the complete radiographic survey.

   E. Perform the clinical aspects of charting.

   F. Following second appointment.
     1. Process and mount radiographs.
     2. Complete radiographic aspects of charting.
     3. Analyze the dietary survey (see page 360).
     4. Make preliminary plans for the Dental Health Education Conference (see page 362).
     5. Plan appointment with the dentist to discuss the case.

III. THIRD APPOINTMENT

   A. Conduct the Dental Health Education Conference with parents and child (see pages 363–365).

   B. Provide specific written instructions for the diet plan to be carried out during the following weeks.

   C. Following third appointment: telephone patient in 5 days to a week to offer encouragement and to clarify any questions about the expected procedure.

IV. FOURTH APPOINTMENT (after interval of 2 to 3 weeks when patient has been on special diet)

   A. Obtain saliva sample.

   B. Review dental health instruction.

   C. Describe 3 to 6 months' recall plan.

V. FIFTH CONTACT

A. Telephone to tell patient the results of the final dental caries activity test.

B. Encourage patient to continue the special dietary and personal oral care procedures.

THE DENTAL CARIES CONTROL STUDY CASE HISTORY

The written history of the dental caries control study relates and integrates the events which have occurred and observations made during the study. Interpretation of the facts should be done objectively.

The case history becomes a part of the patient's permanent record. Careful and complete recording is important in order that the text of the report will be meaningful and clear to all who read it.

I. GENERAL INSTRUCTIONS

A. **Date each recorded entry.**

B. **Record events as soon as possible after they occur.**

1. Take notes during the appointments as an aid to writing the case history. Note taking should be done inconspicuously so it does not distract the patient.
2. Record in the history all contacts with the patient during the study, including telephone conversations.
3. Include specific quotes from conversations if they reflect meaningful attitudes, habits, or acquired knowledge.
4. Record report in ink (typewritten if possible).

C. **Be objective in observations.**

D. **Use correct terminology** in writing history and avoid meaningless abbreviations.

E. **Use well constructed, concise sentences** with correct spelling, punctuation and grammar.

II. RECORDING OBSERVATIONS OF PATIENT'S PERSONALITY AND DEVELOPMENT

The study provides an excellent opportunity to gain insight into the personality and development of the child. Knowledge acquired can greatly augment understanding of the young patient and the parental influences. Suggested questions for consideration while making observations are listed below.

A. **Observing Intellectual Development**

1. Is patient's vocabulary average, below average, or above average for his age? Quote sample sentences in the patient's record.
2. Does he understand what is told him when words that he should understand are used? How does he show this?

    3. Does he show intellectual curiosity about the techniques and services which are performed for him? What questions does he ask?

    4. What does he tell about his success in school?

B. **Observing Physical Development**

    1. Does anything in the patient's medical history indicate abnormal physical development?

    2. Is he apparently of normal height and weight for his age, structure and heredity?

    3. Is his coordination good? Does he learn to brush his teeth readily as might be expected for his age group?

    4. Does he have enough hours of sleep and rest?

C. **Observing Emotional Development**

    1. What is the patient's reaction to his parents' authority? To the authority of dentist or dental hygienist when no parent is present? Is he at ease, apprehensive, obedient, or submissive? How does he show this?

    2. What does he say about his family?

    3. Does he express affection toward his parents? How?

    4. What fears, if any, does he exhibit?

    5. Does he show indications of self-discipline? Does his parent indicate that he brushes his teeth without being told? Did he help to complete the dietary survey? Does he accept the services done for him with a pleasant and cooperative attitude?

OBTAINING THE DATA

Information from the patient history, oral inspection, dental charting, radiographic survey, dental caries activity tests, dietary survey and observations of behavioral patterns is integrated and analyzed to provide the basis for the preventive program. Factors which influence the clinical procedures, educational requirements and recommendations for action are determined from the data.

I. **PATIENT HISTORY** (see pages 69–76)

A. Provides introductory information for considering the *total* health of the patient.

B. Reveals general health conditions under the care of a physician.

C. Identifies allergies or systemic diseases already requiring a special diet which can limit the dietary recommendations for dental caries prevention.

D. Relates the magnitude of the oral health problems to the other health needs of the patient.

E. Relates current dental caries activity to frequency of past dental care.

II. **CLINICAL SURVEY: ORAL INSPECTION AND DENTAL CHARTING** (see pages 81–85 and 255–260)

A. Defines state of oral health as related to personal oral care habits.

B. Reveals problems of personal oral care procedures which require special emphasis because of their relationship to the occlusion, condition of the gingiva, or habits.

C. Relates composition of the current diet to existing conditions of the oral cavity.

D. Provides data for analysis of dental caries activity.

III. **COMPLETE ORAL RADIOGRAPHIC SURVEY**

A. Provides information needed to complete the accurate recording of existing restorations and carious lesions.

B. Provides a visual aid for patient instruction.

CLINICAL PROCEDURES AND INSTRUCTION IN PERSONAL CARE

I. **ORAL PROPHYLAXIS AND TOPICAL FLUORIDE APPLICATIONS**

The oral prophylaxis and topical applications of fluoride solution become educational experiences for the patient along with the special procedures of the caries study. The topical fluoride applications provide a useful motivating agent to supplement the patient's own effort to control dental caries by daily dietary and personal oral care procedures.

II. **RESTORATIVE DENTISTRY**

Specific needs for dental treatment are presented to the patient by the dentist. The dental hygienist may need to interpret suggestions made. Many educational opportunities are available when discussing the need for restorative work, particularly related to the prevention of tooth loss.

A. **Private Dental Office Patient:** Motivation already will have been provided for the continuation of required appointments. Explanation of the probability of lowered incidence of dental caries as a result of following the requirements of the dental caries control study, can provide encouragement for the need for fewer appointments in the future.

B. **Clinic Patient:** The patient is advised of the need for restorative care and its relation to the success of the study. No specific report of the clinical findings from the charting and radiographs are supplied the patient who will be referred to a private dental office, although frequently it is possible for the clinic to provide the dentist with the duplicate set of radiographs.

III. **INSTRUCTION IN PERSONAL ORAL CARE PROCEDURES**

Teaching of purposes and procedures of toothbrushing and related daily care procedures becomes an integral part of each appointment during the series. Brushing promptly after eating and the relation to the removal of fermentable carbohydrates takes on particular significance when there is a dental caries problem. For personal oral care procedures see Chapters 26 and 27 and Table 11 on page 286.

DENTAL CARIES ACTIVITY TESTS

A dental caries activity test may be used as an educational device to guide the patient toward practicing habits conducive to the prevention of dental caries. Available tests have proved most effective in the determination of caries activity in groups, and the accuracy decreases when applied to the individual case.[8,9,10] Test results, therefore, should be used with full recognition of their limitations.

The use of test results for a visual aid for patient instruction is helpful since changes in results of a series of tests can show dramatically the effects of the patient's personal efforts in carrying out dietary and oral care preventive procedures. A real motivation can be provided for certain patients when the purpose for making the test is explained and related to the results of the clinical inspection for dental caries.

The relationship of carbohydrates and acid-forming bacteria to the initiation of dental caries has been outlined on page 114. With the removal of fermentable carbohydrates from the diet or the immediate removal of them from the tooth surface after eating, lowered dental caries activity usually can be expected.

To appreciate fully the use of the caries activity tests, it is important to recognize that it is not possible to assume from the numbers of carious, missing or restored teeth whether the caries process is active or arrested. Neither does the caries activity test result indicate the number of cavities present at any particular time. A positive test result may be apparent when there is no clinical evidence of caries and may forecast possible future dental caries.

I. PURPOSES OF THE CARIES ACTIVITY TEST

A. Serves as a visual aid to illustrate for the patient the need for participation in a program for dental caries prevention.
B. Classifies the patient's relative degree of caries activity at the beginning of the study.
C. Provides information for correlation with clinical and radiographic evidences of dental caries.
D. Motivates the patient to carry out preventive procedures.
E. Evaluates progress throughout the study after personal care procedures and dietary regimen have been initiated.
F. Indicates the degree of cooperation being obtained from the patient in following instructions.
G. Evaluates at recall appointments the continuing effects of the study.

II. OBTAINING THE SALIVA SAMPLES

The patient must understand each step in collecting the sample if cooperation which will assure consistency in the samples obtained is to be gained. The average patient has limited knowledge of scientific facts related to sterile procedure and microbiology; therefore, the instructions must be presented accordingly.

A. **When the Samples Should be Taken**
1. Principles
    a. Single sample test results are not considered reliable. When possible, 2 or 3 tests should be made not more than a week apart to obtain an average result.
    b. For consistent results, samples throughout a series must be taken under similar circumstances of time and its relation to the patient's eating, drinking, smoking, and tooth-brushing.
2. Time of day for obtaining individual sample
    a. Preferred time: The most typical sample is insured when it is obtained upon rising in the morning, before eating, drinking, smoking or toothbrushing.
    b. Alternate time: If the oral cavity is left undisturbed for 2 to $2\frac{1}{2}$ hours, the oral flora settles to nearly its natural distribution. When the saliva sample is to be taken in a clinic or dental office, careful instructions must be given the patient in order that food, drink, tobacco, and toothbrushing will be omitted during the 2- to $2\frac{1}{2}$-hour period prior to the appointment. This system has an advantage in that the sample collection can be supervised.

B. **How the Sample is Taken**
1. Equipment
    a. Sterile saliva collection bottle (20 to 30 milliliter size).
    b. Stick of paraffin.
    c. Instruction and data sheet and mailing tube (when sample is to be sent to a laboratory).
2. Procedure (instructions for patient)
    a. Place paraffin in mouth; chew vigorously, moving the paraffin around.
    b. Collect saliva in mouth and expectorate into the bottle until it is half full. Ordinarily this takes from 3 to 5 minutes.
    c. Do not touch the rim or inside of the collecting bottle at any time.
    d. Discard paraffin. Do not put it in the bottle with the saliva.
    e. Screw top tightly on bottle.
    f. If to be mailed: pack in tube and post promptly.

III. **TYPES OF TESTS**

Tests have been designed to determine the number of acid-forming bacteria in the saliva, a specialized activity of the oral bacteria, or a component or capacity of the saliva. References are provided for a review of the research pertinent to the various tests that have been developed.[9,11,12,13]

The ideal requirements of a caries activity laboratory test to meet dental office needs are that it (1) measure a factor involved in the caries process, (2) have maximum correlation with clinical findings, (3) be accurate with respect to duplication of results, (4) produce results in a short time, (5) not require complicated apparatus or great technical skill, and (6) be inexpensive.[11,13]

Two commonly used tests, the Lactobacillus Plate Count and the Snyder Colorimetric Test are outlined in this chapter. Results of the

Lactobacillus Plate Count show the number of bacteria per milliliter of saliva, whereas the Snyder Test demonstrates the acid produced by the bacteria. Dental office facilities can be adapted to accomplish the laboratory procedures required in the Snyder Test, but the Lactobacillus Plate Count should be made in a well-equipped laboratory. In a number of states the public health department laboratory provides free service to dentists of the state for making Lactobacillus Plate Counts.

A. **Lactobacillus Plate Count**

The oral bacterial flora includes a number of kinds of acid-forming microorganisms and among these are many types of lactobacilli. A direct count is made from colonies grown on special agar.

1. Laboratory procedures
   a. The saliva sample is shaken to distribute the bacteria and from this are made diluted samples which are mixed with a selective lactobacillus medium and poured into a Petri plate.[14,15]
   b. After 4 days' incubation the number of lactobacilli colonies are counted. By multiplying by the dilution factor, the number of lactobacilli in a milliliter of saliva is estimated.
2. Interpretation of results

   A zero or very low count indicates little or no caries activity, whereas counts of 50,000 or greater indicate tendency toward rampant caries activity. The significance of the different levels of counts is summarized as follows:

Number of Lactobacilli Per Milliliter Saliva	Suggested Degree of Caries Activity or Susceptibility
0 — 1,000	Little or none
1,000 — 5,000	Slight
5,000 — 10,000	Moderate
10,000 — 50,000	Marked
More than 50,000	Rampant

3. Causes of unexpected variations in a series of counts[14,16]

   When the patient adheres to a dietary regimen for the elimination of fermentable carbohydrates, a definite lowering of the lactobacillus count could be expected in 2 to 3 weeks. Occasionally in a series of counts there tends to be a wide variation unrelated to the dietary regimen. It is important to recognize some of the factors which tend to contribute to deviations. A number of the factors listed below have application to other caries susceptibility tests than the Lactobacillus Count.
   a. Variable factors in obtaining the saliva sample
      (1) Small children: samples usually are considered unreliable because of child's difficulty in chewing paraffin so that all exposed tooth surfaces are included, as well as in collecting all of the saliva produced.
      (2) Time element: uniform time for obtaining samples may not have been used.

       (a) There is a normal rise and fall in numbers of lacto-
bacilli in the oral cavity during the day and during
different months of the year.

       (b) Saliva varies in viscosity and quantity at different
times. Increased saliva flow may dilute the bacterial content, whereas decreased flow would concentrate it.

       (c) Instructions may have been given inadequately or
misunderstood by the patient concerning time of
collection in relation to eating, drinking, smoking,
or toothbrushing.

    (3) Paraffin chewing cannot be expected to dislodge the same
number of organisms from the teeth each time a sample
is taken.

  b. Variable factors in laboratory procedures

    (1) Uneven distribution (clumping) of bacteria in the original
sample; inadequate shaking before diluting.

    (2) Careless handling of sample before culturing.

       (a) Sample may not have been mailed to laboratory
promptly.

       (b) Too long storage at too high or too low temperatures
so that lactobacilli have either multiplied or died.

    (3) Need for consistency of medium used and procedures of
inoculation and incubation.

    (4) Need for laboratory workers to standardize the counting
of the plates when more than one person carries out
this phase of the work.

B. Snyder Colorimetric Test[17]

The Snyder Test Agar contains the indicator brom-cresol-green
and is adjusted to a pH of 5.0. Acid formation by bacteria from the
saliva sample added to the medium lowers the pH. At lowered pH
the brom-cresol-green changes from green to yellow.

  1. Laboratory procedures

    a. Obtain tubes of standardized Snyder Test Agar from a scien-
tific supply house.

    b. Place tube in boiling water until agar melts; cool until it can
be held comfortably against the cheek.

    c. Shake saliva sample well to distribute the bacteria.

    d. Pipette 0.2 ml. into the agar and mix by gentle rotation.

    e. Allow to solidify and incubate at 37°C.

    f. Examine daily for 3 days and record changes in color com-
pared with uninoculated control. Hold tube against a white
background when making observations.

  2. Interpretation of results

The rate of color change from green to yellow is related to
the degree of caries activity. In the process of changing color
the agar will appear light green, then greenish-yellow, and
finally appear a definite yellow.

No change in color indicates little or no caries activity whereas
a prompt change to yellow within 24 hours indicates marked acid
formation or caries activity. The significance of the color
changes is summarized as follows:

Color of Snyder Test Agar After Incubation			Suggested Degree of Caries Activity or Susceptibility
24 hrs	*48 hrs*	*72 hrs*	
Green	Green	Green	Little or none
Green	Light green	Yellow	Slight
Green	Yellow		Moderate
Yellow			Marked or rampant

THE DIETARY SURVEY

The dietary survey or history is used as a means for understanding the patient and as a guide for patient instruction. For the rampant caries case, the survey shows the frequency of use of retentive, fermentable carbohydrates. It also reveals which of the essential foods for oral development and maintenance are lacking and which foods contribute to oral cleanliness through their detergent action.

The type of survey used is sometimes referred to as *qualitative*. It takes into consideration the general food groups essential or detrimental to good oral health and does not pretend to show precise mathematical calculations of the chemical constituents, as does the *quantitative* type of dietary analysis. The nutritionist is skilled in making detailed quantitative diet analyses and works under the direction of the physician to provide specific therapeutic diets for physiological and pathological conditions. Therapeutic diets are also prescribed by dentists, particularly periodontists, to supplement clinical treatment when a disease of the periodontium has contributing factors due to a nutritional deficiency. A dietary analysis for *therapy* contrasts with a dietary study for patient instruction or *guidance*.

I. OBJECTIVES FOR OBTAINING A DIETARY SURVEY

A. To obtain an over-all picture of the types of food in the patient's dietary, food preferences, and the approximate quantity of food eaten.

B. To study the eating habits with particular reference to frequency and regularity of eating and the order in which food is taken.

C. To compare the frequency of eating carbohydrates with the caries activity test results and clinical and radiographic findings.

D. To determine which detergent foods are routinely included in the diet and the relationship of their position in the diet to the position of fermentable carbohydrates.

E. To provide a basis for making individual recommendations for changes in the dietary important to the prevention of dental caries.

F. To give the patient an opportunity to study objectively his own dietary habits.

II. PROCEDURE FOR OBTAINING THE DIETARY SURVEY

A. When the Dietary Should Be Taken

1. Length of survey: 1 week to 10 days.
2. Circumstances: should be typical of ordinary daily living (unaffected by illness, holidays, fasting, visiting).

B. Suggested Characteristics of Form to Be Used

1. Simple, with ample spacing.
2. Space indicated for patient's name, the day and the date on each page.
3. Blocked off areas for each meal and between-meal.
4. Space to indicate time of eating.
5. Column to record food item and amount (Figure 73).
6. Cover page with sample procedure for entering items (Figure 74).

C. Presentation to Patient

Result obtained can be expected to be directly proportional to the care taken in presentation.

1. Explain the purpose of the survey, avoiding mention of any specific foods and their relationships to oral health: the patient may not provide a true dietary if he knows what will be checked.
2. Explain the form, the cover page where suggestions are given for listing various foods, and the use of household measurements for indicating quantity.
3. Complete the current day's dietary with the patient to illustrate how to itemize and how to list the foods in the order in which they were eaten.
4. Emphasize importance of completing each meal's record as soon after eating as possible to avoid forgetting.
5. Explain need for recording what was actually eaten in contrast to recording everything served.
6. Review details of recording individual items of a combination dish such as a salad, sandwich, casserole.
7. Indicate need for recording vitamin concentrates, prescribed medicines, water.
8. Request that meals eaten other than at home be identified by writing "restaurant," "guest at friend's home" or "party."

D. Receiving Completed Dietary from Patient

1. Question the patient and record additional information.
   a. Whether the dietary represents that of a typical week.
   b. Appetite.
   c. Food likes and dislikes; preferences.
   d. Allergies.
   e. Specially prescribed diets for the patient or other members of the family.
2. Review with the patient each day's recorded food list and supplement details which have been omitted.
   a. Identify additions by using ink if the dietary has been kept in pencil or *vice versa*.
   b. Common omissions
      (1) Garnishes: frosting, whipped cream, butter on vegetables, salad dressings?
      (2) Size of drinking glass: 4-ounce, 8-ounce?
      (3) Bread or toast: white, enriched, wheat?
      (4) Chewing gum: sugarless, amount?
      (5) Canned fruit: packed in water or heavy or light syrup?
      (6) Fruit salad: canned, fresh?

UNIVERSITY OF WASHINGTON
DEPARTMENT OF DENTAL HYGIENE

THE DAY'S FOOD INTAKE

NAME ______

DAY ______ DATE ______

	AMOUNT		AMOUNT
BREAKFAST ______ A.M. Finished ______ A.M.		BETWEEN LUNCH AND DINNER ______ P.M.	
BETWEEN BREAKFAST AND LUNCH ______ A.M.		DINNER ______ P.M. Finished ______ P.M.	
LUNCH ______ A.M. Finished ______ P.M.		BETWEEN DINNER AND RETIRING ______ P.M.	

FIGURE 73.—Dietary survey: form used by patient to record daily diet. A booklet for a week's record is made by fastening seven of these forms together. The cover for the booklet is shown in FIGURE 74.

UNIVERSITY OF WASHINGTON
DEPARTMENT OF DENTAL HYGIENE

NAME _____

AGE ____ CHART # ____ WEEK OF ____

<u>EXAMPLE OF HOW FOODS SHOULD BE LISTED</u>

SUMMARY

BREAKFAST 7:30 A.M.

Oatmeal	1 cup
with milk	$\frac{1}{2}$ cup
with brown sugar	2 teasp.
Milk	1 8 oz. glass
Toast - whole wheat bread	2 slices
with butter	generous
Egg - Boiled	1
with butter	$\frac{1}{2}$ teasp.
Doughnut - glazed	1
Prunes - stewed -- with syrup	6 large

Finished <u>7:45 A.M.</u>

BETWEEN BREAKFAST AND LUNCH 10:00 A.M.

Coffee	1 cup
with cream	1 teasp.
with sugar	2 teasp.
Water (around 11:00)	1 paper cup

Food eaten at lunch and dinner should be listed just as carefully as the breakfast shown above. If sandwiches are eaten, list the contents of the filling, such as egg, beef, lettuce, dressing.

Please show the approximate amounts of every kind of food that you ate. Do not mention any food that is served unless you ate it.

Please record all candy, cough drops, milk shakes, soft drinks, ice cream cones, popcorn, fruit (kinds), cookies, that you ate between meals. Also record vitamin concentrates or other medicaments related to diet.

FIGURE 74.—Dietary survey: cover page for patient's dietary record. Examples of how to list foods and indicate household measurements are provided on the left. The blank space on the right is for summary. The cover is fastened with seven copies of the form for recording a day's food diary as shown in FIGURE 73.

(7) Cereal: kind, milk, cream, sugar, quantity?
(8) Potato: baked, buttered, fried?
(9) Doughnut: sugared, glazed, plain?

III. SUMMARY AND ANALYSIS OF THE DIETARY

The three principal parts to analyze are the fermentable carbohydrates, the detergent foods, and the basic food groups for adequate nutrition. For convenience, check sheets should be devised for recording the frequency of use of each of the three.

A. Basic Food Groups

Analysis of over-all content of the diet in relation to dental caries control is made to identify deficiencies. Thus when recommendations are made for an anti-cariogenic diet with adequate detergent foods for chewing, the suggestions made can contribute also to basic nutritional needs.

1. Factors to be considered
   a. Comparison with *Essentials of an Adequate Diet:* Four Basic Food Groups.[18]
   b. Quantity of food eaten.
   c. Approximate proportion of foods containing fermentable carbohydrate compared with proportion of protective foods.
2. Suggested procedure: use check sheet which permits checking daily portions of each food group (Figure 75).
   a. Total for the week may be summarized for each category.
   b. Gross excesses and deficiencies can be identified readily.

B. Fermentable Carbohydrate

1. Factors to be considered
   a. Types of sugar-containing foods included.
   b. Frequency of use
      (1) Daily or occasionally.
      (2) Number of between-meal sweets.
   c. Time of use.
   d. Consistency of sugar-containing foods: related to probable length of time food might remain on the tooth surfaces.
   e. Quantity: related to frequency more than size of individual serving.
   f. Water taken at times when it could aid in rinsing.
2. Suggested visual aid for use with patient: in addition to making check sheet recording, underline in red on patient's dietary survey the foods containing fermentable carbohydrate.

C. Detergent Foods: Factors to Be Considered

1. Types of detergent foods used.
2. Frequency of use: daily or occasionally.
3. Time of use
   a. Meal or between-meal.
   b. Relation to providing cleansing mechanism for fermentable carbohydrates left on the teeth.

D. Analysis

1. Identify desirable and undesirable diet practices.
2. Compare findings with clinical and radiographic inspection and results of caries activity test.

UNIVERSITY OF WASHINGTON
DEPARTMENT OF DENTAL HYGIENE

NAME _____

AGE _____ DATE _____

THE WEEK'S FOOD ANALYSIS

FOODS	MONDAY	TUESDAY	WEDNESDAY	THURSDAY	FRIDAY	SATURDAY	SUNDAY		ADEQUATE	DEFICIENT	EXCESS
Dairy Foods (cheese, butter,etc.)											
Milk (2-4 glasses daily)											
Meat Group (2 or more daily)											
Eggs (3-5 weekly)											
Vegetables and Fruits (4 or more daily)											
Potatoes											
Breads and Cereals (4 or more daily)											
**Detergent Foods											
Refined CHO											

Place check in appropriate column each time the food appears in the Survey.

Synopsis of Dietary Survey:

**Usually found also in Vegetable-and-Fruit Group

Figure 75.—Dietary survey: form used to summarize and analyze the patient's diet. The amount and frequency of use is recorded. The analysis serves as a basis for patient instruction. (Courtesy of Alice Tronquet.)

THE DENTAL HEALTH EDUCATION CONFERENCE

I. **PREPARATION**

A. **Define Objectives for the Patient**
1. To help the patient and his parents study his individual oral problems and understand the need for changing habits.
2. To define and explain specific dietary changes for the elimination of fermentable carbohydrates and the substitution of protective foods.

B. **Think Through Factors Which Influence Presentation of Recommendations**[19,20]
1. Consider patient's willingness and ability to cooperate in relation to other demonstrations, such as conscientiousness in keeping appointments and following personal oral care procedures.
2. Identify problems which arise in presenting dietary changes as they apply to this particular patient.
   a. Difficulty in change of any habit.
   b. Patient may feel dissatisfied without the foods to which he is accustomed.
   c. Lack of appreciation of need for change because of limited knowledge concerning diet, nutrition and their relation to oral health.
   d. Common misconception that concentrated sugar is an indispensable source of energy.
   e. Degree of emphasis: dental disease doesn't kill anyone and nothing drastic is going to happen if minor deviations from the recommended diet occur.
   f. Social prejudices against coarse, raw or unrefined foods.
   g. Cultural patterns.
   h. Financial considerations.
   i. Emotional disturbances which have led to or contributed to the craving for sweets.
   j. Parental attitude that removal of sweets from a child's diet would be depriving him of normal childhood pleasures.

C. **Outline Recommendations to be Made:** List recommendations for dietary changes with suggestions for foods to use as substitutes. Consider items from the patient's medical history as well as known likes and dislikes.

D. **Select Appropriate Visual Aids**
1. Patient's radiographs, dental charting, dietary survey.
2. Diagrams, models or charts applicable to material to be presented.
3. Instructive leaflets to illustrate patient's special dietary or oral health needs. (*Essentials of an Adequate Diet*[18] useful for discussion of basic food groups).
4. Printed outline of diet plan with specific suggestions for food substitutes.
5. Printed list of snack suggestions.

E. **Review Data and Recommendations with Dentist** for additions, suggestions and final approval.

II. GENERAL CONFERENCE PROCEDURES

A. Participants

1. Patient.
2. Parents. Both parents should be encouraged to be present since both participate in supervising the child. It is particularly important for the person who plans and prepares the family meals to be present.
3. Dentist when possible.
4. Dental hygienist.

B. Setting

1. Location: free from interruptions.
2. Arrangement: comfortably seated in a group. Avoid having desk between dental hygienist and parents as atmosphere of authority is created.

C. Pointers for the Success of the Conference

1. Be prepared—on time.
2. Plan for only a few simple visual aids, as too much material causes confusion and clutter.
3. Encourage parents to exclude small children (other than patient) from the conference, as they create distraction.
4. Develop a permissive atmosphere.
5. Take care not to follow a written outline of recommendations so rigidly that the conference lacks informality.
6. Include all people present in the discussion.
7. Use a conversational tone of voice.
8. Make certain that all questions from patient or parent are discussed adequately.
9. Avoid note taking during the conference as much as possible.

III. PRESENTATION

A. Review of Purposes and Parts of the Study with Summary of Clinical and Radiographic Findings and Caries Activity Test Results.

Extent of detail included depends on whether parents attending conference have already participated in previous appointments. A teen-age patient may have been coming for appointments unattended, hence the need for clear review for understanding of all details by the parents.

B. Examine the Patient's Dietary Survey and Summary.

1. Discuss deficiencies and excesses, defining the role of the various food groups, detergent foods and carbohydrates in dental caries initiation or prevention.
2. Explain need for strict diet regimen for 2- to 3-week period, followed by modified regimen during continuing months.

C. Explain Program for the Elimination of Fermentable Carbohydrates from the Diet.

To make a major change in dietary habits is difficult, if not traumatic, for any individual. Application of the knowledge of the principles of learning (page 267) and the skills of a nutrition counselor are essential. The attempt must be made to retain as much as possible of the patient's present food habits, and to make recommendations which will adapt into the patient's pattern of living.[21]

It should be obvious that the patient cannot be told simply to "cut out the sweets in the diet." The meaning of "sweets" must be made clear, and specific suggestions provided for "cutting them out."

1. Define what is meant by a fermentable carbohydrate and use specific examples from the patient's dietary survey.
2. Discuss principles for understanding the role of fermentable carbohydrates in dental caries initiation.
    a. Sugar on the tooth surface is changed to acid within 5 minutes' time.
    b. Acid left undisturbed is not cleared from the mouth for $1\frac{1}{2}$ to 2 hours.
    c. *Amount* of sugar consumed is not as important as *when* it is consumed; large amounts of sweet foods with a meal are not as detrimental as small amounts at intervals as between-meal snacks.
    d. Natural sugars are just as detrimental as refined ones (examples: maple syrup, honey).
    e. *Significance of length of time food is retained in the mouth.*
        (1) Sugar in liquid form is retained in the mouth for less time than solid.
        (2) Texture of the food which contains the sugar influences the length of time it will stay in the mouth (whether sticky or combined with a sticky substance).
        (3) Vigorous rinsing after eating a concentrated sweet helps to remove it from the mouth.
        (4) Sweet food taken before going to bed is not cleared readily from the mouth since salivary flow decreases during sleep.
3. Presentation of specific dietary procedures
    There are varying degrees of recommendations concerning the elimination of carbohydrates from the diet. The well-known Jay Dietary Program[22] provides for a drastic removal of all types of carbohydrates. In such a plan the patient must be carefully supervised by physician and dentist. A modified plan may best be used when the dental hygienist presents the program under the supervision of the dentist.
    The suggestions listed below represent basic principles to be applied. More specific recommendations should be added as they relate to the individual family. Directions must be simple and specific as the interpretation of many new ideas is difficult for the patient. The printed sheets which list suggestions for the changes to be made should be used throughout the presentation to clarify the points discussed.
    a. Incorporate foods from the basic groups to complete the patient's dietary. A diet high in protective foods frequently implies a diet low in fermentable carbohydrate.
    b. Limit the use of fermentable carbohydrates to mealtimes, paying particular attention to the final food used in the

meal which may remain on the teeth if immediate tooth-brushing is not possible.

    c. Omit sweet foods even at mealtime when a very high dental caries rate is evident, and limit the diet to foods from the meat, milk and vegetable-fruit groups.[18] Selections from the bread and cereals should be limited to dark bread and whole grain cereals.

    d. Select between-meal snacks from protective noncariogenic foods such as milk, fresh fruits and raw vegetables.

    e. Use as little concentrated sweet in the preparation of foods as possible, and observe care in the purchase of prepared foods. Examples: unsweetened fruit juice, dietetically prepared canned fruits, and sugar-free ice cream.

    f. Eat well at mealtime to lessen desire for between-meal snacks. Protein and fat containing foods digest more slowly and need to be included at each meal to prevent between-meal hunger.

    g. Emphasize need for rigid adherence to the diet features: even occasional deviations can affect the results.

    h. Explain that the rigid diet may be required only for 2 to 3 weeks if the next caries activity test shows favorable results.

4. Ask leading questions in the attempt to determine parent and patient understanding.
5. Relate personal oral care procedures to the diet program.
6. Summarize the total program.

IV. POSTCONFERENCE PROCEDURE

    A. **Contact the patient and parent** a few days after the conference.

        1. Determine whether procedures are clear.
        2. Provide opportunity for questions.
        3. Give encouragement.

    B. **Plan for making next caries activity tests.**

    C. **Adapt follow-up procedure** to caries activity test results.

        1. When test result shows no improvement
            a. Study for possible misunderstanding or lack of cooperation on part of patient.
            b. Reassess own presentation of the program.
            c. Review details of the restricted diet and encourage its continuance.
        2. When test result shows improvement
            a. Commend patient.
            b. Suggest slight relaxation in use of food containing fermentable sugars but need for continuation of basic principles.

EVALUATION OF PROGRESS

The success of the dental caries control study is entirely dependent upon learning by the patient. Learning implies a change of habit and progress toward goals which are clearly understood by the learner.

I. IMMEDIATE EVALUATION

    A. A lowered caries activity test result at the end of the 2- to 3-week test period of restricted diet indicates success to that date.

    B. The patient's expressed interest and demonstration of cooperation in the caries control program indicate that at least temporarily the patient is motivated.

II. EVALUATION AT 3 TO 6 MONTHS' RECALL APPOINTMENTS

    A. Continued low caries activity test results indicate that recommended procedures for dietary and personal care have been followed.

    B. Parents' demonstrated interest in applying caries prevention information to all members of the family shows real learning.

III. OVER-ALL EVALUATION

    A. Consistent reduction in dental caries rate in the years following the study shows sustained change in habits.

    B. Patient's and parents' attitudes toward maintaining adequate oral health habits of personal care, diet containing minimum fermentable carbohydrate, and routine professional dental care indicate application of learning.

RECALL OF THE DENTAL CARIES CONTROL STUDY PATIENT

I. THREE MONTHS' FOLLOW-UP

    A. Obtain saliva sample for caries activity test.

    B. Review personal oral care procedures and provide suggestions as needed.

    C. Recommend return to restricted carbohydrate diet when caries activity test has not remained low.

II. FIVE TO SIX MONTHS' RECALL

    A. Obtain saliva sample for caries activity test.

    B. Inspection and clinical procedures
        1. Oral prophylaxis.
        2. Topical application of fluoride solution.
        3. Bite-wing radiographic survey.
        4. Charting.

    C. Compare dental caries incidence with previous chartings and completed restorative dentistry.

    D. Make dietary recommendations in accord with results from the test.

REFERENCES

1. DAVIES, G. N.: The Management of Rampant Dental Caries, Dent. J. Austral., *26*, 57, April, 1954.

2. DeRevere, R. E.: A Comprehensive Treatment Plan for the Control of Dental Caries, Annals Dent., *16*, 1, March, 1957.
3. Goldsworthy, N. E., Sullivan, H. R., and Harris, Robert: Practical Caries Control, Dent. J. Austral., *27*, 45, April, 1955.
4. Nizel, A. E.: *Nutrition in Clinical Dentistry*. Philadelphia, Saunders, 1960, pp. 322–357.
5. Strieff, Mary, Seglins, Biruta, Marshall, Geneanne, Finstad, Sharlene, Borgendale, Glen: The Caries Control Study, Am. Dent. Hygienists' A. J., *29*, 143, October, 1955.
6. Breckenridge, M. E. and Vincent, E. L.: *Child Development*, 4th ed. Philadelphia, Saunders, 1960, pp. 538–553.
7. Spock, Benjamin: *Baby and Child Care*. New York, Pocket Books, 1957, pp. 260–261, 346–356, 357–368, 384–389, 413–421.
8. Burnett, G. W. and Scherp, H. W.: *Oral Microbiology and Infectious Disease*, 2nd ed. Baltimore, Williams and Wilkins, 1962, p. 390.
9. Snyder, M. L., Porter, D. R., Claycomb, C. K., and Sims, W.: Evaluation of Laboratory Tests for Estimation of Caries Activity, Am. Dent. A. J., *65*, 30, July, 1962.
10. Snyder, M. L., Porter, D. R., Claycomb, C. K., Sims, W., and Macho, F. R.: Evaluation of Laboratory Tests for the Estimation of Caries Activity. Correlation with Specific Surfaces, Arch. Oral Biol., *8*, 541, July, 1963.
11. Snyder, M. L.: Laboratory Methods in the Clinical Evaluation of Caries Activity, Am. Dent. A. J., *42*, 400, April, 1951.
12. Muhler, J. C., Hine, M. K., and Day, H. G.: *Preventive Dentistry*. St. Louis, Mosby, 1954, pp. 97–121.
13. Rapp, G. W.: Fifteen Minute Caries Test, Illinois D. J., *31*, 290, May, 1962.
14. Snyder, M. L., Suher, Theodore, Porter, D. R., Claycomb, C. K., and Gardner, M. K.: Evaluation of Laboratory Tests for the Estimation of Caries Activity, J. Dent. Res., *35*, 332, June, 1956.
15. Rogosa, M. L., Mitchell, J. A., and Wiseman, R. F.: A Selective Medium for the Isolation and Enumeration of Oral Lactobacillus, J. Dent. Res., *30*, 682, October, 1951.
16. Permar, Dorothy, Kitchin, P. C., and Robinson, H. B. G.: Variations in Counts of Lactobacilli Made from Single Specimens of Saliva, J. Dent. Res., *25*, 475, December, 1946.
17. Snyder, M. L.: A Simple Colorimetric Method for the Estimation of Relative Numbers of Lactobacilli in the Saliva, J. Dent. Res., *19*, 349, August, 1940.
18. United States Department of Agriculture, Agriculture Research Service: Essentials of an Adequate Diet. Home Economics Research Report No. 3. Washington, United States Government Printing Office, November, 1957. 21 pp.
19. Bruch, Hilde: Social and Emotional Factors in Diet Changes, Am. Dent. A. J., *63*, 461, October, 1961.
20. Harris, R. S.: Cultural, Geographical and Technological Influences on Diet, Am. Dent. A. J., *63*, 465, October, 1961.
21. Young, C. M.: Nutrition Counseling for the Dental Patient, Am. Dent. A. J., *63*, 469, October, 1961.
22. Jay, Philip, Beeuwkes, A. M., Blecha, E. E., and Bust, M. S.: *Dietary Program for the Control of Dental Caries*. Ann Arbor, Michigan, Overbeck, 1950. 39 pp.

SUGGESTED READINGS

American Association of Public Health Dentists, Reference Committee on Research: Role of Fermentable Carbohydrates in the Production of Caries, Pub. H. Dent., *23*, 144, Fall, 1963.
Bibby, B. G.: Caries Prevention Without Fluorides, Dental Clinics of North America, July, 1962, p. 411.
Bibby, B. G.: Cariogenicity of Foods, J.A.M.A., *177*, 316, August 5, 1961.
Blass, J. L. and Thaller, J. L.: Aids in Evaluating the Dietary Intake of the Periodontal Patient, J. Periodont., *31*, 107, April, 1960.
Cox, G. F., Draus, F. F., and Entress, C. P.: How Long Does Sugar Remain in the Mouth? Dent. Prog., *3*, 152, April, 1963.
Dreizen, Samuel: Nutrition Research of Dental Significance, Am. Dent. A. J., *66*, 607, May, 1963.
Everson, G. J.: Bases for Concern About Teenagers Diets, J. Am. Dietetic A., *36*, 17, January, 1960.
Jay, Philip and Bennett, A. S.: Role of Diet in the Control of Dental Caries, Am. Dent. A. J., *52*, 18, January, 1956.
Lauterstein, A. M. and Massler, Maury: Sugar Intake and Caries in Children, Dent. Prog., *1*, 100, January, 1961.

NEWTON, M. E. and ANDERSON, G. K.: An Experience With Two Methods of Dietary Analysis, Am. Dent. Hygienists' A. J., *36*, 69, 2nd Quarter, 1962.

POLLACK, HERBERT: Oral Manifestations of Nutritional Deficiencies as an Aid in Nutritional Diagnosis, Am. Dent. A. J., *63*, 459, October, 1961.

ROARK, K. T., WEISS, R. L., and YOUNG, P. O.: Tennessee Study of Bacteriological Tests for Caries Activity, Am. J. Pub. Health, *53*, 564, April, 1963.

SHAFER, W. G., HINE, M. K., and LEVY, B. M.: *Textbook of Oral Pathology*, 2nd ed. Philadelphia, Saunders, 1963, pp. 308–377.

SHAW, J. H.: Problems in Relationship of Diet and Nutrition to Dental Health, Am. Dent. A. J., *63*, 454, October, 1961.

SOGNNAES, R. F.: Present Status of Caries Research, J. Pros. Dent., *13*, 921, September-October, 1963.

VOLKER, J. F.: Nutritional Control of Dental Disease, J. Pros. Dent., *10*, 341, March-April, 1960.

VOLKER, J. F. and CALDWELL, R. C.: Food and Dental Caries, in Finn, S. B.: *Clinical Pedodontics*, 2nd ed. Philadelphia, Saunders, 1962, pp. 660–680.

WEISS, R. L. and TRITHART, A. H.: Between-meal Eating Habits and Dental Caries Experience in Preschool Children, Am. J. Pub. Health, *50*, 1097, August, 1960.

Chapter 32

ORAL AND GENERAL SURGERY PATIENTS

DENTAL HYGIENE CARE PRIOR TO ORAL SURGERY

A MOUTH is not considered a good surgical risk when the teeth are covered with debris and calculus, and the gingiva shows signs of inflammation and possible nutritional deficiency. It is recommended that unless emergency surgery is required, the appointment be postponed until the mouth is in a better state of cleanliness and health.[1-4]

Objectives and procedures described in this section are primarily with reference to the removal of teeth, but principles apply alike to oral surgery of the soft tissues. Performance of the oral prophylaxis may be complicated by the extent and position of a pathological lesion and the ability of the patient to maintain his mouth in an open position.

The patient's medical history will reveal essential information to guide procedures. Presurgery patients may have extensive oral infection and calculus deposits which may result in considerable tissue trauma associated with scaling. Since the frequency and severity of bacteremias are directly related to the degree of trauma, prophylactic antibiotic therapy for appropriate patients is indicated (see page 161).

I. OBJECTIVES

Dental hygiene care and instruction prior to oral surgery may contribute to the patient's health and well-being by one or more of the following:

A. **Remove Debris and Reduce Oral Bacterial Count**
1. Aid in the preparation of an aseptic field of operation.
2. Make postextraction infection less likely.

B. **Reduce Inflammation of the Gingiva and Improve Tissue Tone**
1. Lessen local hemorrhage at the time of the operation.
2. Promote postoperative healing.

C. **Remove Calculus Deposits**
1. Remove the source of irritation to gingiva and thus improve tissue tone.
2. Prevent interference with placement of surgical instruments.
3. Prevent pieces of calculus from breaking away during tooth removal.
   a. Danger of inhalation particularly when a general anesthetic is used.
   b. Possibility of calculus falling into socket and acting as a foreign body to inhibit healing.

D. **Instruction in Presurgery Personal Oral Care Procedures** which will contribute to reducing inflammation and thus improve tissue tone.

E. **Instruction in the Use of Foods** which provide the elements essential to tissue building and repair during pre- and postsurgery periods.

F. **Interpret the Dentist's Directions** for the immediate preoperative preparation with respect to rest and dietary limitations, particularly when a general anesthetic is to be administered.

G. **Motivate the Patient Who Will Have Teeth Remaining** after the surgery to prevent further tooth loss through routine dental and dental hygiene professional care and personal oral care procedures.

H. **Introduce to the Patient Who Will Have All Teeth Removed** and dentures inserted the importance of a diet containing all essential food groups.

II. PSYCHOLOGICAL CHARACTERISTICS OF THE PATIENT

The extent of the surgery to be performed and previous experiences of tooth removal will affect the patient's psychological attitude. A majority of the patients who are in greatest need for presurgery dental hygiene care and instruction will be people who have neglected their mouths for many years. They have been indifferent toward or unaware of the importance of obtaining adequate care. Their knowledge of preventive measures is very limited. A few of the characteristics which may confront the dental hygienist are suggested below.

A. **Apprehensive and Fearful**
   1. Apprehensive and indifferent toward need for cleaning teeth which are to be removed.
   2. Fearful of all dental procedures, particularly oral surgery and anesthesia.
   3. Fearful of personal appearance after tooth removal.

B. **Impatient:** When teeth have caused discomfort and pain it is difficult to understand need for delay while dental hygiene procedures are accomplished.

C. **Ashamed:** of appearance or of having neglected teeth.

D. **Resigned:** feeling of inevitableness of the situation; lack of appreciation for natural teeth.

E. **Discouraged:** over tooth loss.

F. **Resentful**
   1. Toward time lost from work.
   2. Toward the financial aspects of dental care.
   3. Toward inconvenience and discomfort from a condition which they do not recognize as a result of their own neglect.

III. **APPOINTMENT PLANNING**

Two appointments frequently are needed, but the pending date for the surgery and the patient's attitude may be prohibitive.

A. **First Appointment:** Develop patient rapport, remove gross calculus deposits, demonstrate toothbrushing procedures and make suggestions for diet.

B. **Second Appointment:** Observe response of gingival tissue, continue the scaling, review toothbrushing and dietary procedures.

IV. **ORAL PROPHYLAXIS**

Scaling techniques are of primary importance. Frequently, polishing procedures are contraindicated because of the condition of the gingival tissues.

A. **Removal of Gross Deposits of Materia Alba and Food Debris**
  1. Spray with mouth wash.
  2. Apply 3 per cent hydrogen peroxide with cotton pellet and request patient to rinse thoroughly.
  3. Use dental floss.

B. **Scaling**
  1. Problems
      a. Teeth with large carious lesions.
      b. Mobile teeth.
      c. Edentulous areas.
      d. Sensitive, enlarged gingival tissue which bleeds readily.
  2. Suggestions for technique
      a. Apply all principles for the use of scalers as described in Chapter 15.
      b. Use topical anesthetic when tissue is sensitive and patient is apprehensive (see pages 159–160).
      c. Maintain as clear a field as possible using cotton rolls and gauze wipes.
      d. Use alternate fulcrums to adapt to mobile teeth or edentulous areas.
      e. Stabilize mobile teeth during scaling stroke by exerting slight pressure on occlusal or incisal surface with finger of left hand. Pressure applied should counteract that used to accomplish calculus removal.
      f. Ultrasonic scaling techniques may be particularly appropriate (see pages 157–158).

C. **Polishing**
  1. Contraindications
      a. Enlarged, inflamed, sensitive gingiva.
      b. Deep gingival sulci.
      c. Profuse hemorrhage.
  2. Effects
      a. Irritation to tissue by polishing abrasive and action of rubber polishing cup.
      b. Movement of rubber cup forces abrasive particles into the gingival sulcus.

3. Recommended procedure

For patients whose anterior teeth will not be removed, improvement of appearance by polishing labial surfaces may provide encouragement and motivation for attention to future personal and professional care. The use of the porte polisher is recommended to prevent abrasive from being forced into the gingival sulcus.

An oral prophylaxis should be planned for a few weeks after surgery to complete the procedures. Such an appointment should not be scheduled until the sockets have closed and healing has progressed favorably.

V. PATIENT INSTRUCTION IN PERSONAL ORAL CARE PROCEDURES

A. Toothbrushing

1. Brush: a soft-textured brush usually is recommended depending on the condition of the tissues.
2. Technique: the Rolling Stroke technique (see pages 285–287) is usually recommended because it is easier for the patient to adapt. It should be kept in mind that many of these patients would not have established a brushing routine previously.

B. Rinsing (see pages 195 and 311)

1. Objective: To promote healing of tissues following scaling.
2. Rinsing solution: warm mild hypertonic salt solution.

VI. PATIENT INSTRUCTION IN DIET SELECTION[5,6,7]

A. Nutritional and Dietary Needs

1. Essentials for promotion of healing: protein and vitamins, particularly Vitamin A, Vitamin C, and Riboflavin.
2. Essential for building gingival tissue resistance: a varied diet which includes adequate portions of all essential food groups.
3. Essential for providing gingival stimulation: detergent foods which require mastication, especially fresh fruits and vegetables. Possibilities for making recommendations in this area are limited by the patient's masticatory deficiencies.
4. Essential for dental caries prevention: foods without fermentable carbohydrate. When a patient has not been able to masticate properly, the diet employed frequently has included many soft carbohydrate foods.

B. Suggestions for Instruction

1. Provide printed instruction sheets which show specific meal plans for pre- and postsurgery.
2. Express nutritional needs in terms of quantity or servings of foods so that the patient clearly understands.
3. For the patient who will receive dentures.

Extensive and careful instruction must be provided over a period of time. At the presurgery appointment only an introduction can be given, particularly because the patient is probably more concerned about the operation than about the after effects.

When the patient will lose the teeth because of dental caries, the diet has likely been high in fermentable carbohydrates. Emphasis should be placed on helping the patient include nutritious foods for the general health of the body and more specifically the health of the alveolar processes which will support the dentures.

DENTAL HYGIENE CARE FOR THE PATIENT WITH A FRACTURED JAW

The limited access to the gingiva for personal oral care procedures and the effect of the liquid diet which fails to stimulate and cleanse the oral tissues, define the need for special dental hygiene care for the patient with a fractured jaw. Attention to rehabilitation of the oral tissues during the period following the removal of appliances takes on particular significance lest permanent tissue damage result or inadequate oral care habits be continued indefinitely.

Many fractured jaw cases are hospitalized. A dental hygienist employed in a hospital would be called upon to assume a part of the responsibility for patient care and instruction. After dismissal from the hospital, the patient may require special attention in the private dental office for a long period of time.

I. GENERAL INFORMATION CONCERNING FRACTURED JAWS

Fractured jaw cases may be very complex and the patient may suffer considerably, both physically and mentally. Some basic knowledge of the nature of fractures and their treatment is helpful in understanding the patient's needs.

A. Causes
1. Exciting: trauma.
2. Predisposing: pathological conditions such as tumors, cysts or osteomyelitis weaken the bone, thus permitting slight trauma to cause fracture.

B. Types
The fracture or fractures are classified by using any combination of those listed below under mandibular and maxillary, and described by their nature and severity.
1. Mandibular (described by location)
   a. Condyle
   b. Angle
   c. Body
   d. Symphysis
2. Maxillary
   a. Horizontal
   b. Pyramidal
   c. Transverse Facial
3. Classification by nature of the fracture
   a. Closed (simple): has no communication with outside.

      b. Open (compound): has communication with outside.

      c. Multiple: two or more distinct fractures of the same bone.

      d. Comminuted: shattered.

      e. Incomplete: "Greenstick" fracture occurring in incompletely calcified bones (young children usually). The fibers tend to bend rather than break.

C. First Aid

When the cause of the fracture is an accident, immediate attention must be paid to first aid measures for care of the patient's general condition. First aid care is given for hemorrhage, impaired airway, shock, and skull or internal head injuries, in that order. Almost any category of first aid may be required (see pages 468–472). Although treatment for the fractured jaw must not be postponed for any great length of time, its immediate care takes second place in the light of the vital aspects of patient care.

D. Treatment by the Oral Surgeon

1. Objective of treatment: to permit healing through reduction and immobilization of the parts in correct anatomical relationship with the teeth in functional occlusion.

2. Types of treatment

    The descriptions given below are incomplete and only suggestive of the complexity and variety of treatment used. Appreciation of this complexity is important to recognition and understanding of the patient's problems.

    Each fracture differs from the next, and the methods used in treatment vary with the individual case. Many factors are involved when the oral surgeon selects the methods to be used, particularly the location of the fracture or fractures, the presence or absence of teeth, existing injuries to the teeth, other head injuries, and the general health and condition of the patient.

    Maxillary fractures are more difficult to handle because of the number of bones, the associated anatomy and the complications of basal skull fractures. Undisplaced maxillary or mandibular fractures occasionally require no fixation but the patient must avoid all masticatory stresses. Treatment methods may be divided into the three general groups listed below.

    a. Indirect: intermaxillary wiring: securing each jaw with direct wiring or arch bars and then holding jaws in occlusion by wires or elastic bands.

    b. Direct: bone wiring with open surgical reduction.

    c. Skeletal fixation: use of headcaps, external pin fixation, splints or circumferential wiring. Splints may be metal or acrylic.

E. Healing

Union is affected by the location and character of the fracture. Much depends on the patient's general health and resistance, and cooperation. Six weeks is considered the average for the uncomplicated mandibular case and 4 to 6 weeks for the maxillary. The major cause of complication is infection.

II. EFFECTS CONTRIBUTING TO THE NEED FOR DENTAL HYGIENE CARE

Fixation apparatus, however carefully placed to prevent tissue irritation, interferes with normal function. The length of time the appliances must be in place is sufficient for considerable disturbance of tissue metabolism. Identification of possible effects of treatment provide the basis for planning dental hygiene care.

A. Development of Gingivitis or Periodontal Complications

1. Rapid calculus formation in susceptible patients and debris accumulation resulting from a nondetergent diet and saliva stagnation, provide sources of irritation to the gingiva.
2. Lack of normal stimulation to the circulation of the periodontium usually provided by the excursion of food lowers tissue resistance.
3. Tender, sensitive gingiva makes toothbrushing more difficult even on available surfaces.

B. Difficulty in Planning Interesting Diet with limited use of fermentable carbohydrates contributes to dental caries initiation in the susceptible patient.

C. Loss of Appetite related to monotonous liquid or soft diet leads to weight loss and lowered physical resistance. Secondary infections, including those of the oral tissues, may result.

D. Difficulty in Opening the Mouth

1. When there has been injury to the temperomandibular joint, the patient wearing fixation appliances involving only the mandible has difficulty in applying a toothbrush to the lingual surfaces of teeth.
2. After removal of appliances, all patients have a degree of muscular trismus which hinders toothbrushing and mastication.

III. ORAL PROPHYLAXIS

A. Presurgery: Gross calculus is removed insofar as possible before wiring or the placement of metal or acrylic splints.

B. At Time of Removal of Appliances: Scaling to remove cement and gross calculus deposits is required.[8,9]

C. After Removal of Appliances: A few weeks after removal of appliances, when the patient can open his mouth normally and the gingiva has responded to the use of solid foods, an oral prophylaxis is recommended.

IV. DIET

A. Nutritional Needs

After any surgery the diet must be planned to promote tissue building and repair.[7]

1. All essential food elements.

2. Emphasis on protein, vitamins, particularly A and C, and minerals, particularly calcium and phosphorus.

3. Usual caloric requirements for patient's age, taking into consideration lack of physical exercise and loss of appetite while ill.

B. **Types of Diets**

In a hospital the dietetics department plans the menus from orders provided by the oral surgeon. Special suggestions may be made; for example, foods containing high content of fermentable carbohydrate should be limited for the caries susceptible individual.

1. Liquid diet
   a. Indications
      (1) All patients with jaws wired together.
      (2) All patients with no appliance or single jaw appliance who have:
         (a) Difficulty in opening mouth due to condition such as temperomandibular joint involvement.
         (b) Tongue or lip injury which will hinder insertion of food or manipulation of food in the mouth.
   b. Examples of foods: fruit juices; milk; eggnog; meat juices and soups; cooked thin cereals; canned baby foods. Strained vegetables and meats (baby foods) may be added to meat juices and soups.

2. Soft diet
   a. Indications
      (1) Patients with no appliance or with single jaw appliance without complications in opening mouth or in movement of lips and tongue.
      (2) Patient who has been maintained on liquid diet throughout treatment period: after appliances are removed the soft diet is recommended for several days to a week.
         (a) For providing the stomach with foods which are readily digestible rather than making drastic change to regular diet.
         (b) For protecting tender oral tissues from rough textures of regular diet until tissues have a chance to respond to softer foods and regular toothbrushing routine.
   b. Examples of foods: soft poached, scrambled or boiled eggs; cooked cereals; mashed soft cooked vegetables including potato; mashed fresh or canned fruits; soft, finely divided meats; custards, plain ice cream.

C. **Methods of Feeding**

1. Glass drinking tube: liquid is sucked from the tube through the teeth, or the tube can be inserted through an edentulous area.
2. Cup or bowl, small pitcher or teapot.
3. Spoon-feeding: when patient's arms are not functional.
4. Oropharyngeal, nasopharyngeal, or rectal feeding for severely injured or unconscious patients.

D. **Hints for Diet Planning With the Nonhospitalized Patient**

1. Provide printed instruction sheets which show specific meal plans.

2. Express nutritional needs in quantities or servings of foods.
3. Show methods of varying the diet. A liquid or soft diet is at best monotonous because of sameness of texture.
4. Suggest limitation of foods containing high content of fermentable carbohydrate as an aid to prevention of dental caries.

V. PERSONAL ORAL CARE PROCEDURES

Every attempt to keep the patient's mouth as clean as possible and provide some degree of tissue stimulation should be made for both health and comfort. The extent of possible care depends on the appliances, the condition of the lips, tongue and other oral tissues, and the cooperation of the patient. Encouragement must be given to the patient to begin toothbrushing as soon as possible after the surgery, but until he is able, a plan for care is outlined for his attendant.

A. While Appliances Are in Place
1. Irrigation
   a. Indications
      (1) During first few days after surgery while mouth is too tender for brushing, frequent irrigations are required.
      (2) As an adjunct to toothbrushing.
   b. Method: spray bottle or suction tube. Power spray 2 or 3 times a week aids in removing debris which has accumulated interproximally.
   c. Mouth wash used
      (1) Physiologic saline solution as an aid to healing.
      (2) Sodium bicarbonate as a detergent to thick mucous plaque which forms.
      (3) Flavored mouthwashes may improve the comfort of the patient.
      (4) Oral surgeon may recommend an astringent or oxidizing mouthwash for special cases.
2. Cleansing before a toothbrush can be used: a cotton roll can be wiped over gingiva, exposed tooth surfaces and appliances.
3. Use of toothbrush with suction
   This method can be effective particularly during the early days after the appliances are placed. When the patient is ready to care for his own mouth, procedures can be supplemented by the toothbrush with suction. For method of use see page 334.
4. Toothbrushing by the patient
   As soon as possible the patient is instructed in personal care. A toothbrushing method such as is used for orthodontic appliances is recommended and demonstrated (see page 312). The patient must be shown why care must be taken not to entangle the toothbrush bristles with the wires. When the patient's tongue is not injured he can be instructed to use his tongue as an aid in cleaning the lingual surfaces of the teeth and massaging the gingiva.
5. Massage: in addition to the massage provided by the cotton roll and toothbrush, the patient may be instructed in digital massage for the gingival tissue.

B. **After Appliances Are Removed**

A thorough review of toothbrushing procedures should be provided as soon as the oral tissues are accustomed to a regular diet and the patient can open his mouth normally.

DENTAL HYGIENE CARE PRIOR TO GENERAL SURGERY[10]

An oral prophylaxis prior to general surgery has significance particularly when a general inhalation anesthetic is to be administered, and when a long recovery period and convalescence are anticipated. Providing a clean mouth with gingival irritants removed is one means of treating the patient as a whole: it contributes to comfort and protection against complications.

The oral prophylaxis aids in reducing the oral bacterial count. Since the mouth is the entrance to the respiratory chamber there is always the possibility of the inhalation of debris and fluids from the mouth. This could occur during the administration of an anesthetic, or when the patient coughs.

When the patient has a clean mouth initially, the problems of postoperative oral care are lessened. If a patient is very ill he will not be attending to his own personal oral care for some time. Certain types of surgery require that the patient remain immobile for a long period. In these cases oral care must be provided by an attendant, and at best the results are limited.

When emergency surgery is performed, procedures of dental hygiene care are obviously impossible. However, when surgery is planned in advance, the patient should be informed of the importance of a clean mouth, and be encouraged to have an appointment. The dental hygienist in private practice has an important role to play in this phase of dental hygiene care.

REFERENCES

1. MEAD, S. V.: *Oral Surgery*, 4th ed. St. Louis, Mosby, 1954, p. 37.
2. THOMA, K. H.: *Oral Surgery*, 4th ed., Vol. I. St. Louis, Mosby, 1963, p. 127.
3. MAXWELL, M. M.: Aspects of Oral Diagnosis and Oral Surgery of Interest to the General Practitioner, Am. Dent. A. J., *40*, 425, April, 1950.
4. BELTING, C. M.: Dental Treatment Planning, Am. Dent. A. J., *53*, 288, September, 1956.
5. ARCHER, W. H.: *Oral Surgery*, 3rd ed. Philadelphia, Saunders, 1961, pp. 68–70, 915–916.
6. MEAD: op. cit., pp. 1411–1414, 1436–1443.
7. NIZEL, A. E.: Diet in Oral Surgery, Oral Surg., Oral Med., & Oral Path., *14*, 539, May, 1961.
8. MEAD: op. cit., p. 664.
9. GEHRIG, J. D.: Seattle, School of Dentistry, University of Washington, personal communication.
10. BEDER, O. E.: Seattle, School of Dentistry, University of Washington, personal communication.

SUGGESTED READINGS

General Information About Fractures

ARCHER, W. H.: *Oral Surgery*, 3rd ed. Philadelphia, Saunders, 1961, pp. 696–814.
CLARK, H. B.: *Practical Oral Surgery*. Philadelphia, Lea & Febiger, 1955, pp. 262–313.
FREID, M. G. and BADEN, E.: Management of Fractures in Children, J. Oral Surg., *12*, 129, 1954.
GEHRIG, J. D.: Preoperative and Postoperative Care of the Dental Surgery Patient, Dental Clinics of North America, November, 1959, p. 637.
IVY, R. H. and CURTIS, LAWRENCE: *Fractures of the Jaws*, 3rd ed. Philadelphia, Lea & Febiger, 1945. 174 pp.
JOHNSTON, W. J.: Some Thoughts on the Treatment of Facial Injuries, Dental Clinics of North America, July, 1963, p. 527.
KRUGER, G. O.: *Textbook of Oral Surgery*, St. Louis, Mosby, 1959, pp. 273–355.

MEAD, S. V.:   *Oral Surgery*, 4th ed.   St. Louis, Mosby, 1954, pp. 640–780.

PARKER, D. B.:   Jaw Fractures and Methods of Treatment, Oral Surg., Oral Med., & Oral Path., *3*, 1211, October, 1950.

THOMA, K. H.:   *Oral Surgery*, 4th ed., Vol. I. St. Louis, Mosby, 1963, pp. 367–571.

THOMA, K. H.:   Treatment of Jaw Fractures, Past and Present, J. Oral Surg., Anes. & Hosp. D. Serv., *17*, 30, September, 1959.

Diet

IVY: op. cit., pp. 168–172.

KRUGER: op. cit., pp. 338–339.

MEAD: op. cit., pp. 1213–1215, 1436–1445.

PANAGOPOULOS, A. P. and ELFENBAUM, ARTHUR: Nutritional Needs in Fractures of Jaws in Children and Healing Processes, Oral Surg., Oral Med., & Oral Path., *9*, 578, June, 1956.

ROTH, H.:   Diet, Nutrition, and Dentistry, Oral Surg., Oral Med., & Oral Path., *12*, 830, July, 1959.

Chapter 33

CLEFT LIP AND PALATE PATIENTS

The patient with a cleft lip or palate or both may be a dental cripple. Understanding of the physical defects and resulting speech and personality problems shows why treatment and care require the integrated efforts of nearly all of the dental specialists as well as the plastic surgeon, speech therapist, psychologist, otolaryngologist, social worker, and vocational counselor. The dental hygienist is an important member of the team, to assist the patient with oral cleanliness and health of the tissues through dental hygiene care and instruction.

Cleft lip, cleft palate or both are found in one out of approximately 800 live births. Speaking ability and appearance are necessarily the first factors considered when the long-range treatment program is planned since the objective is to help the patient lead a normal life. Dental personnel need to maintain a current list of the health agencies, clinics, and other community resources where the patient and his family may obtain assistance for the various phases of treatment and habilitation.

I. ORAL CHARACTERISTICS

Patients present a variety of oral conditions depending on the extent of the cleft and other factors suggested below.

A. Classification of Cleft Lip and Palate[1,2]

The classification is based on the interference with embryologic development of the palate which occurs from the premaxillary region toward the uvula in a definite pattern related to the tendency for bilateral development. There may be an interference with normal development of the palate at one age level of the embryo and the normal pattern may be reestablished at a later age. Such interferences would modify the classification suggested below.

All degrees are found from an insignificant notch in the mucous membrane of the lip or uvula which produces no functional disability, to the complete cleft defined by Class 6 of this classification. The first 6 classes are illustrated in Figure 76.

Class 1. Cleft of the tip of the uvula.
Class 2. Cleft of the uvula (bifid uvula).
Class 3. Cleft of the soft palate.
Class 4. Cleft of the soft and hard palates.
Class 5. Cleft of the soft and hard palates which continues through the alveolar ridge on one side of the premaxilla; usually associated with cleft lip of the same side.
Class 6. Cleft of the soft and hard palates which continues through the alveolar ridge on both sides, leaving a free premaxilla; usually associated with bilateral cleft lip.

Class 7. Submucous cleft in which there is imperfect muscle union across the soft palate. The palate is short, the uvula often bifid, a groove is situated at the midline of the soft palate, and the closure to the pharynx is incompetent.

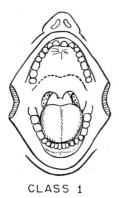

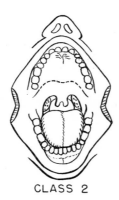

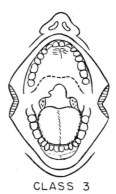

CLASS 1

CLASS 2

CLASS 3

Cleft of the tip of the uvula.

Cleft of the uvula (bifid uvula).

Cleft of the soft palate.

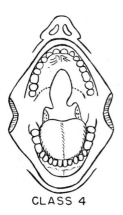

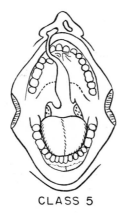

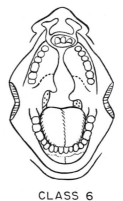

CLASS 4

CLASS 5

CLASS 6

Cleft of the soft and hard palates.

Cleft of the soft and hard palates which continues through the alveolar ridge on one side of the premaxilla. Usually associated with cleft lip of the same side.

Cleft of the soft and hard palates which continues through the alveolar ridge on both sides, leaving a free premaxilla. Usually associated with bilateral cleft lip.

FIGURE 76.—Classification of cleft lip and palate. (Courtesy of O. E. Beder.)

B. **Disturbance of Normal Development of Tooth Buds,** more marked in complete lip clefts, with one or more missing teeth, or supernumerary teeth.

C. **Malocclusion and Malalignment of Teeth.**

D. **Open Area in Palate** with direct communication with nasal cavity.

E. **Lack of Coordinated Movements** of lips, tongue, cheeks, floor of mouth, palate and throat with compensatory habits formed in the attempt to produce normal sounds while speaking.

F. **Gag Reflex Diminished.**[3]

G. **Gingival Disturbances** resulting from malocclusion, difficulties in accomplishing adequate personal oral care procedures, and masticatory interferences.

H. **Marked Dental Caries** related to lack of dietary control in turn related to eating difficulties.

I. **Treated Case**
1. Suture lines from surgery.
2. Removable prosthesis.

II. GENERAL PHYSICAL CHARACTERISTICS

A. **Other Congenital Anomalies:** incidence is higher than in non-cleft people.

B. **Facial Deformity:** depression of nostril on the side with the cleft lip; deficiency of upper lip in which it may be short or retroposed, lower lip may be over-prominent.

C. **Predisposition to Upper Respiratory and Middle Ear Infections**

D. **Hearing Loss:** may result from improper ventilation and drainage of the eustachian canals which can lead to infection. The cleft exposes the nasopharynx region to oral debris and microorganisms which can enter the eustachian canals. Adenoid tissue sometimes grows over the openings of the canals and prevents drainage. Approximately 20 to 25 per cent have hearing loss of one degree or another.[4,5]

E. **Speech:** difficulty in making certain sounds; nasal tones produced. Anatomical structure is not considered the only contributing factor to the speech problem. It may be related to the hearing loss or psychological factors related to inferior feelings or parental attitude.

F. **Undernourishment:** may result when feeding problems continue for a long period.

III. ETIOLOGY

A. **Embryology**[6]
1. Partial or complete failure of normal fusion of embryonic processes. Normal fusion begins in the premaxillary region at about the sixth week in utero, and continues backward toward the uvula. The soft palate and uvula are fused by about the twelfth week.
2. Cleft lip: epithelial fusion may occur, but because of lack of perforation by mesoderm, the epithelial attachment may rupture.

B. Predisposing Factors
Heredity is believed the major factor.[7] A number of other influences have been considered and some of these have been shown effective in animal experimentation. Examples are infectious diseases in the mother, nutritional deficiencies, or mechanical interferences in the fetus.

IV. PSYCHOLOGICAL CHARACTERISTICS

Most cleft lip and palate patients do not have personality problems but realization of the social effects of speech and appearance makes it easy to understand why some of them exhibit evidences of maladjustment. The ridicule of contemporaries soon teaches even the small child that he is "different." Parental acceptance or rejection no doubt can be a strong influence in adjustment. A few possible characteristics are suggested here.

A. **Self-consciousness:** hypersensitivity to taunts or obvious pity.

B. **Feelings of Inferiority:** result may be a person who is quiet, unresponsive and withdrawn or one who is openly brash or rebellious until rapport is established.

C. **Interference with Educational Adjustment:** some drop out of school when they reach high school age because of personality difficulties.[7,8]

D. **Handicap in Competition** with normal persons in earning a living.

V. TREATMENT

A. Cleft Lip
Surgical union of the cleft lip is made early, frequently within a few days after birth, provided the infant's general health permits. The closure aids in feeding, helps development of the premaxilla and growth of the lip, and may also help to close partially the palatal cleft. The psychological effect on parents and family members can be more favorable when the lip operation is performed before the infant is taken home from the hospital.

B. Cleft Palate
It is generally agreed that treatment should be undertaken as soon as technically possible during the preschool years. The combined efforts of many specialists are required. A few are mentioned here.
1. Purposes for Early Treatment[1]
    a. Improve child's well-being.
    b. Aid child's mental development.
    c. Prevent malnourishment by improving the feeding apparatus.
    d. Aid in development of the speech pattern.
    e. Reduce possibilities of repeated infections of the nasopharyngeal region.
2. Maxillofacial Surgery: Closure of the palate is accomplished by surgery or prosthodontics or both. Surgery provides direct

union of the existing tissue that has been moved to a more desirable position for function.

3. Prosthodontics: a removable appliance is designed to provide closure of the palatal opening and/or to complete the palatopharyngeal valving required for speech.

   a. Definitions

      (1) Prosthesis: artificial replacement for a missing part.

      (2) Obturator: removable appliance designed to close an opening such as a cleft of the hard palate.

      (3) Speech Aid: a removable appliance related to the soft palate which provides a means for palatopharyngeal valving for speech.

   b. Purposes of the appliance (it may be designed to accomplish one or all of the factors below)

      (1) Closure of the palate.

      (2) Replacement of missing teeth.

      (3) Scaffolding, to fill out the upper lip.

      (4) Masticatory function.

      (5) Restoration of vertical dimension.

      (6) Postorthodontic retainer.

4. Orthodontics: treatment may be initiated as early as 3 years of age depending on the problems of dentofacial development.

5. Speech Therapy: training may be started with very young children and is particularly emphasized after the surgical or prosthodontic treatment has been accomplished.

6. Operative Dentistry (pedodontist or general dental practitioner): a major problem can be dental caries leading to tooth loss. With missing teeth, major difficulties arise related to all phases of treatment particularly the retention of the prosthesis. Preservation of the primary teeth is very important.

VI. APPLIED DENTAL HYGIENE CARE

Preventive measures for preservation of the teeth and their supporting structures are essential to the success of the special care needed for the habilitation of the cleft palate patient. Each phase of dental hygiene care and instruction which is important for all patients takes on even greater significance in the light of the magnified problems of the dental cripple.

Every attempt should be made to avoid the need for removal of teeth since this patient has enough oral problems without also being edentulous. Primary and permanent teeth are needed for the stabilization of the speech aid or obturator and success of all treatment procedures. Understanding by the patient and the parents of the value of preventive procedures is accomplished through explanation and instruction.

When the patient has not had specialized care, the dental hygienist has a responsibility in working with the dentist to arrange referral to an available agency, clinic, or private practice specialist.

A. Objectives for Appointment Planning

Frequent recall appointments, scheduled every 3 or 4 months, are usually needed during the maintenance phase of the patient's care.

1. To perform the oral prophylaxis as a supplement to the patient's personal daily care procedures.
2. To make topical fluoride applications at proper intervals for both primary and permanent dentitions.
3. To review personal oral care techniques and provide encouragement for the patient in maintaining the health of the supporting structures and the cleanliness of the obturator or speech aid.

B. **Appointment Psychology**
1. Speech may be almost indiscernible, although with repeated contact, understanding is developed.
   a. Avoid embarrassment produced by constantly asking the patient to repeat what has been said.
   b. Provide pencil and paper for the older child to write his requests or comments.
   c. Let parent or other person accompanying small child interpret.
2. Hearing loss: depending on severity, approach is similar to that for speech difficulties listed above. (See also page 423.)
3. Avoid solicitousness or obvious pity. Approach as to a normal patient.
4. Provide motivations for the quiet, unresponsive or bold, rebellious types which will help them gain an objective approach to the care of their mouths.

C. **Sterile Techniques**
Although procedures should be the same for all patients, it should be remembered that the open fissure lines make the cleft palate patient more susceptible to infections.

D. **Oral Prophylaxis**
Techniques are adapted to the oral characteristics. All objectives of the oral prophylaxis have particular implications for the cleft palate patient (see page 102).
1. Malaligned teeth: adjust scaling and polishing procedures.
2. Free premaxilla related to bilateral cleft of alveolar ridge: avoid undue pressure with fulcrum or instrument to prevent movement of the part.
3. Area of recent surgery: avoid pressure.
4. Sensitive, enlarged gingival tissue which bleeds readily.
   a. Maintain as clear a field as possible by using cotton rolls and gauze wipes.
   b. Arrange follow-up appointment to check response of tissue.
5. Open fissures: prevent debris, pieces of calculus or polishing abrasive particles from passing into or being retained in the clefts.
6. Lack of coordinated movements: small children especially may need instruction in how to rinse when this is a new procedure for them.
7. Prosthesis or speech aid: use same procedures and precautions as for cleaning a removable denture (see pages 181–183).

E. **Topical Application of Fluoride Solution:** Free premaxilla or short upper lip may complicate cotton roll placement.

VII. **PATIENT INSTRUCTION**

A. **Personal Oral Care Procedures**

The self-conscious patient with an inferiority complex may actually fear or exhibit rejection toward his oral cavity. With a small child the parents may be afraid of damaging the deformed areas or hurting the child if cleansing methods are employed. The dental hygienist must have an empathetic and sympathetic approach and plan for continued instruction over a long period of time.

1. Teeth and gingiva
   a. Select toothbrush, brushing method and auxiliary aids according to the individual needs (see Chapters 26 and 27).
   b. Adapt techniques for patient with free premaxilla to prevent its movement. A soft brush may be indicated.
   c. Suggest rinsing procedures (see pages 195 and 311).
      (1) Mild hypertonic salt solution for tissue healing.
      (2) Solution of bicarbonate of soda when there is a tendency for heavy mucinous plaques to form.
2. Prosthesis or speech aid
   Halitosis may be a real problem when the prosthesis forms the soft palate and the floor of the nasal cavity because of the accumulation of mucous secreted by the nasal surface.[9]
   a. Instruct patient in the need for frequent removal of appliance for cleansing, particularly following eating.
   b. Method for cleaning prosthesis: same as for removable partial denture (see page 314).

B. **Diet**

1. Need for building gingival tissue resistance: a varied diet which includes adequate proportions of all essential food groups.
2. Need for providing gingival stimulation: detergent foods, particularly fresh fruits and vegetables. Patient's malocclusion and cleft may present difficulties, but usually the patient can adapt.
3. Need for prevention of dental caries: limitation of foods containing fermentable carbohydrates, particularly for between-meal snacks. Procedures of the dental caries control study are recommended (see pages 363–365).

VIII. **DENTAL HYGIENE CARE RELATED TO ORAL SURGERY**

A. **Presurgery Oral Prophylaxis** (see pages 371 and 378)

Objectives have particular significance because the cleft palate patient is unusually susceptible to infections of the upper respiratory area and middle ear. Every precaution should be taken to prevent complications.

B. **Postsurgery Personal Oral Care**[10]

In certain of the palate operations, arm restraints are applied to prevent accidental damage to the repaired region. After each feeding (liquid diet for several days, soft diet for the next week) the mouth must be rinsed carefully. Brushing must be accomplished with great care, usually by the parent or hospital attendant, to avoid damage to the healing suture lines. In certain cases the toothbrush with suction attachment may be useful (see page 334).

REFERENCES

1. Beder, O. E. and Saporito, L. A.:   The Orofacial Cripple, Am. J. Orthodont. and Oral Surg. (Oral Surg. Sect.), *32*, 351, June, 1946.
2. Beder, O. E.:   *Surgical and Maxillofacial Prosthesis.* Seattle, University of Washington Press, 1959.
3. Sharry, J. J.:   Treatment of the Handicapped Child, in Finn, S. B.: *Clinical Pedodontics.* 2nd ed. Philadelphia, Saunders, 1962, pp. 445–454.
4. MacCollum, D. W.:   Habilitation of the Cleft Palate Patient, New Eng. J. Med., *254*, 299, February, 1956.
5. Whaley, J. B.:   The Otolaryngologist's Role in the Care of the Cleft Palate Patient, Canad. Dent. A. J., *23*, 574, October, 1957.
6. Sicher, Harry: *Orban's Oral Histology and Embryology,* 5th ed. St. Louis, Mosby, 1962, pp. 28–30.
7. Curtis, Elizabeth: Genetical and Environmental Factors in the Etiology of Cleft Lip and Cleft Palate, Canad. Dent. A. J., *23*, 576, October, 1957.
8. Kessler, H. E.:   A Study of Cleft Palate and Harelip Cases in the Cleveland Public School System, Oral Surg., Oral Med., & Oral Path., *4*, 1381, November, 1951.
9. Cooper, H. K.:   Integration of Services in the Treatment of Cleft Lip and Cleft Palate, Am. Dent. A. J., *47*, 27, July, 1953.
10. Archer, W. H.:   *Oral Surgery,* 3rd ed.   Philadelphia, Saunders, 1961, p. 632.

SUGGESTED READINGS

Beder, O. E.:   Congenital Cleft Lip and Palate Treatment Plan, J. Pros. Dent., *11*, 184, January–February, 1961.
Beder, O. E., Coe, H. E., Braafladt, R. P., and Houle, J. D.:   Factors Associated with Congenital Cleft Lip and Cleft Palate in the Pacific Northwest, Oral Surg., Oral Med., & Oral Path., *9*, 1267, December, 1956.
Beder, O. E., Carrell, J., Coe, H. E., and Moore, A. W.:   Problem of the Premaxilla in Bilateral Cleft Lip and Cleft Palate, Oral Surg., Oral Med., & Oral Path., *12*, 156, February, 1959.
Bzoch, K. R.:   Current Treatment Procedures for Cleft Lip and Cleft Palate Rehabilitation: A Symposium, Am. Dent. A. J., *60*, 695–726, June, 1960.
Kobes, H. R. and Pruzansky, S.:   Cleft Palate Team—A Historical Review, Am. J. Public Health, *50*, 200, February, 1960.
MacKay, C. D.:   Survey of Cleft Lip and Palate, Am. Dent. Hygienists' A. J., *37*, 203, 4th Quarter, 1963.
Neaderland, R. B.:   The Pedodontist and the Cleft Palate Patient, J. Dent. Child., *24*, 258, 4th Quarter, 1957.
Ricketts, R. M.:   Present Status of Knowledge Concerning the Cleft Palate Child, Angle Orthodont., *26*, 10, January, 1956.
Seide, L. J.:   Early Treatment of Cleft Palate, Dent. Radiog. & Photog., *35*, 51, #3, 1962.
Webster, R. B.:   Cleft Palate, Oral Surg., Oral Med., & Oral Path., *1*, 647, July, 1948; *1*, 943, October, 1948; *2*, 99, January, 1949; *2*, 485, April, 1949.
White, M. F.:   Cleft Lip and Cleft Palate, in Cohen, M. M.: *Pediatric Dentistry,* 2nd ed. St. Louis, Mosby, 1961, pp. 306–319.
Whitlock, Marilyn: Cleft Palate Story, Am. Dent. Hygienists' A. J., *29*, 50, April, 1955.

Chapter 34

MENTALLY RETARDED PATIENTS

The most challenging aspect of dental hygiene care for the mentally retarded is their need for oral health. Mental retardation is handicap enough without added oral problems which can even further reduce the already limited potential.[1]

Mental deficiency or retardation means that a defect in mental competency makes adequate and independent social adjustment impossible. The term *mental deficiency* is used more to designate those children whose potential is below normal, and even though everything possible is done to help them, the deficiency remains evident. The term *mental retardation* refers to the child who has the possibility, with optimal training and treatment, to approximate the normal range of intelligence. Approximately 3 per cent of the population in the United States are mentally retarded.

The background for understanding the problems and needs of the mentally retarded is a clear knowledge of what constitutes normal growth and development and the behavioral manifestations of normal children at each age level. The approach to any dental patient depends on his physical, mental, and emotional capabilities for cooperation and comprehension. Dental hygiene care for the mentally retarded requires patience and ingenuity for a skillful application of clinical and educational techniques. The dental hygienist's efforts contribute to the over-all habilitation of the patient in order that he may become more useful and effective.

I. CLASSIFICATION OF MENTAL RETARDATION BY ETIOLOGY

Mental retardation represents a more or less important symptom in well over 100 different conditions. Many of these are rare. Although a variety of means of classification is found in the literature, the most generally accepted is to divide the causes into factors operating before birth, at birth, and after birth before mental development has been completed. Percentagewise, a majority result from prenatal influences, whereas only a small number are effected as injuries at birth. It should be appreciated that diagnosis may be very complicated and difficult and many cases can only be classified as of unknown etiology.

The classification given below provides general etiological categories and is not all-inclusive. More comprehensive study of references is recommended when further detail is needed.[2-5]

A. Prenatal

1. *Familial:* physiological heredity; factors inherent in genes which transmit intelligence in everyone.
2. *Metabolic:* effected by genes responsible for absence of or interference with enzymatic activity related to metabolism of specific carbohydrates, proteins, or lipids. Phenylketonuria

is a disorder in which the amino acid phenylalanine is inadequately metabolized. Galactosemia is a condition in which galactose is improperly utilized.

3. *Prenatal infections:* toxoplasmosis, rubella (German measles) and congenital syphilis.
4. *Kernicterus:* high level of bilirubin in infant's blood, one cause of which is erythroblastosis fetalis due to Rh factor (when fetus is Rh positive and mother Rh negative).
5. *Endocrine deficiency:* particularly thyroid: cretinism.
6. *Mongolism:* cause unknown; higher incidence associated with advanced maternal age.

B. Natal

1. Cerebral birth injury: it should be realized that approximately one-half the children with evidence of brain injury are mentally retarded.
2. Asphyxia with resulting anoxia.

C. Postnatal

1. Inflammations of central nervous system: meningitis, encephalitis.
2. Cerebral trauma: accidents of infancy (rare).
3. Prolonged toxemia, malnutrition or vitamin deficiency (rare).
4. Accidental poisoning: lead, carbon monoxide, or coal-tar derivatives (rare).
5. Congenitally blind and deaf: because of lack of stimulation from environment a degree of mental retardation may result unless special training is initiated.

II. MENTAL CAPABILITIES AND LIMITATIONS[6,7,8]

The degree of subnormal intelligence or mental deficiency ranges from borderline deficiency down to an intellectual level too low to measure.

Various criteria have been used to classify the mentally retarded including the following: scholastic educability, mental ability test scores, social capacity, that is, to what degree he is able to support himself, and legal definitions. Probably the most descriptive and useful classification is based on educability, trainability, and dependency as described below.

A. Educable: mildly retarded (approximately 83% of all mentally retarded)

1. I.Q. above 50.
2. Make slow progress in elementary grades in school; may complete fourth grade, or continue in special classes.
3. Usually learn to read and write.
4. Do not have mental capacity for successful independent social adjustment.
5. Not capable of consistent planning.
6. Low capacity for sustained effort under pressure.
7. With supervision can perform simple routine work to contribute towards own support, provided competition is kept at a minimum.

B. **Trainable:**   moderately retarded (approximately 13% of all mentally retarded).

1. I.Q. between 25 and 50.
2. Capable of learning to walk and talk.
3. Poor motor control: awkwardness increases with severity of mental defect.
4. Many show constant overactivity.
5. May develop special motor tics with age: performed deliberately when not interested in surroundings.
    a. Frowning or knitting of the eyebrows.
    b. Blinking.
    c. Grimacing.
    d. Head nodding, shaking, rolling or bumping.
    e. Shoulder shrugging.
    f. Rocking and swaying of the body.
    g. Oral habits: tongue thrusting and sucking, thumb sucking, nail biting.
6. Can learn to recognize and avoid ordinary physical dangers such as fire and traffic.
7. May be trained to follow simple instructions and assist in simple tasks but cannot contribute to own support.
8. Will always need a protective, supportive environment.

C. **Dependent:** severely retarded (approximately 3% of all mentally retarded)

1. I.Q. below 25.
2. Cannot guard against common physical dangers; need continuous care.
3. Do not learn to form sentences; rarely form articulate words; many cannot speak at all.
4. Many remain inert and placid throughout early years; later movements are slow and clumsy; many never learn to sit up.
5. Usually have to be fed.

III. PHYSICAL CHARACTERISTICS

No particular set of characteristics can be ascribed the mentally retarded. Anomalies of physical development are observed somewhat more frequently than in other groups, but characteristic anomalies are confined to specific conditions such as Mongolism which will be described separately. Signs of nutritional deficiencies are frequently observed which may be due to lack of interest in eating or factors related to the inability to eat.

IV. ORAL CHARACTERISTICS

In the retarded, a higher incidence of oral developmental malformations has been observed, some specifically associated with a particular condition such as Mongolism.[9]

A. Dental Caries

High caries rate as might be expected considering the soft, carbohydrate diet used when there are masticatory and feeding problems. Personal oral care is difficult for many and impossible for the severely retarded. Research has shown that the dental caries rate in Mongoloids is much lower than for other retardates.[10]

B. **Periodontal Conditions:** common; associated with local irritation from deposit accumulations.

1. Masticatory difficulties prevent inclusion of detergent foods in diet thus preventing gingival massage by natural mechanisms.
2. Inability to perform regular personal oral care.

C. **Gag Reflex:** hypersensitive.[11]

V. PSYCHOLOGICAL FACTORS

Many factors affect the patient's approach to the dental appointment including environment, training, and parental attitude. Mentally retarded children present no constant personality pattern since some are quiet, subdued, and easily managed whereas others are restless, unstable, and aggressive.[12] Fear is generally the basis for behavioral difficulties in the dental office. Problems of the patient, parents, and the dental personnel need identification when dental hygiene care is planned. The generalities suggested below require thought and adaptation.

A. **The Mentally Retarded Patient**

1. Fears and anxieties: intensified because of slow development, limited comprehension, and previous medical care experiences.
2. Emotional immaturity
   a. No capacity for setting long-range goals and exercising self-discipline in achieving them; lives in immediate present.
   b. Desires are simple and pass quickly.
   c. Lacks control of emotions if desires are thwarted.
   d. Instability: upset by trivial difficulties.
   e. Lack of self-confidence.
3. Lack of feeling of security: apprehensive; needs attention and praise.
4. Feeling of dependence and helplessness: a reaction to parental overprotection.
5. Easily discouraged: particularly when goals are set too high for his capabilities.
6. Irritability with tenseness and aggression: if attempt is made to push him beyond his abilities.
7. Older patient
   a. Needs feeling of adequacy and usefulness as do other adolescents but frequently lives in atmosphere of frustration and rejection.
   b. May become increasingly lonely.
   c. Discouragement and lowered morale may result when not employed regularly.

B. **The Parents**[13-15]

Everything that applies to normal parent-child relationships applies alike to parents and their subnormal children. Parents of the mentally retarded have additional emotional problems since the child is so completely dependent on parental care. Some of the difficulties mentioned below are more characteristic while the child is very young.

1. Sense of shame or guilt: disappointment over having a retarded child: in part at least, this characteristic is socially determined. Found more in intelligent parents; less intelligent ones tend to accept the child more readily.
2. Overprotectiveness and overindulgence: failure to realize that although the mentally retarded child needs attention and love as does any child, an excess can seriously affect the child's future.
3. Failure to accept the child for what he is; need to limit goals set for the child to those which can be accomplished.

C. The Dental Personnel

The emotional reaction toward the mentally retarded will vary with a person's cultural and educational background and the amount of experience in working with the handicapped. The relationship of dental personnel to the patient will be reflected by attitudes and behavior as well as the sincere desire to help. Some may experience one or more of the psychological reactions listed below.[14] Dental personnel must guard against manifesting their own anxieties and will need to analyze their own feelings as they attempt to overcome any reactions which may interfere with the progress and success of dental and dental hygiene care.

1. Curiosity: diminishes with added experience.
2. Pity: need for understanding the problems and needs of the patient.
3. Oversolicitousness.
4. Mild dislike; feeling of discomfort or uneasiness.
5. Rejection.
6. Fear: of doing or saying something offensive.
7. Sympathetic understanding.

VI. THE MONGOLOID[16-17]

Approximately 20 per cent of institutionalized mentally retarded patients are mongoloids. It is rare for more than one mongoloid to be born within a family.

Mongoloids represent a distinctive group with a combination of characteristic abnormalities which are relatively constant. They tend to resemble one another.

A. **Mental Characteristics:** greatest per cent are moderately retarded, in the trainable group.

B. **General Physical Characteristics**

1. Infants
    a. Quiet and placid.
    b. Development: retarded.
    c. Speech: frequently delayed.
2. Head
    a. Skull: small, flattened on facial and occipital sides.

   b. Eyes: slanting, Asiatic appearance.
   (1) Widely spaced.
   (2) Opening between eyelids narrow.
   (3) Fold of skin continues from upper eyelid over inner angle of eye.
   c. Nose: short, broad with depressed bridge.
   d. Hair: at first soft, later dry and scanty.
3. Hands: broad, flat, clumsy-looking; fingers spread, short incurved little finger.
4. Abdomen: large.
5. Joints: unusual range of movement.
6. Circulation: poor.
7. Respiration: shallow, irregular; frequent mouthbreathing.
8. Vitality and resistance: low, subject to infections.
9. Disease incidence
   a. High incidence of congenital heart disease.
   b. High incidence of leukemia.

C. Oral Characteristics[18,19,20]

1. Lips: often thickened, cracked.
2. Jaws: prognathic profile.
3. Palate: high and narrow.
4. Tongue
   a. Large, protruded.
   b. Fissured.
   c. Papillæ hypertrophied.
5. Teeth
   a. Eruption: delayed, partial anodontia.
   b. Microdontia; peg shaped teeth.
   c. Poor alignment.
   d. Enamel hypoplasia.
6. Periodontal disturbances: high incidence, even in very young.[21,22,23]
7. Dental caries: low incidence.[10,24]

D. Psychological Characteristics: Personality[25]

1. Lovable; affectionate.
2. Like attention; require affection for feeling of security.
3. Cheerful disposition: rarely irritable.
4. Sociable: social development is ahead of physical; easily amused.
5. Tendency to imitate; mischievous.
6. Full of initiative; observant.
7. Fondness for music: have sense of rhythm (not usually observed in other mentally retarded).
8. Stubbornness: related to their inability to shift quickly from one object to another.

VII. DENTAL AND DENTAL HYGIENE CARE FOR THE SEVERELY RETARDED PATIENT

A. Use of General Anesthesia

The severely retarded are difficult to handle and in most instances impossible without general anesthesia. Treatment of the severely retarded has to be limited in certain cases to the removal of diseased teeth. This is extremely unfortunate since with loss of teeth, diminished masticatory efficiency may lead to nutritional deficiencies.

B. **Radiographs:** may require assistance of parent, use of drug relaxant, or general anesthesia.[26]
   1. Extraoral and occlusal views used to supplement intraoral.
   2. Modified technique required for patient in prone position.

C. **Restorative Dentistry**
   Restoration of teeth including endodontic treatment is possible under general anesthesia. Several carious lesions or an entire quadrant may be restored at an appointment.[11,27–29] Such procedures are conducted by the dentist in a hospital with the assistance of a competent anesthetist, registered nurse and dental assistant in constant attendance.

D. **Oral Prophylaxis:** when a complete oral prophylaxis is not possible because of time limitation, at least scaling procedures should be completed.

VIII. APPLIED DENTAL HYGIENE CARE FOR THE LESS SEVERELY RETARDED

Procedures used depend upon the cooperation which the patient is able to give. Experience helps to define necessary adaptations.

A. **Objectives:** All of the principles for care of the normal patient apply with greater intensity.
   1. Oral cleanliness contributes not only to oral health through prevention of periodontal diseases, but to appearance; the mentally retarded have difficulty in being accepted by society. An untidy, slovenly person with debris-covered teeth and halitosis is much less socially desirable.
   2. Improvement of oral appearance helps to minimize the patient's self-consciousness.
   3. All objectives related to prevention of tooth loss leading to malocclusion and/or the need for dentures have particular importance. Dentures are difficult for the normal person to wear, and with limited patient cooperation and sensitive gag reflex, problems are increased for the mentally retarded.

B. **Appointment Planning**
   1. Recall intervals: ideally, 3 or 4 times each year.
      a. To prevent development of acute conditions.
      b. To help the patient adjust to dental and dental hygiene procedures.
      c. To provide repetition and encouragement for patient's personal care.
   2. Time of appointment: best planned in the morning when the patient, parent and dental hygienist are in the most responsive state.

3. Length of appointment
   a. Patient's lowered vitality and increased fatiguability indicate need for shorter appointments. However, with premedication, appointment time may be extended.
   b. Allow time for proceeding slowly as patient becomes confused when hurried.

C. Preparation for the Appointment

1. Parental preparation of child: prior to appointment instruct parent to talk about the anticipated visit; repetition of statements concerning the dentist and dental hygienist as friends who are kind and helpful, description of the chair that goes up and down, and the practice by the parent of putting fingers in the patient's mouth may aid in alleviating fears. The parent's own attitude toward going to the dental office reflects in the mentally retarded as in the normal child.[11]
2. Patient history
   a. Determine other health problems: many will have multiple complications; for example, heart disease is not uncommon and indicates possible need for premedication.
   b. Determine drugs used in treatment: some patients may be heavily medicated.
   c. Need for close integration of services with physician.
   d. Be a good listener: parent may be reluctant to talk at first, but after rapport is established may offer background information of importance to the various phases of care, management and instruction.[30]
3. Premedication to produce sedation and relaxation: used upon prescription by dentist for highly active or inadequately trained patients of any degree of deficiency.

D. General Suggestions for the Appointment

1. Never hurry but be direct. Patient should not be rushed.
2. Be cheerful and hopeful; work to develop child's confidence; exhibit confidence in child's ability to cooperate.
3. May assist in child's general training.[31]
   a. Questioning at time of taking patient's medical history may bring out possibilities.
   b. Example: child being trained to speak; effort may be being made to have child state what he wants instead of pointing.
4. Observe interaction of child and parent: may get clues to ways of obtaining cooperation.
5. Presence of parent in operatory: overprotected, completely dependent child may be impossible to handle without parent's presence and assistance.
6. Training of patient to open his mouth: may accomplish by mimicry.
7. Child may hold something in his hands to keep him busy.
8. Praise the patient at the end of the appointment.

E. **Radiographic Technique**[26]

1. Premedicated or quiet, docile patients: parent may hold intra-oral films successfully.
2. Active patient: parent may hold film and stabilize head.
3. Gag reflex: may limit possibility of obtaining complete intra-oral survey.

F. **Oral Prophylaxis**

1. Use of instruments at first may be contraindicated. Retract lips with fingers and inspect oral tissues until patient becomes accustomed to the idea.
2. Introduce each instrument slowly: avoid surprise or "sneak" procedures.
3. Motor-driven handpiece may be particularly terrifying to the patient: if so, use of porte polisher is indicated.
4. When necessary to postpone completion of prophylaxis, parent may be loaned a mouth mirror to practice placing it in patient's mouth daily until the next appointment.
5. Use of compressed air or water syringe can be very frightening to the unsuspecting patient or even to the forewarned one.[30]

G. **Topical Application of Fluoride**

1. Use of cotton roll holder is frequently contraindicated because of lack of understanding leading to resistance by patient.
2. May be advisable to make separate applications for each quadrant, using the fingers to hold the cotton rolls. This also aids in stabilizing the head. Parent may assist in holding the cotton rolls.

IX. PATIENT INSTRUCTION

A. **Toothbrushing:** Suggestions for Instruction.

Personal daily oral care ordinarily will be limited to toothbrushing, and a simple method is advised. Instruction for the person who cares for the patient is often more important than instruction given to the patient. The mentally retarded learn by constant drilling on a day-to-day basis, as a part of their regular schedule. Some parents may have an organized plan of instruction, working from goal to goal.

For the severely retarded, manipulation of the toothbrush is far beyond his capability so that the cleansing of the oral cavity must be accomplished by the parent or, when the child is in an institution, by an attendant. The toothbrush with suction attachment may be used effectively for institutional care (see page 334). An automatic toothbrush has been shown to be particularly adaptable for this group of patients.[32]

1. For the patient[15]
   a. Short attention span: present only a little instruction at a time.
   b. Coordination is acquired with difficulty.
      (1) Repetition important: teaching of a procedure may take 5 to 6 visits; need for continuous supervised practice.
      (2) Plastic toothbrush handles may be bent if a better grasp can be provided; when the patient uses a curved handled

spoon for eating, the toothbrush handle curved in the same manner may be helpful.
   c. Teaching must be specific: mentally retarded patients cannot grasp generalities.
      (1) Give directions in simple parts.
      (2) Demonstrate slowly, letting the patient participate.
2. For the parent
   a. Help the parent integrate toothbrushing into the child's daily routine: immediately after eating, particularly after eating foods containing fermentable carbohydrates.
   b. Parent may have developed special methods of teaching for the individual child: teach principles to the parent for working with the child.
   c. Repetition for the mentally subnormal parent: repeated visits with review and redemonstration.
   d. Training for the child who will not tolerate toothbrush.[11]
      (1) Take cotton-tipped applicator dipped in a commercial sweetening agent (containing no sugar) and touch child's tongue: do this at the usual times for toothbrushing throughout the day for several days, gradually increasing from a touch to moving the swab over the tongue.
      (2) Run applicator over tongue and over anterior teeth.
      (3) Add more and more areas until all of the teeth are covered, several times each day, particularly after meals and before going to bed.
      (4) Continue after a week with soft bristled toothbrush with a small head: go over each area, gradually working up to using a Rolling Stroke technique.
      (5) Gradually work toward using a stiffer bristled brush.
      (6) May experiment with child's acceptance of a mild flavored dentifrice or use bicarbonate of soda.

B. Diet

1. For dental caries control
   a. Help parent and older, mildly retarded child to understand role of fermentable carbohydrates in caries initiation.
   b. Make specific suggestions for the use of foods which do not contain concentrated sweets, particularly for between meals (see pages 363–365).
2. For gingival health and cleansing effect on teeth
   a. Dietary suggestions should be checked with the physician to determine any specially prescribed diet and to insure consistency in teaching.
   b. Detergent foods are recommended within the child's capability for mastication.

REFERENCES

1. DEISHER, R. W.: Seattle, University of Washington Child Health Center, personal communication.
2. YANNET, HERMAN: Classification and Etiological Factors in Mental Retardation, J. Pediat., *50*, 226, February, 1957.
3. NOYES, A. P. and KOLB, L. C.: *Modern Clinical Psychiatry*, 6th ed. Philadelphia, Saunders, 1963, pp. 282–290.

4. FRENCH, E. L. and SCOTT, J. C.: *Child in the Shadows*, Philadelphia, Lippincott, 1960, pp. 39–47.
5. BAKWIN, HARRY and BAKWIN, R. M.: *Clinical Management of Behavior Disorders in Children.* Philadelphia, Saunders, 1953, p. 264.
6. NOYES and KOLB: op. cit., pp. 280–281.
7. WECHSLER, DAVID: *Measurement and Appraisal of Adult Intelligence*, 4th ed. Baltimore, Williams & Wilkins, 1958, pp. 49–58.
8. FRENCH and SCOTT: op. cit., pp. 47–48.
9. SPITZER, RICHARD and MANN, IDA: Congenital Malformations in the Teeth and Eyes in Mental Defectives, J. Ment. Sci., *96*, 681, July, 1950.
10. JOHNSON, N. P., YOUNG, M. A., and GALLIOS, J. A.: Dental Caries Experience of Mongoloid Children, J. Dent. Child., *27*, 292, 4th Quarter, 1960.
11. ADELSON, J. J.: Dental Care and Home Training of the Mentally Retarded Child, Am. J. Ment. Defic., *59*, 434, January, 1955.
12. KLEISER, J. R.: Psychological Approach to Mental Retardation in Dental Practice, J. Dent. Child., *28*, 199, 3rd Quarter, 1961.
13. BAKWIN and BAKWIN: op. cit., pp. 274–275.
14. BAKWIN, R. M. and BAKWIN, HARRY: Cerebral Palsy in Children, J. Pediat., *39*, 113, July, 1951.
15. HAUSER, M. R.: Working with Mentally Retarded People, Am. J. Nurs., *53*, 822, July, 1953.
16. NOYES and KOLB: op cit., pp. 288–289.
17. BENDA, C. E.: *The Child With Mongolism.* New York, Grune & Stratton, 1960, pp. 4–8, 23–44, 63–66.
18. COHEN, M. M.: *Pediatric Dentistry*, 2nd ed. St. Louis, Mosby, 1961, pp. 490–493.
19. McMILLAN, R. S.: Relation of Human Abnormalities of Structure and Function to Abnormalities of the Dentition. II. Mongolism., Am. Dent. A. J., *63*, 368, September, 1961.
20. BENDA: op. cit., pp. 28–30.
21. BROWN, R. H. and CUNNINGHAM, W. M.: Some Dental Manifestations of Mongolism, Oral Surg., Oral Med. & Oral Path., *14*, 664, June, 1961.
22. COHEN, M. M., WINER, R. A., SCHWARTZ, S. and SHKLAR, G.: Oral Aspects of Mongolism. Part I. Periodontal Disease in Mongolism, Oral Surg., Oral Med. & Oral Path., *14*, 92, January, 1961.
23. JOHNSON, N. P. and YOUNG, M. A.: Periodontal Disease in Mongols, J. Periodont., *34*, 41, January, 1963.
24. WINER, R. A. and COHEN, M. M.: Dental Caries in Mongolism, Dent. Prog., *2*, 217, April, 1962.
25. BENDA: op. cit., pp. 67–68.
26. ADELSON, J. J.: Handicapped and Problem Patient—Radiodontic Examination and Treatment, Dent. Radiog. & Photog., *34*, 27, #2, 1961.
27. ADELSON, J. J.: Dental Care and Management of the Mentally Retarded Child, Am. J. Ment. Defic., *61*, 399, October, 1956.
28. MICHELS, P. J.: Seattle, University of Washington, Department of Pedodontics, and Buckley, Rainier State School for Mentally Retarded, personal communication.
29. SPRAGUE, B. F.: Simplified Management Technic for the Physically or Mentally Handicapped Dental Patient, Am. Dent. A. J., *59*, 1169, December, 1959.
30. GODFREY, K.: Dental Services for Handicapped Children, Dent. J. Austral., *27*, 118, June, 1955.
31. GRAVES, W. S.: Psychological Development of the Mentally Retarded Child: A Training Course for Attendants, Am. J. Ment. Defic., *62*, 912, March, 1958.
32. KELNER, MORRIS: Comparative Analysis of the Effects of Automatic and Conventional Toothbrushing in Mental Retardates, Penn. D. J., *30*, 102, April, 1963.

SUGGESTED READINGS

CHATHAM, J. W.: Role of the Dentist in a School for Mental Defectives, Am. J. Ment. Defic., *61*, 341, October, 1956.
FOALE, MARTHA: The Special Difficulties of the High Grade Mental Defective Adolescent, Am. J. Ment. Defic., *60*, 867, April, 1956.
GODFREY, K.: Childhood Mental Subnormality and Dentistry, Austral. D. J., *2*, 25, February, 1957.
LESSER, A. J.: New Program for Mentally Retarded Children, Am. J. Pub. Health, *48*, 9, January, 1958.
MASLAND, R. L.: Prevention of Mental Retardation—A Survey of Research, Am. J. Ment. Defic., *62*, 991, May, 1958.
SPOCK, BENJAMIN: *Baby and Child Care.* New York, Pocket Books, 1957, pp. 587–593.
THOMAS, D. H. H.: Cultural Attitudes to Mental Subnormality, Am. J. Ment. Defic., *61*, 467, January, 1957.

Chapter 35

EPILEPTIC PATIENTS

EPILEPSY is not a disease entity, but rather is a term used to describe a symptom or group of symptoms of disordered function of the central nervous system. An epileptic person is one who is susceptible to recurrent involuntary loss of consciousness, with or without convulsive movements or spasms.

The incidence of epilepsy in the United States is estimated at approximately one in 200 of the population, with a greater incidence in males. Less than 5 per cent are institutionalized.

The patient's medical history should reveal his susceptibility to seizures and his physician must be contacted when additional information other than that provided by the patient is required. Seizures tend to recur with a slight degree of predictability, which permits appointments to be planned when the patient may be unaffected. A knowledge of symptoms is important in all cases whether diagnosed or undiagnosed, and dental personnel should know and be able to apply first aid measures in or out of the dental office.

Except for effects left by accidents occurring during a seizure, oral manifestations are limited to epileptics being treated with dilantin sodium which may produce a gingival hyperplasia. All patients are advised by their physicians to live a moderate life and pay strict attention to general health rules. Care of the oral cavity becomes important both for its relationship to general health and to oral accidents which may occur during a severe convulsion.

I. PHYSICAL SYMPTOMS[1,2]

The three major types of seizures are *grand mal, petit mal* and psychomotor. There are many variants, some of which go unrecognized, but loss of consciousness is a criterion. The course of attacks varies from several a day to one every few years.

A. Grand Mal

1. The aura or warning: lasts from a moment to several seconds and may consist of one of a number of sensations suggested below. Approximately one-half of the patients experience the aura.
   a. Numbness or tingling.
   b. Strange feeling over stomach.
   c. Hallucination of a special sense: flashes of light, noises, peculiar taste.
   d. Twitching or stiffness of certain muscles.
2. The Seizure
   a. Loss of consciousness: sudden and complete; patient falls. If patient is in dental chair he may slide out.

  b. Entire voluntary musculature experiences continuous contraction: lasts from 10 to 20 seconds; bladder, and rarely rectum, may be emptied.

  c. Muscles of chest and pharynx may contract at same time thus forcing air out which results in a peculiar sound known as the "epileptic cry."

  d. Color: pale at first, then superficial veins become gorged; chest becomes fixed and aeration of blood ceases, leading to cyanosis of face.

  e. Pupils dilate.

  f. Intermittent muscular contractions follow, rapidly at first, then less frequently. If tongue is between the teeth it may be bitten.

  g. Respiration begins to return. Saliva which could not previously have been swallowed may become mixed with air and appear as foam.

  h. Postconvulsive coma
   (1) Rigid pupils.
   (2) Noisy respiration.
   (3) Profuse perspiration.
   (4) Cyanosed lips.
   (5) Complete relaxation of body muscles.

  i. Patient emerges in a cloudy state.

 3. Postconvulsive phase: headache and drowsiness; usually falls into a deep sleep.

 4. Occurrence: most frequently during the night just as patient is falling asleep, or may be in morning an hour or so after rising.

 5. *Status Epilepticus:* series of seizures without gaining consciousness between; danger to life.

B. Petit Mal

 1. The Seizure
  a. Loss of consciousness for 5 to 30 seconds.
  b. Patient does not fall; posture becomes fixed; may drop whatever he has in his hand.
  c. May become pale.
  d. May have rhythmic twitching of eyelids, eyebrows, or head.
  e. Resumes activities: may or may not be aware of attack.

 2. Occurrence: most common in children 10 to 18 years, and with increasing age may disappear or be replaced by other type of seizure. Two out of three children with *petit mal* subsequently develop *grand mal.* Individual *petit mal* seizures occur more frequently than *grand mal.*

C. Psychomotor

 1. The Seizure
  a. Trance-like state with confusion: usually for few minutes, sometimes for hours or days.
  b. No loss of consciousness.
  c. May manifest emotional excitement.
   (1) Fear, rage.
   (2) Irritability, depression, ill humor, bad temper.

(3) Ecstatic mood with religious exaltation.

(4) May commit acts of violence.

2. Occurrence: may occur with *grand mal* seizure; frequency increases with age.

II. ETIOLOGY[3,4]

Epilepsy is a symptom of a disorder of the central nervous system, the explanation for which has not been clearly defined.

A. Idiopathic or Cryptogenic Epilepsy

1. May have innate flaw in brain which causes nerve cells to effect the seizure.
2. Includes approximately 77 per cent of all epilepsies.
3. Tends to manifest early in life; majority of cases between ages 10 and 20.
4. Heredity may be a predisposing factor.

B. Symptomatic or Acquired Epilepsy

1. Known cerebral lesion brings about dysfunction leading to seizures.
    a. Tumor.
    b. Trauma.
    c. Inflammation.
    d. Degenerative brain disease.
2. Occurrence: not related to age, but generally a symptomatic cause is suspected in epilepsy which manifests after age 20.

III. ORAL MANIFESTATIONS[5-9]

Epilepsy in itself has no oral manifestations. Patients being treated with the anticonvulsant, dilantin sodium, are subject to a noninflammatory hyperplasia of the gingiva. Other oral structures may show the effects of accidents following severe seizures.

A. Gingiva: Dilantin Hyperplasia

1. Occurrence
    a. Approximately one-half patients treated with the drug develop hyperplasia.
    b. Begins approximately 3 months after initiation of the drug.
    c. Size of lesion unaffected by duration of treatment or dosage.
    d. Does not occur in edentulous areas.
2. Clinical appearance and symptoms of the uncomplicated case
    a. Primary lesion
        (1) Hyperplasia of isolated interdental papillæ.
        (2) Granular, highly stippled.
        (3) Firm, pale coral pink, resilient.
        (4) Size
            (a) Gradual increase to form an elevated mass (bulb-like).
            (b) Clefts may form between individual papillæ.
        (5) No tendency to hemorrhage.
        (6) No pain.

   b. Advanced
      (1) Massive tissue fold partially obstructs tooth from view.
      (2) Level of gingival attachment not disturbed.
   c. Most severe
      (1) Attached gingiva becomes involved.
      (2) Hyperplasia appears continuous from tooth to tooth.
      (3) Interference during mastication: pain.
3. Complications
   a. Secondary increase in size
      (1) Cause: local irritants
         (*a*) Calculus and soft deposits.
         (*b*) Overhanging restorations.
         (*c*) Large carious lesions.
      (2) Effects
         (*a*) Inflammation.
         (*b*) Hemorrhage.
   b. Halitosis: resulting from debris and bacterial accumulation in crevices and clefts between and under areas of hyperplasia.

B. Other Oral Structures: Effects of Accidents

1. Scars of lips and tongue.
2. Fractured teeth.
3. Cuspal wear due to bruxism.

IV. PSYCHOLOGICAL CHARACTERISTICS[10-12]

There is no characteristic personality of epileptics. A good part of any maladjustment exhibited by the noninstitutionalized patients can be blamed on the attitude of society toward them. They react individually according to their feelings toward themselves and how others look upon their illness.

Occupation is limited as the epileptic cannot be permitted to participate in activities which provide hazards in the event of a seizure. This is particularly depressing to adults who have acquired epilepsy since reaching the working age and who must change their vocation.

In studying the behavior and personality of the epileptic, it should be clear that the symptoms suggested below may appear in part or may not appear at all.

A. Characteristics Related to Disease or Injury of Central Nervous System

1. Variability of mood without apparent cause; changes in disposition.
2. Restlessness; overactivity; at times has seeming excess energy; difficulty at times in sitting still.
3. Irritability: related to impatience and ease in becoming aroused to aggressive activity.
4. Short attention span
   a. Varying difficulty in powers of concentration and remembering what has been learned previously.
   b. Distractibility; difficulty in continuous application to task at hand.

5. Difficulty in reasoning, problem-solving situations: difficulty in mathematics for school age child.

B. **Characteristics Related to Attitude Toward Illness**
1. Dread or anxiety toward having a seizure.
2. Irritation: oversolicitousness of parents or others hampers activity and provides aggravation.
3. Despair and resentment: over being excluded from school and community activities; may create antisocial tendencies.
4. Aggressiveness: reaction to parental rejection.
5. Shyness: related to state of insecurity.

V. **APPLIED DENTAL HYGIENE CARE**

A. **Appointment Planning**
1. Recall intervals
   a. Sufficient to maintain tissues in optimum health.
   b. Patient with dilantin hyperplasia may require frequent appointments.
2. Length of appointment: adjust time to degree of illness.
   a. Patients are advised by physician to avoid fatigue.
   b. Recognize restlessness, particularly in children.
3. Time of day: patients with controlled epilepsy frequently know when seizures may be expected and may plan appointments to avoid those hours.
4. Appointment keeping: drugs used in treatment, if hypnotic, tend to make patient drowsy; may sleep more than an average person.
   a. Be understanding when patient is late or misses an appointment.
   b. Plan telephone reminder at opportune time if patient is chronically late.

B. **Patient Approach**
   Each of the physical and possible psychological characteristics should be given consideration during the appointment.
1. Treat as an ordinary individual with patience, sympathy, but avoid oversolicitousness.
2. Impress the patient with his importance and responsibility; express confidence in him.
3. Avoid discussions or actions which may create anxiety; explain procedures to be used.
4. Encourage self-expression particularly if the patient tends to be quiet and withdrawn and has narrowed interests.
5. Do not mistake drowsiness (effect of drugs) for inattentiveness.
6. Recognize possible impairment of memory when reviewing personal oral care procedures.
7. Plan instruction for short periods, in accord with patient's shortened attention span.
8. Appeal to patient's lagging interest in personal appearance: develop interest in caring for his mouth; commend his successes.

C. **Special Objectives in Dental Hygiene Care and Instruction**
1. Maintain oral health as a part of general health. One fundamental in the treatment of epileptics by the physician is the maintenance of optimum physical health.
2. Prevent tooth loss leading to need for dentures.
   a. Severe bruxism causes wear and fracture of the denture.
   b. Denture is a hazard during seizures.
3. For epileptics with dilantin hyperplasia: strict oral care.
   a. To prevent complications of inflammation and hemorrhage resulting from deposits on the teeth which cause irritation to the gingival tissue.
   b. To prevent halitosis resulting from debris accumulation in clefts and crevices of the hyperplastic gingiva.

D. **Oral Prophylaxis:** Adapt instrumentation and rinsing procedures to unusually deep gingival sulci resulting from dilantin hyperplasia.

VI. PATIENT INSTRUCTION

A. **Oral Physical Therapy for Dilantin Hyperplasia**
1. Rigid toothbrushing routine to aid in preventing accumulation of deposits which encourage hyperplasia and secondary effects.
2. Use of interdental stimulator when prescribed by dentist as special cleansing and massaging agent (see pages 306–307).

B. **Diet**
1. Physician's recommendations
   a. Normal diet: same as for other members of the family.
   b. Moderate amount of food; no alcohol.
   c. Avoid long periods without food: low blood sugar may precipitate a seizure.
2. Dental caries control: since patient may eat frequently, need for suggestions for foods which do not contain excessive fermentable carbohydrates.
3. Gingival health: need for helping patient understand nutritive foods of basic groups and detergent foods for gingival massage.

C. **Special Instruction Related to Seizures**
1. Preservation of natural teeth: to prevent need for removable dentures which may provide a hazard during a *grand mal* seizure.
2. Removable dentures should be removed at night as seizures frequently occur shortly after patient retires.

VII. FIRST AID[8,13,14]

No attempt should be made to stop the convulsion. An outline for procedure appears in Table 15 on page 471. Some additional suggestions for application to the dental office are included here. First aid is generally required only for *grand mal* seizures.

A. Objectives

1. To prevent body injury.
2. To prevent accidents related to the oral structures.
   a. Tongue bite.
   b. Broken or dislocated teeth.
   c. Dislocated or fractured jaw.
   d. Broken fixed or removable dentures.

B. Preparation at Beginning of Appointment

When patient's medical history indicates epilepsy, precautions may prevent complications should a seizure occur.

1. First aid equipment should be readied in a convenient place.
   a. Rubber mouth prop such as used in general anesthesia administration. This should be part of the first aid equipment in every dental office. A towel wrapped around a blunt instrument or tongue depressor may also be used.
   b. Suture with needle.
2. Have patient remove dentures for duration of appointment.

C. First Appearance of Signs of a Seizure

1. Lower the dental chair so that patient may be assisted to open area on floor away from furniture. The many metal parts of the dental equipment offer hazards.
2. Use of a couch is dangerous because of the possibility of falling off or bumping against adjacent wall.
3. Insert rubber mouth prop between the teeth.
4. Hold tongue to prevent its falling into the throat.
   a. Use tongue forceps.
   b. Dentist may insert suture with needle and tongue may be held by the suture.
5. Place pillow or other soft object beneath patient's head to prevent bumping.
6. Loosen tight belt or collar.
7. Call physician when seizure is prolonged.
8. Postconvulsive phase: allow patient to sleep.
9. Check oral cavity for accident: dentist will attend to appropriate treatment.

REFERENCES

1. NOYES, A. P. and KOLB, L. C.: *Modern Clinical Psychiatry*, 6th ed. Philadelphia, Saunders, 1963, pp. 230–235.
2. WECHSLER, I. S.: *A Textbook of Clinical Neurology*, 8th ed. Philadelphia, Saunders, 1958, pp. 592–596.
3. NOYES and KOLB: op. cit., pp. 226–230.
4. WECHSLER: op. cit., pp. 588–592.
5. GLICKMAN, IRVING: *Clinical Periodontology*, 2nd ed. Philadelphia, Saunders, 1958, pp. 86–90.
6. ORBAN, B. J. and WENTZ, F. M.: *Atlas of Clinical Pathology of the Oral Mucous Membrane*, 2nd ed. St. Louis, Mosby, 1960, p. 87.
7. GRANT, D., STERN, I. B., and EVERETT, F. G.: *Orban's Periodontics*, 2nd ed. St. Louis, Mosby, 1963, pp. 220–222.
8. DUMMETT, C. O.: Oral Tissue Reactions from Dilantin Medication in the Control of Epileptic Seizures, J. Periodont., *25*, 112, April, 1954.
9. BURKET, L. W.: *Oral Medicine*, 4th ed. Philadelphia, Lippincott, 1961, pp. 333–335.

10. BAKWIN, HARRY and BAKWIN, R. M.: *Behavior Disorders in Children.*   Philadelphia, Saunders, 1953, pp. 130–135.
11. BRADLEY, CHARLES: Behavior Disturbances in Epileptic Children, Am. Med. A. J., *146,* 436, June 2, 1951.
12. NOYES and KOLB: op. cit., pp. 236–237.
13. GOLDMAN, A. M.: The Epileptic Seizure in the Dental Chair, N. Y. S. Dent. J., *15,* 224, April, 1949.
14. American Red Cross: *First Aid Textbook,* 4th ed.   New York, Doubleday, 1957, pp. 90–91.

SUGGESTED READINGS

ADELSON, J. J.:   Dental Management of Epileptic Children, J. Dent. Child., *28,* 52, 1st Quarter, 1961.
BERNIER, J. L.: *Management of Oral Disease.*   St. Louis, Mosby, 1955, pp. 269–272.
BEUBE, F. E.: *Periodontology.*   New York, Macmillan, 1953, pp. 662–663.
BROWN, A. F.: *Medical and Surgical Nursing,* II.   Philadelphia, Saunders, 1959, pp. 487–497.
KELLN, E. E. and GORLIN, R. J.:   Healing Qualities of an Epilepsy Drug, Dent. Prog., *1,* 126, January, 1961.
KELLN, E. E.:   Further Studies of an Epilepsy Drug, Dent. Prog., *3,* 271, July, 1963.
PANUSKA, H. J., GORLIN, R. J., BEARMAN, J. E., and MITCHELL, D. F.:   Effect of Anticonvulsant Drugs Upon the Gingiva—A Series of Analyses of 1048 Patients, J. Periodont., *32,* 15, January, 1961.
WALSHE, F. M. R: *Diseases of the Nervous System,* 8th ed.   Baltimore, Williams and Wilkins, 1955, pp. 121–137.
WARD, H. L. and LITWIN, HERMAN: Current Medico-Dental Status of Epilepsy, Ann. Dent., *20,* 1, March, 1961.

Chapter 36

PATIENTS WITH PHYSICAL AND SENSORY HANDICAPS

It is not possible to describe in detail the many diseases of the locomotor system, nervous system, and organs of special senses which have as a symptom or leave as a chronic after-effect, loss of sensory or motor function in the form of a handicap. The purposes of this chapter are to outline a few of the classic manifestations of handicapped patients, to provide brief descriptions of selected diseases to illustrate the types of manifestations, and to suggest adaptations which may be required in dental hygiene care and instruction for an afflicted patient. References and suggested readings are included for additional information.

It is expected that imagination and ingenuity will help to develop applications for procedures for handicapped patients in addition to those included in this chapter. The objective should be to make the dental hygiene appointment as pleasant and comfortable an experience as possible for each patient and to motivate the patient to practice personal oral care habits conducive to health within his range of ability.

Oral health for the handicapped takes on more than usual significance and presents a challenge to dental personnel. The handicap provides enough of a burden without additional oral problems which can reduce an already lowered potential for normal living. Preventive measures, particularly fluoridation and other means for supplying the teeth with fluoride (see pages 197 to 200), must be encouraged and promoted through community effort and personal instruction.

General health, to which oral health contributes and is an integral part, is important for several reasons. One is that the basic disease condition may be aggravated by such conditions as malnutrition and lack of resistance to infection, and more than that, with adequate general health the patient may be able to cope with his disease and overcome some of the difficulties encountered. Appearance contributes to social acceptance which may be difficult for a person with a marked deformity. An untidy person with unclean teeth and halitosis is much less acceptable socially than one with a clean mouth. Furthermore, maintenance of oral health prevents the need for extensive dental or periodontal care which the patient may not be able to undergo because of his lowered physical stamina or ability to cooperate. Dentures can be a hazard for certain patients or impossible for others.

Psychological and emotional factors enter into the picture with greater intensity. Knowledge of the characteristics of the variety of handicapping conditions can prevent personal, emotional reactions to a patient's distorted appearance, postural deformity, or inability to cooperate with the usual procedures. Calmness, patience, and kindness are key words in defining the approach to the patient.

Physical and sensory handicaps may be hereditary, congenital, or the result of trauma or disease. Of the diseases of the locomotor system, muscular dystrophy and arthritis, which are diseases of the muscles and joints respectively, will be described briefly in this chapter. Examples of diseases of the nervous system included are multiple sclerosis and cerebral palsy. Disturbances of the special senses are represented by blindness and deafness.

I. GENERAL CHARACTERISTICS OF PATIENTS WITH PHYSICAL DISABILITIES

No specific list can be designated which would describe the symptoms of all physically handicapped patients. The list below is suggestive of types of characteristics which may be observed in certain patients.

A. **Lowered Physical Stamina:** fatigue easily.

B. **Lowered Resistance to Infection.**

C. **Signs and Symptoms Associated with Neurological Diseases**
 1. Speech disturbances (aphasia).
 2. Convulsive states: example, epilepsy (see Chapter 35).
 3. Narcolepsy: uncontrollable desire for sleep or sudden attack of sleep.
 4. Headaches.
 5. Paralysis
  a. Hemiplegia: paralysis of one side of the body; most frequent cause is cerebral vascular accident.
  b. Paraplegia: paralysis of lower extremities or lower part of body; caused by trauma or diseases including poliomyelitis and multiple sclerosis.
  c. Quadriplegia or triplegia: 4 or 3 extremities involved.

D. **Symptoms Associated with Muscular Diseases**
 1. Weakness and atrophy of muscles.
 2. Limitation of motion.
 3. Pain: spontaneous or evoked by movement or pressure.

II. PSYCHOLOGICAL FACTORS

Handicapped people show the same wide range of individual differences found in others of the same ages. Patients with handicaps may have intellectual and emotional disabilities because of the attitudes of other people toward them and acceptance by their family. Loss or lack of ability to function independently or predict one's movements is psychologically traumatizing. Lack of esthetic appearance may have a tremendous influence on a person's life. The general factors suggested below may apply to a child, an adult, or in most instances, either.[1-5]

A. **Factors Affecting Emotional Problems of Patient**
 1. Overprotection by family
  a. Decreases incentive to make full use of own abilities.
  b. Prevents acceptance of new situations such as would confront patient in dental office; may react aggressively or may be retiring.
  c. May be apprehensive or undisciplined.
  d. May have resistance against assuming responsibility.

2. Rejection by family and others: may feel inadequate and inferior.
3. Parents may deny existence of disability; patient may be pushed beyond his capabilities which can lead to frustration.
4. Inability to act independently and control movements may lead to irritability, defensiveness or fear.
    a. Most difficult time to adjust is frequently when symptoms are relatively slight.
    b. Anxiety from increasing helplessness; fear of helplessness.
    c. Frustration from limitation and restriction of activities.
    d. Increased desire for attention, affection and protection.

B. **Suggestions for Patient Approach**[1]
1. Avoid oversolicitousness.
2. Respect personal pride of patient: encourage patient's interest in personal appearance.
3. Avoid mention of patient's symptoms.
    a. Help patient from becoming self-centered.
    b. Prevent embarrassment or self-consciousness.
4. Encourage patient in all achievements, however small.
5. Maintain cheerful atmosphere: contribute to patient's happiness and peace of mind.

III. GENERAL APPOINTMENT SUGGESTIONS

A. Appointment Planning
1. Time of appointment
    a. Morning: less fatiguing while patient is rested. When medication is to be administered, early afternoon may be preferable since some of the patient's early morning alertness has worn off. A child would be more relaxed prior to nap time.[6]
    b. Hour: convenient to patient's daily care schedule.
2. Allow sufficient time so that patient does not feel rushed; many handicapped people cannot hurry.
3. Recall: frequent
    a. To decrease length of single appointment.
    b. To assist patient whose handicap limits ability in personal oral care procedures.

B. Reception and Seating
1. Assist patient only as needed: he wants to feel independent.
2. Learn the way to help patient as he walks which will contribute most to his support.
3. Position chair to give patient feeling of security.
4. Wheel chair patient
    a. Lower or detach arm of dental chair to permit transfer of patient.
    b. Obtain portable headrest which can be attached to back of wheel chair; more effective stabilization may be obtained when patient remains in his own chair.

C. **Techniques**

1. Skillful adaptations are required for all techniques when the patient is unable to cooperate because of muscular involvement of the face or tongue or disturbance of temperomandibular joint function.
2. Radiographs: films may need to be held by patient's attendant when the hands and arms are involved or there is lack of coordination. Drug relaxants or general anesthesia may be indicated.[7]
3. Rinsing: use emesis basin, depending on limitations of movement by the patient.

D. **Procedures for Bedridden Patient:** see pages 330–333.

E. **Instruction**

1. Personal oral care procedures: instruction must be given to person caring for patient when patient is not able to manipulate toothbrush.
   a. Adaptations of the toothbrush handle for patients with limited control: an enlarged handle is easier to grasp, or a device to attach the handle to the patient's hand may be prepared.[8]
   b. Automatic toothbrush: ease of manipulation permits improved care.[9,10,11]
2. Diet: a varied diet with all essential food elements is important to the general health of the patient; prevention of dental caries has particular significance since performance of techniques required for dental care is extremely difficult.

MUSCULAR DYSTROPHY

Muscular dystrophy is a hereditary disease characterized by progressive loss of use and atrophy of symmetrical groups of muscles with eventual involvement of practically the entire voluntary musculature. Pain is rarely evident until the late stages of the disease when there is muscular contracture. Muscular dystrophy is one of the many diseases of the muscles for which the etiology is unknown and therefore treatment is impossible.

I. CHARACTERISTICS

As many as 5 different types of muscular dystrophy are identified, but classification does not imply any differences in the underlying pathologic processes. Classification is based on the distribution of muscles affected most in the early stages, the presence or absence of pseudohypertrophy of muscles, and the age of onset. The two types described below illustrate characteristics and classification.[12,13] Most of the afflicted are males.

A. **Pseudohypertrophic Muscular Dystrophy:** most severe type.

1. Age of onset: childhood, usually from 2 to 5 years.
2. Effects of muscular involvement
   a. Enlargement (pseudohypertrophy) of certain muscles, particularly the calves, is present in early years.

b. Weakness of hips: child falls frequently, has increasing difficulty in erecting himself.

c. Lordosis; abdominal protuberance.

d. Progressive muscular wasting: eventual involvement of thighs, shoulders, trunk; inactivity is detrimental and increases helplessness.

3. Prognosis: disablement severe by age of 15; patients rarely live to reach third decade.

B. Facioscapulohumeral Muscular Dystrophy

1. Age of onset: between 7 and 30, most commonly between 15 and 20.

2. Effects of muscular involvement

a. Facial muscles weak: expression impaired.

(1) Lips: prominent, gaping; patient cannot whistle or purse lips.

(2) Eyes: cannot be closed completely.

b. Shoulder muscles weakened; shoulders slope.

c. Upper arms: difficulty in raising arms above shoulders.

d. Forearms: frequently show marked hypertrophy.

3. Prognosis: progresses more slowly than pseudohypertrophic form of the disease; occasional case may become arrested after 6 to 12 years leaving permanent disability in proportion to severity of disease in its active stage.

C. General Physical Characteristics[14]

1. Appearance: 2 types

a. Thin, emaciated: typical of majority of ambulatory patients.

b. Heavy, obese, flabby: typical of nonambulatory.

2. Gait

a. Waddling: either walk on toes or flatfoot: results from muscle contracture.

b. Balance: precarious; patient arches back in attempt to find center of gravity; gait is slow as balance must be attained with each step.

3. Fatigue readily and do not recover promptly.

D. Occlusion[15]

1. Shifting, spreading or protrusion of teeth; openbite common.

2. Effect: disproportionate function of weak muscles of cheeks and lips in contrast to tongue which may be hypertrophied; loss of molding effect of muscles of lips.

II. APPOINTMENT SUGGESTIONS

Adaptations will depend on the patient's disability. Patients may have slight muscular involvement, be ambulatory but have balancing difficulties, be in a wheel chair or bedridden. All factors listed for general consideration of handicapped patients (see page 409) have application. Suggestions listed below will be useful for certain patients.

A. **Patient Reception and Seating**[14]
  1. Assistance while patient is walking
     a. Certain patients are better without assistance as they have developed their own method of balancing and the merest touch may upset them.
     b. Many gain balance by holding both hands on partially flexed forearm of person walking beside them.
  2. Seating
     a. Prior to seating
        (1) Raise chair: patient does not have strength to lower himself into chair.
        (2) Remove chair arm: allow patient to sit directly; climbing steps is difficult.
     b. After seating patient: tilt chair back: balance is precarious while sitting as well as standing; patient may fall forward.
  3. Assistance for patient while rising from chair
     a. Stand directly in front of him: lock arms around lower back and pull forward near hips.
     b. Allow patient to sway upper trunk back as he rises to standing position.
     c. Provide support until he obtains balance for walking.

B. **Patient Instruction**
  1. Problems of oral cleanliness
     a. Facial muscle weakness
        (1) Interferes with self-cleansing mechanisms.
        (2) Prevents adequate rinsing.
     b. Gaping lips: effect on oral tissues similar to that of mouth-breathing.
     c. Weakness of arm and shoulder: difficulty in applying toothbrush.
  2. Patient response to instruction
     a. Tendency to sluggishness in mental response.
     b. Speech is slow; word forming difficult.
     c. Lack of facial expression: not necessarily an indication of lack of attention or understanding.
  3. Toothbrushing instruction
     a. Instruct parent or other person who cares for patient.
     b. When patient is receiving physical therapy treatments, solicit assistance and advice from the physical therapist.

ARTHRITIS

Rheumatism and rheumatic diseases including arthritis are the most common causes of chronic illness in the United States. Because a large number of cases involve temporary or permanent, partial or complete disability, dental and dental hygiene care for this group of patients is complicated.

Arthritis means inflammation in a joint. It may occur in the acute or chronic form. The etiology varies and is not completely defined, which makes classification difficult. A patient may suffer from more than one type at the same time. Causes relate to a variety of conditions including specific infectious diseases such as tuberculosis, syphilis, gonorrhea or rheumatic fever; disturbances of metabolism such as gout; direct trauma; or neoplasms of the joints.   In addition there are rheumatoid arthritis of unknown etiology, and osteoarthritis, a degenerative joint disease associated with the aging process.   The latter two are the most prevalent types of arthritis and a few of the symptoms and characteristics of these are listed in this chapter.   For detailed information concerning these and the many other forms the reader is referred to textbooks of medicine, general and oral pathology, and nursing.[16-20]

There is no specific oral manifestation in arthritis except in cases where the temperomandibular joint is affected.   Such involvement presents difficulty in performing techniques for the patient who has limited ability in opening his mouth or has temperomandibular joint pain.

Maintenance of oral health contributes to general health, which in turn may increase the patient's ability to combat arthritis.[21]   In the past the theory that either periodontal or periapical infections might serve as a focus in the cause of arthritis, led to the extraction of many teeth.   Research has not proved that the theory of focal infection relates to arthritis.   Excellent reviews of the literature on this subject are available.[22-24]

I. CHARACTERISTICS OF MAJOR TYPES OF ARTHRITIS

A. Rheumatoid

1. Occurrence: more common in females; onset in early adulthood more frequent although it may occur at any age; tendency to recurrence.
2. Early symptoms
    a. Migratory swelling and stiffness of the joints particularly fingers, hands and knees; varying degree of pain when exercised.
    b. Weakness, fatigue, loss of weight, anemia.
3. Subsequent symptoms
    a. Joint symptoms tend to be symmetrical; painful.
    b. Subcutaneous nodules in elbows, wrists, or fingers in approximately 15 per cent of the patients.
    c. Temperomandibular joint involvement occurs in some patients; may have pain with movement of the jaw; ankylosis may develop.[25]
    d. Atrophy of muscles leads to deformities; progressive disability; eventually may be bedridden.

B. Osteoarthritis or Degenerative Arthritis

1. Occurrence: onset in middle-aged or elderly; associated with aging process.
2. Early symptoms: insidious, with slight stiffness in a single joint.
3. General physical characteristics: obesity, poor posture, limping.
4. Joint symptoms
    a. Hips, knees, fingers, vertebræ affected most frequently.
    b. Swelling is rare; ankylosis does not occur.
    c. Stiffness after rest, diminishes with exercise.
    d. Pain aggravated by temperature changes, bearing body weight.

    e. Temperomandibular joint usually not involved.[25]
        (1) Changes that do occur may be result of disturbed occlusal balance due to loss of teeth.
        (2) Crepitation, clicking or snapping may occur when the joint is exercised.

C. Psychological Factors

With long-range illnesses patients are frequently discouraged or apprehensive. Certain patients may be worried, pessimistic or resigned. Some may be impatient and tend to harm themselves by overexercise. A few are irritable, a characteristic related to the pain which has been suffered.

II. SUGGESTIONS FOR DENTAL HYGIENE CARE

Although the characteristics of all types of arthritis are not the same, the general suggestions provided below can be applied.

  A. **Room Temperature:** adjust, prevent drafts; patients are susceptible to cold and dampness.

  B. **Patient Positioning:** make adaptations for limited and painful movement.
    1. Lower arm of chair to permit patient to sit directly rather than having to step up to foot rest.
    2. Arrange chair seat so that flexion of knees and hips is at a minimum.
    3. Adjust foot rest so that feet may be placed squarely to avoid strain on knee joints.
    4. Suggest that patient flex and extend knees a few times before rising from chair: joints become stiff after being seated for a while.
    5. Offer hand to patient as he rises from chair: provides secure hold and usually is more helpful than assistance under the arms since many patients are used to devices for pulling themselves up.

  C. **Instrumentation:** for patient with temperomandibular joint involvement.
    1. Adapt instrumentation to minimal opening of jaws: do not expect patient to strain, particularly since pain may result.
    2. Avoid traumatizing joint by pressure on mandible.

MULTIPLE SCLEROSIS

Multiple sclerosis is an acute or chronic, remittent or progressive disease of unknown origin. It is characterized by nervous dysfunction. Pathologically the white matter of the central nervous system degenerates in patches and is replaced by sclerotic tissue. There is interference with the transmission of nervous impulses.

The marked variability in onset, course, and degree of dysfunction means that the illness is not a disease entity but a syndrome. There are no specific oral manifestations but the muscles of the tongue and face are involved in some cases.

I. CHARACTERISTICS

A. **Occurrence:** in cold and temperate climates primarily; affects males and females alike.[26]

B. **Onset:** in young adulthood between 20 and 40 years of age; rarely before 15 or after 50.[26]

C. **Initial Symptoms:** vary.[27]

1. May be minor visual impairment, tremor, fatigue, weakness or numbness of a part of the body; tend to disappear without treatment.
2. May have a sudden onset of severe illness with paralysis or marked weakness.

D. **Course of Disease:** characterized by attacks and remissions; patient may live for 20 years or much longer after first attack; bronchopneumonia is the most common immediate cause of death.

E. **Physical Symptoms**
There is a wide distribution of areas affected which results in a variety of symptoms. Symptoms fluctuate and there may be several years between attacks. They may be brought on by infections, particularly with fever, fatigue, psychological or emotional disturbances, malnutrition, or chilling. With extended rest, symptoms usually subside.

1. Involuntary motion of eyes (nystagmus); may later become partially or completely blind.
2. Speech disorders: possible loss of speech in advanced stages.
3. Changes in muscular coordination and gait: one side of body usually affected more than the other; loss of balance.
4. Paralysis of one or more extremities; occasionally facial paralysis.
5. Autonomic derangements such as urinary frequency and urgency; later urinary incontinence.
6. Susceptibility to infection, particularly upper respiratory.

F. **Personality Factors**[28,29]

1. Optimism and cheerfulness out of proportion to the degree of disability and seriousness of the illness; euphoria.
2. Subject to sharp deviations of mood: emotional outbursts with spells of laughing and crying.
3. Poor memory; poor judgment.
4. Passive dependency; lack of responsibility.

II. TREATMENT[27]

A. No specific treatment since the cause of the disease is unknown.
B. General hygienic care: adequate nutrition, rest, avoidance of strain, prevention of infections.
C. Physical therapy; exercise is very important.
D. Psychotherapy for personality problems and morale building: frequently necessary.
E. Drugs: primarily prescribed for alleviation of symptoms.
F. Patient should continue in his usual occupation as long as possible; activity should be encouraged.

III. **APPOINTMENT SUGGESTIONS**

Knowledge of physical, personality and treatment factors listed above is applied during appointment procedures. Since attacks may be initiated by infection, dental hygiene care for the prevention of oral infection assumes particular significance.

A. **Psychological Considerations**[30]

1. Provide a quiet, comfortable atmosphere: the patient needs to remain relaxed mentally and physically, therefore people around him cannot be tense and restless.
2. Prepare for emotional outbursts of laughing or crying by the patient.
   a. May be initiated by something as simple as the sudden introduction of hot or cold into the mouth, or being startled by a sudden air blast from the compressed air syringe.
   b. When an outburst occurs, change the subject of conversation to something impersonal: suggest something sad if the patient is laughing or something humorous if the patient is crying.

B. **Patient Instruction**

1. Problems of personal oral care
   a. Involvements of the tongue and facial muscles interfere with the self-cleansing mechanisms.
   b. Involvements of hands or arms make grasping and manipulating a toothbrush difficult or impossible.
2. Factors affecting teaching
   a. Slow response of patient: give instruction slowly and simply.
   b. Poor memory: instruction should be reviewed frequently.
   c. Visual disturbances: (see pages 420–422).

CEREBRAL PALSY

Palsy means paralysis and cerebral palsy means a condition in which injury to parts of the brain has resulted in paralysis or disruption of motor parts. Such a condition can occur at any age as a result of brain injury from a variety of causes, and therefore cerebral palsy is not really a disease entity. Through common usage, however, the term has come to be applied to cases of congenital spastic paralysis in children.

Causes relate to cerebral birth injuries, diseases *in utero*, or, less frequently, a developmental anomaly. Symptoms usually can be observed during the first year but may not appear for a number of years. Deafness, visual disturbances, speech problems or lowered mentality may accompany the paralysis, weakness, and incoordination of the motor system.

I. **GENERAL CHARACTERISTICS**[31]

The three main types of cerebral palsy are described briefly below. Two other types, rigidity and tremor, have mixed symptoms and frequently are associated with the major classifications. In each type different parts of the brain are affected and the symptoms vary respectively.

A. **Spastic Paralysis**
  1. Condition characterized by spasms which are sudden, involuntary contractions of single muscles or groups of muscles.
  2. Muscles have excess tone, tension, and activity.
  3. Patient has complete or diminished ability to control muscular movement, therefore movements are awkward; mental effort toward control results in less control.
  4. Activity: lack of control causes patient to fall easily; tends to avoid activity; may put on weight; caloric requirement is therefore low.[32]

B. **Athetosis**
  1. Condition characterized by constant involuntary unorganized muscular movement.
  2. Patient lacks ability to direct his muscles in the motions he desires; probably the most difficult dental patient.
  3. Factors influencing movements
      a. May be initiated and aggravated by stimuli outside body.
      b. Made worse by attempts of patient to control them.
      c. Intensity influenced by emotional factors: patient is at his worst in an emotionally charged environment such as the dental office.
  4. Activity: constantly in motion; burns up energy; usually very thin; caloric requirement of diet is therefore high.[32]

C. **Ataxia**
  1. Loss of equilibrium: balance and orientation difficult; walk uncertain; has difficulty in sitting straight.
  2. Difficulty in control of eye muscles; some dizziness and nausea.
  3. Activity: inactive because of balance disturbance; tends to put on weight; caloric requirement in diet is therefore low.[32]

II. ORAL CHARACTERISTICS[33,34]

A. **Disturbance of Facial, Masticatory, and Tongue Musculature**
  1. Prevents normal chewing pattern and swallowing process.
  2. Intraoral forces produce varying degrees of orthodontic involvements.
      a. Tongue thrusting may result from faulty swallowing reflex: may tend to push maxillary anterior teeth forward.
      b. Mouth breathing and tissue biting may occur.
  3. Interferes with voluntary opening of mouth.
  4. Drooling may result from inability to swallow and control facial muscles.
  5. Hyperactive reflexes cause patient to clamp jaws together suddenly.

B. **Increased Periodontal Involvements**
  1. Evidences of dietary deficiencies: foods essential to health are omitted from diet because of inability to chew.
      a. Gingival tissues show signs of malnutrition.
      b. Use of soft foods rather than detergent prevents tissue stimulation.

2. Lack of effects of natural self-cleansing mechanisms in cleansing the teeth; increased food retention.
3. Increased calculus deposits may be observed as an effect of mouth breathing, lack of self-cleansing processes, and inability to carry out personal care.
4. Inability to manipulate toothbrush: abnormal movements of arms, lack of control of hands, disturbance of facial and tongue musculature prevent success in personal care procedures; difficult for others to accomplish for patient because of involuntary movements.

C. **Attrition:** severe; constant, involuntary grinding of teeth wears down tooth structure and restorations.

D. **Fractured Teeth:** patients fall frequently; accidents to anterior teeth result.

E. **Hyperactive Gag Reflex**

III. SUGGESTIONS FOR DENTAL HYGIENE CARE AND INSTRUCTION[33,35]

Dental hygiene care is complicated by the difficulties which the patient has in cooperating and by the oral manifestations listed above. Psychological factors have been listed on page 408. Understanding of the physical characteristics is particularly necessary to the success of the appointment. Athetoid movements should not be interpreted as lack of cooperation and a patient's inability to communicate does not mean lack of comprehension.[36] Dentists use general anesthesia in a hospital situation for the unmanageable patient.[37,38,39]

There are dangers for both the patient and dental personnel which may result from the uncontrolled movement of the patient. The sudden forceful closure of the mouth on the finger of the operator or on a glass mouth mirror, or movement of the patient which diverts a sharp instrument into the patient's tissues, are examples. Skill, alertness, patience, and application of principles from the experience of others as listed below are needed. Assistance usually is required and it may be advisable to solicit the aid of the parent or other person who accompanies the patient since he would be familiar with the characteristics of the patient. Overprotective parents, particularly if they are not cooperative dental patients themselves, would be of limited help.

A. **Preparation for the Appointment:** Premedication to obtain a degree of relaxation would be given on recommendation of the dentist and advice of the patient's physician.

B. **Patient Positioning:** to help patient overcome feeling of insecurity.
1. Tilt chair back so patient cannot slide forward.
2. Use canvas or leather bands or belts.
   a. Place around patient under arms, around abdomen and attach to back of the chair.
   b. When patient wears leg braces, tie them to the chair.
   c. Arm restraint: restraint can serve as an irritant which could result in increased involuntary movement.

    (1) Have parent or assistant hold arms.

    (2) Arm splint made of cloth: not a straight jacket, but a simple enclosure for the arms; must be fully understood and approved by the patient.

  3. Wheel chair patient: may be best to keep patient in his own chair and attach portable headrest.

C. Techniques

1. Position of operator: may be effective to operate standing with arm around patient's head; use crotch of elbow for stabilization.
2. Mouth mirror: use metal-surfaced mirrors.
3. Avoid placing fingers between patient's teeth: use facial surfaces for fulcrum rests. Improvised finger protectors may be used such as a metal thimble covered with a rubber finger cot.[40]
4. Mouth prop: may be effective with a few patients, but lateral uncontrolled movements of jaw will dislodge it; long wooden wedge wrapped in gauze may be held by assistant.
5. Avoid sudden movements, noises, blasts of compressed air, bright light in patient's eyes or other effects which may startle the patient and cause muscle reaction.

D. Instruction

1. Give instruction in simple toothbrushing method to parent or other person who cares for the patient; training the patient is a long-range process.
2. Parents can be shown how to use a mouth prop placed on one side of the mouth while brushing teeth on opposite side.
3. Patient with some coordination may be able to use a toothbrush with a built-up or large handle, or an automatic brush.

BLINDNESS

Limitations of sight cover a broad spectrum from the slightly affected to the completely blind with no perception of light. Adaptations during the appointment vary then, from a procedure as simple as providing the patient with his eyeglasses before demonstrating a toothbrushing procedure, to those required for the nearly or completely sightless as described in this section. Loss of sight is a major physical deprivation. In many people blindness is only secondary to a primary condition which may have been the cause of the blindness and in itself may be disabling.

I. CAUSES OF BLINDNESS[41]

In children there is a higher percentage of cases of prenatal origin or which result from infectious diseases or accidents.[42] In the aging population major causes are cataracts, glaucoma, senile degenerative changes and effects of general diseases such as arteriosclerosis involving parts of the eyes. Well over half of those who are blind have lost their vision after the age of 65.[43] Because of the increasing population in the older age group, the incidence of blindness is likely to increase.

II. PSYCHOLOGICAL CONSIDERATIONS FOR PATIENT UNDERSTANDING

Each blind person must be considered in relation to his aptitudes, interests, abilities, and potentialities, with blindness only one factor involved and frequently not the most important. No pattern of patient attitudes and personality characteristics can be described. The only thing this group of patients has in common is difficulty in seeing. A few suggestions of factors involved are mentioned below.

A. Child

1. Learning ability
   a. Sensory defects often mask the child's intellectual capacity since he cannot respond as other children.
   b. Blind children learn to speak later than seeing children and frequently start school when they are a year or two older.
   c. It takes a blind child longer to cover the same amount of material, therefore there may be a different educational level than for the seeing child of the same chronologic age.
   d. Blind children are deprived of the opportunity to learn by imitation.
2. Personality factors
   Environment influences the child's adjustment and parental attitude affects the blind child as it does the seeing child. When the parent is overindulgent and protective, the child may be self-centered, dependent, and emotionally less stable.[42]

B. Adult

The adult who has been blind all his life or since childhood has made adjustments and may be employed in a limited but useful occupation. The greater number who become blind after adulthood experience an immediate natural reaction of depression and feeling of helplessness. When there is incipient loss of vision there usually is less shock and upheaval, but there may be many years of dread, worry, and anxiety in anticipation. When the patient begins to accept the handicap, efforts for rehabilitation are made easier.[44] He needs to develop independence and self-confidence, and must be helped not to become helpless.

III. SUGGESTIONS FOR THE DENTAL HYGIENE APPOINTMENT

A. Totally Blind

1. Factors to consider for adaptation of procedures and instruction.
   a. A blind person can perceive a new experience readily if he is told about it in detail.
   b. Because of the visual handicap, the patient must rely more on his other senses and so he cultivates them.
   c. A blind person has to be neat and orderly: if he puts something down he has to know where to find it.
   d. A blind person does things deliberately and slowly to gain perception and prevent accidents.
   e. Effective conversation with a blind person can best be accomplished by speaking as on the telephone.
   f. A blind person learns to interpret tone of voice and put more

reliance on this than people with sight who can watch facial expressions.

2. Patient reception and seating
   a. Lower dental chair prior to receiving patient; move other dental equipment such as bracket table, motor arm, operating stool from pathway.
   b. Guide to dental chair: patient holds dental hygienist's arm and is lead without being held.
   c. Provide forewarnings of potential hazards in the pathway.
      (1) Instruct patient of step up to dental chair.
      (2) For recall patient: when patient has become familiar with office arrangement from previous appointments, changes should be mentioned to prevent embarrassment.
   d. When leaving operatory during the appointment
      (1) Explain absence; prevent embarrassment of patient speaking to someone who isn't there.
      (2) Speak when reentering the room.

3. Techniques
   a. Describe each step in detail before proceeding: instruments, materials, and how each will be applied; mention flavors.
   b. Permit patient to handle instruments before they are used while describing how each will be used; this applies particularly to child patient who is not familiar with dental procedures.
      (1) Use second set of instruments in order to maintain sterile procedures.
      (2) Use other instruments of a similar size and shape when describing scalers or explorers since handling sharp instruments would be dangerous for the patient.
      (3) Moving rubber cup may be applied to child's finger: if motor-driven instruments disturb the patient, use porte polisher for entire procedure.
      (4) Avoid surprise applications of compressed air, water from syringe or motor-driven instruments.
   c. Speak before touching the patient: by maintaining contact of a finger on a tooth or through retraction while changing instruments, repeated orientation is avoided.
   d. Rinsing
      (1) When water syringe is not available it is advisable to place rinsing cup in patient's hand each time rather than expect him to pick it up from unit: help avoid patient's embarrassment if water is spilled.
      (2) Relation to cuspidor: after original orientation an older child or adult will have no difficulty; if chair position is changed, patient needs reorientation. Use of emesis basin is easier for small child or adult who has become blind recently.

4. Patient instruction
   a. Give instructions clearly and concisely.
   b. Visual aids such as models may be used if described in detail and given to the patient to handle.
   c. Toothbrushing: demonstration in patient's mouth.

B. **Partially Blind**

People with sight often underestimate degree, and fail to realize how useful a little vision can be. Patience in helping a patient make full use of available vision, without oversolicitousness, is important. Although many of the procedures described for the totally blind can be applied to the partially blind, a few additional hints are suggested below.

Elderly patients with failing sight will rarely admit such a handicap. Sight failure in the aged or lowered vision at any age may be suspected from the patient's unusual squinting, blinking, or lack of persistent attention. Techniques can be adapted without mention of sight to the patient.

1. Avoid glare of operating light in patient's eyes: this is true of all patients in helping to preserve sight.
2. Do not expect patient to see fine detail as in a radiograph or on a small model.
3. Work patiently and give instruction slowly: patient may have slow accomodation.
4. Give patient his eyeglasses before beginning instruction.

DEAFNESS

When there is impairment of hearing to the extent that it is no practical value for the purpose of communication, a person is considered deaf. When hearing is defective but functional with or without a hearing aid, the terms "hard of hearing" or partially deaf are used.

I. CAUSES OF HEARING IMPAIRMENT

Inability to hear may be temporary or permanent. There is a wide variety of factors which contribute to deafness. These include physical injuries; communicable diseases, particularly meningitis, scarlet fever, diphtheria and measles; infections of the inner ear; mastoiditis; foreign bodies; congenital defects or malformations; noise, chemicals used in industry, or other occupational hazards; and the aging process and the chronic diseases associated with aging.[45]

II. CHARACTERISTICS

A. Major Types

1. Conduction or bone deafness.
   a. Part involved: middle ear, external canal or drum membrane.
   b. Hearing aid: plate behind ear; sound is conducted by bone.
   c. Speech: soft and low; person hears himself louder than others.
2. Perception or nerve deafness.
   a. Part involved: inner ear; injury to nerves.
   b. Hearing aid: button in ear; sound conducted by air.
   c. Speech: loud; person cannot hear himself.

B. Characteristics Suggesting Hearing Impairment

Partial deafness may not have been diagnosed or certain patients, particularly the elderly, may not admit hearing limitation. Clues to the identification of a hearing problem are listed below.

1. Lack of attention; fails to respond to conversational tone.
2. Intentness; strained facial expression; stares at others.
3. Turns head to one side; hearing may be good on one side only.
4. Gives unexpected answer unrelated to question; does one thing when told to do another.
5. Frequently asks others to repeat what was said.
6. Unusual speech tone.
7. Inaccurate pronounciation: characteristic in child who repeats what he hears; with defective hearing certain sounds are missing in his hearing range.

C. Psychological Factors

People with hearing loss tend to have more emotional difficulties than those with sight loss. It is more devastating to live in a silent world than in darkness.[46] Hard of hearing people are inclined to withdraw. They are bothered when they do not know what others are saying. This is mostly true of older people who develop paranoid tendencies and believe that when they cannot hear other people are talking about them. Children do not have this problem but live in their own little world and watch others. General characteristics described for handicapped people (pages 408–409) may apply to the hard of hearing.

III. SUGGESTIONS FOR PATIENT APPROACH DURING THE DENTAL HYGIENE APPOINTMENT[46–49]

A. Patient With Hearing Aid: Allow time for adjustment.

B. Patient With Partial Hearing Ability

1. Speak clearly and distinctly; direct speaking to side of "good" ear if hearing is impaired on one side only.
2. Eliminate interfering noises: from street outside or saliva ejector suction.

C. Lip Reader

1. Be sure patient is looking; do not turn to side; speak directly.
2. Speaker's face must be lighted so patient can read lips easily; difficult because dental light is directed to patient's face; operator may have back to window.
3. Speak in normal tone; do not accentuate words.
4. Do not raise voice; raising voice aggravates the situation; patient may be inclined to withdraw.
5. When patient cannot understand: use different words to express the same thought; many letters and combinations of letters look the same on the lips; others are not visible at all.
6. Be sure patient understands; he will be troubled if he thinks he did not understand correctly.
7. Keep calm; display of irritation or annoyance over difficulties in conversing will discourage or upset the patient.
8. Write proper names or unusual words which the patient fails to understand.

D. Patient Without Hearing Aid Who Does Not Lip Read:
Use gestures and written notes.

E. General Instructions

1. Do not startle the patient by tapping him to gain attention.
2. Watch for patient's motions and facial expressions to determine reaction or discomfort during oral prophylaxis techniques.
3. Teach by demonstration.
   a. Open mouth wide each time patient is to open.
   b. Small child may be taught to rinse by watching and imitating.
4. Appointment making: hard of hearing person should always have written appointment card to assure complete understanding; appointments made by telephone should be confirmed by mail.
5. Use judgment in prolonging conversation with deaf person: certain patients are under tension and tire easily whereas others enjoy the opportunity to be the center of attention.

REFERENCES

1. RIPLEY, H. S.: Understanding Emotional Reactions to Disability, Phys. Therapy Rev., *39*, 13, January, 1959.
2. BAKWIN, HARRY and BAKWIN, R. M.: *Behavior Disorders in Children.* Philadelphia, Saunders, 1953, pp. 125–127.
3. GODFREY, K.: Dental Services for Handicapped Children, Dent. J. Austral., *27*, 118, June, 1955.
4. KAUFFMAN, J. H.: Psychological Aspects of Dentistry for Children with Cerebral Palsy, J. Dent. Child., *23*, 69, 2nd Quarter, 1956.
5. TRACHT, V. S.: Psychological Adjustment of the Family to the Handicapped Child, J. Dent. Child., *23*, 92, 2nd Quarter, 1956.
6. SPRAGUE, B. F.: Simplified Technic for the Physically or Mentally Handicapped Dental Patient, Am. Dent. A. J., *59*, 1169, December, 1959.
7. ADELSON, J. J.: Handicapped and Problem Patient—Radiodontic Examination and Treatment, Dent. Radiog. & Photog., *34*, 27, #2, 1961.
8. BUSH, B. A.: Toothbrushing Aids for Handicapped Children, Am. Dent. Hygienists' A. J. *38*, 76, 2nd Quarter, 1964.
9. GREEN, A., ROSENSTEIN, S. N., PARKS, A., and KUTSCHER, A. H.: Electric Toothbrush as an Adjunct in Maintaining Oral Hygiene in Handicapped Patients, J. Dent. Child., *29*, 169, 3rd Quarter, 1962.
10. KELNER, M.: Use of an Electrically Powered Toothbrush in the Home Dental Care of Handicapped Children, Penna. Dent. J., *28*, 3, November, 1961.
11. VOWLES, J. K.: Assessment of an Automatic Action Toothbrush (Broxodent) in Spastic Children, Brit. Dent. J., *115*, 327, October 15, 1963.
12. BEESON, P. B. and McDERMOTT, WALSH: *Cecil-Loeb Textbook of Medicine,* 11th ed. Philadelphia, Saunders, 1963, pp. 1451–1453.
13. DENNY-BROWN, D. E.: Diagnosis and Treatment of Muscular Dystrophy, Postgrad. Med., *22*, 558, December, 1957.
14. WRATNEY, M. J.: Physical Therapy for Muscular Dystrophy Children, Phys. Therapy Rev., *38*, 26, January, 1958.
15. WHITE, R. A. and SACKLER, A. M.: Effect of Progressive Muscular Dystrophy on Occlusion, Am. Dent. A. J., *49*, 449, October, 1954.
16. BESSON and McDERMOTT: op. cit., pp. 1467–1483.
17. ANDERSON, W. A. D.: *Synopsis of Pathology,* 5th ed. St. Louis, Mosby, 1960, pp. 780–786.
18. BURKET, L. W.: *Oral Medicine,* 4th ed., Philadelphia, Lippincott, 1961, pp. 294–300.
19. SHAFER, K. N., SAWYER, J. R., McCLUSKEY, A. M. and BECK, E. L.: *Medical-Surgical Nursing,* 2nd ed. St. Louis, Mosby, 1961, pp. 803–815.
20. THOMA, K. H.: *Oral Pathology,* 5th ed. St. Louis, Mosby, 1960, pp. 851–864.
21. FREYBERG, R. H.: Focal Infection in Relation to Rheumatic Diseases: A Critical Appraisal, Am. Dent. A. J., *33*, 1101, September 1, 1946.
22. SHAFER, W. G., HINE, M. K., and LEVY, B. M.: *A Textbook of Oral Pathology,* 2nd ed. Philadelphia, Saunders, 1963, pp. 417–423.
23. EASLICK, K. A.: An Evaluation of the Effect of Dental Foci of Infection on Health, Am. Dent. A. J., *42*, 615, June, 1951.

24. MITCHELL, D. F. and HELMAN, E. Z.:   The Role of Periodontal Foci of Infection in Systemic Disease: An Evaluation of the Literature, Am. Dent. A. J., *46*, 32, January, 1953.
25. SHAFER, HINE, and LEVY: op. cit., pp. 593–594.
26. KURLAND, L. T.:   Epidemiological Characteristics of Multiple Sclerosis, Am. J. Med., *12*, 561, May, 1952.
27. BEESON and McDERMOTT: op. cit., pp. 1670–1672.
28. DENNY-BROWN, D. E.:   Multiple Sclerosis—The Clinical Problem, Am. J. Med., *12*, 501, May, 1952.
29. LANGWORTHY, O. R. and LeGRAND, DAVID: Personality Structure and Psychotherapy in Multiple Sclerosis, Am. J. Med., *12*, 586, May, 1952.
30. BOYCE, H. E.:   Rehabilitation in Multiple Sclerosis, Nurs. Outlook, *3*, 549, October, 1955.
31. BEESON and McDERMOTT: op. cit., pp. 1581–1582.
32. PHELPS, W. M.:   Dietary Requirements in Cerebral Palsy, J. Am. Dietetics A., *27*, 869, October, 1951.
33. LEONARD, R. C.:   Dentistry for the Cerebral Palsied, Am. Dent. A. J., *41*, 152, August, 1950.
34. EISENFELD, IRWIN and FRIEDMAN, E. U.:   Observations on the Dental Treatment of Cerebral Palsied Children, Am. Dent. A. J., *47*, 538, November, 1953.
35. GELLIN, M. E.:   Is Dental Treatment for the Handicapped Child a Special Problem? J. Dent. Child., *22*:26, 1st Quarter, 1955.
36. ADELSON, J. J.:   Erroneous Concepts in the Dental Treatment of Children with Cerebral Palsy, J. Dent. Child., *24*, 247, 4th Quarter, 1957.
37. ALBUM, M. M.:   Dentistry for the Handicapped Child, Dent. Radiog. & Photog., *27*, 57, No. 4, 1954.
38. JORGENSEN, N. B., LEVINE, M. G., and HURLEY, C. T.:   Dental Management of Adult Patients with Cerebral Palsy, Am. Dent. A. J., *57*, 843, December, 1958.
39. JORGENSEN, N. B.:   Restorative Dentistry for Adult Cerebral Palsy Patients, J. Pros. Dent., *12*, 366, March-April, 1962.
40. NAISMITH, R.:   Dental Care of Handicapped Children in the Hospital, J. Dent. Child., *26*, 149, 2nd Quarter, 1959.
41. deROETTH, ANDREW and DORMAN, PURMAN: Role of the General Practitioner in Prevention of Blindness, Am. Med. A. J., *164*, 1525, August 3, 1957.
42. BAKWIN and BAKWIN: op. cit., pp. 140–146.
43. BELLOC, N. B.:   Blindness Among the Aged, Pub. Health Rep., *71*, 1221, December, 1956.
44. AYCOCK, H. B.:   Rehabilitation of the Blind, Postgrad. Med., *23*, 636, June, 1958.
45. PRICE, A. L.:   *Art, Science and Spirit of Nursing*, 2nd ed. Philadelphia, Saunders, 1959, p. 603.
46. NICHOLS, R. E.:   The Newly Deafened Patient, Am. J. Nurs., *46*, 223, April, 1946.
47. SHAFER, SAWYER, McCLUSKEY, and BECK: op. cit., pp. 498–501.
48. PRICE: op. cit., pp. 828–830.
49. COPESTAKE, E.:   Some Observations on the Dental Treatment of Deaf Children, Brit. Dent. J., *103*, 78, August 6, 1957.

SUGGESTED READINGS

Handicapped—General

ALBUM, M. M.:   Providing Dental Care for the Handicapped Patient, Am. J. Pub. Health, *50*, 1727, November, 1960.
ALBUM, M. M., COHEN, M. M., and WHITE, M. F.:   The Handicapped Child, in Cohen, M. M.: *Pediatric Dentistry*, 2nd ed. St. Louis, Mosby, 1961, pp. 286–302.
BRAMER, M. L.:   Portable Auxiliary Headrest in Dentistry for Children, Am. Dent. A. J., *51*, 718, December, 1955.
BRAUER, J. C., HIGLEY, L. B., LINDAHL, R. L., MASSLER, MAURY, and SCHOUR, ISAAC: *Dentistry for Children*, 5th ed. New York, Blakiston, 1964, pp. 577–595.
LYONS, D. C.:   Dental Health of a Group of Handicapped Adolescent Children, J. Periodont., *31*, 52, January, 1960.
SHARRY, J. J.:   Treatment of the Handicapped Child, in Finn, S. B.:   *Clinical Pedodontics*, 2nd ed. Philadelphia, Saunders, 1962, pp. 439–459.
SPOCK, BENJAMIN: *Baby and Child Care*, New York, Pocket Books, 1957, pp. 578–587.

Muscular Dystrophy

HENLEY, T. F. and ALBAM, B.:   A Psychiatric Study of Muscular Dystrophy; the Role of the Social Worker, Am. J. Physical Med., *34*, 258, February, 1955.

Arthritis

COLLINS, L. H., and CRANE, M. P.:   *Internal Medicine in Dental Practice*, 5th ed. Philadelphia, Lea & Febiger, 1960, pp. 373–419.

Multiple Sclerosis

BROWN, A. F.:   *Medical and Surgical Nursing*, II. Philadelphia, Saunders, 1959, pp. 542–552.
SCHUMACHER, G. A.:   Multiple Sclerosis, Am. Med. A. J., *143*, 1059, July 22, 1950; *143*, 1146, July 29, 1950.
SHAFER, K. N., SAWYER, J. R., McCLUSKEY, A. M., and BECK, E. L.:   *Medical-Surgical Nursing*, 2nd ed. St. Louis, Mosby, 1961, pp. 742–745.

Cerebral Palsy

ALBUM, M. M.:   Effect of Vitamins on the Gingival Tissue of Handicapped Children, Oral Surg., Oral Med., & Oral Path., *10*, 148, February, 1957.
BUCKLEY, R. R.:   Acrylic Mouthpiece for Poliomyelitis and Cerebral Palsy Patients, J. Dent. Child., *26*, 248, 3rd Quarter, 1959.
Committee on Child Health, American Public Health Association and American Academy for Cerebral Palsy: *Services for Children with Cerebral Palsy*, New York, American Public Health Association, 1955.
HOLSER, P. and MICHAELSON, B. W.:   Self-help Adaptations for the Adult Cerebral Palsied Woman, Am. J. Occupational Therapy, *13*, 64, March-April, 1959.
KASTEIN, SHULAMITH: Oral, Dental and Orthodontic Problems of Speech in Cerebral Palsy, J. Dent. Child., *24*, 243, 4th Quarter, 1957.
SHMARAK, K. L. and BERNSTEIN, J. E.:   Caries Incidence among Cerebral Palsy Children: a Preliminary Study, J. Dent. Child., *28*, 154, 2nd Quarter, 1961.
SILVERMAN, S. I.:   Partial and Complete Denture Prosthesis for Patients with Cerebral Palsy, J. Dent. Child., *26*, 135, 2nd Quarter, 1959.
TOBIS, J. S.:   Physiologic Basis for the Clinical Management of Patients with Cerebral Palsy, J. Dent. Child., *26*, 132, 2nd Quarter, 1959.
WALLACE, H. M., LOSTY, M. A., SANDERS, D., SIFFERT, R. S., TOBIS, J. S. and RICH, H.:   Children with Cerebral Palsy, Pediatrics, *20*, 703, October, 1957.
World Health Organization, Joint Expert Committee on the Physically Handicapped Child: First Report, W.H.O. Technical Report Series, No. 58, December, 1952. 26 pp.

Blindness

BINDT, JULIET: *A Handbook for the Blind.* New York, Macmillan, 1952. 244 pp.
Committee on Child Health, American Public Health Association and the National Society for the Prevention of Blindness: *Services for Children with Vision and Eye Problems*, New York, American Public Health Association, 1956.
DAVIS, K. L. and STEWART, F. A.:   Dental Health Material for Blind Children, Am. Dent. A. J., *67*, 118, July, 1963.
ROUSE, D. D., GRUBER, K. F., and BLEDSOE, C. W.:   Occupational Therapy for Blind Patients, Am. J. Occupational Therapy, *10*, 252, September-October, 1956.
SHAFER, SAWYER, McCLUSKEY, and BECK: op. cit., pp. 700–715.

Deafness

BAKWIN, HARRY and BAKWIN, R. M.:   *Behavior Disorders in Children.* Philadelphia, Saunders, 1953, pp. 147–162.
Committee on Child Health, American Public Health Association: *Services for Children with Hearing Impairment*, New York, American Public Health Association, 1956.
KESSLER, H. E.:   Hearing—as Related to Dentistry, Dent. Radiog. & Photog., *34*, 3, #1, 1961.

Chapter 37

PATIENTS WITH DISEASES OF THE CIRCULATORY SYSTEM

THE circulatory system includes the heart, blood vessels, blood, and the lymphatics. A wide variety of complicated diseases may affect these vital parts. Since many of the conditions are prolonged or even incurable, maintenance of oral health through preventive care assumes particular significance. There should not be further complications of the already existing general health problems by the addition of oral diseases, particularly dental caries or periodontal involvements. In certain instances the physical condition of the patient is not such that he could withstand the complicated, time-consuming oral or dental operations which might be required if the health of the mouth were neglected. The oral comfort of the patient is also important, particularly when there may be a long period of disability involving confinement.

The patient's medical history may reveal the existence of a circulatory disease although frequently the patient may not know the specific nature or seriousness of the disorder. Undiagnosed cases may be suspected by the general physical or oral symptoms observed, and the dental hygienist may have the opportunity to assist in the recognition of conditions which should be referred to a physician. In either the diagnosed or suspected case, consultation with the patient's physician must precede dental and dental hygiene procedures. When the physician is called it is necessary to explain the details of the techniques to be performed and to inquire concerning medication which the patient may be receiving. The physician will suggest precautions which should be observed and the extent of treatment which the patient can be expected to withstand.

Application of knowledge of the characteristics of the particular disease can aid in the prevention of complications which may arise from, for example, excessive hemorrhage, the patient's lowered resistance to infection, or emergencies requiring first aid. Premedication may be mandatory, as in the case of the patient with a damaged heart valve.

CARDIOVASCULAR DISEASES

Cardiovascular, as the name implies, includes diseases of the heart and blood vessels. Heart disease is the leading cause of death in the United States. Patients are encountered frequently in the dental office since the course of the disease is long and the incidence high, particularly in the age group over 50 years. Heart disease may exist for many years prior to the time symptoms are recognized. The patients seen in the dental office range, therefore, from those with no obvious symptoms to the nearly disabled. In severe cases, the nonambulatory patient may require care in the home (see pages 330–333).

Classification of the diseases is made either on an anatomic or etiologic basis. In the anatomic system diseases of the pericardium, myocardium, endocardium, heart valves and blood vessels are defined. In the etiologic system the diseases are named by the cause, as for example, congenital, rheumatic, arteriosclerotic or hypertensive. Characteristics and symptoms are complex and overlapping. A few of the more common conditions are listed and defined here with major symptoms. Additional reading is recommended for detail and clarification.[1-4]

I. GENERAL COMPLICATIONS OF HEART DISEASE

A. **Arrhythmia:** variation in the normal rhythm of the heart beat.

B. **Congestive Heart Failure:** the heart is no longer able to circulate the amount of blood required by the body.

   1. Causes
      a. Degenerative changes in the muscles of the heart.
      b. Increased demand on a damaged heart.
      c. Insufficient return of blood to the heart because of failure in the peripheral vessels.
   2. Symptoms
      a. Shortness of breath following moderate exertion.
      b. Swelling of ankles.
      c. Cough.
      d. Oral: cyanosis of the lips, tongue, oral mucosa; marked distention of veins on undersurface of tongue.

II. MAJOR TYPES OF CARDIOVASCULAR DISEASES

A. **Congenital Heart Disease:** abnormalities in the anatomic structure of the heart or major blood vessels due to faulty or arrested development during fetal life.

   1. Major symptom: cyanosis involving lips and tissues of the oral cavity.
   2. Susceptibility of damaged heart to infection may predispose to subacute bacterial endocarditis (see pages 430–431).

B. **Rheumatic Heart Disease:** a complication of rheumatic fever which frequently results in heart valve damage. As with the damaged heart valve of congenital heart disease, there is susceptibility to infection predisposing to subacute bacterial endocarditis.

C. **Arteriosclerotic Heart Disease:** hardening and thickening of the arteries which diminishes their capacity to supply blood, thus requiring additional work by the heart.

   1. Causes: evidence not conclusive; related to aging, elevated blood pressure and lipid metabolism.
   2. Major clinical types
      a. Angina pectoris.
         (1) Transient sharp pain in the chest over the region of the heart accompanied by sense of suffocation; pain may radiate to left arm and to neck and mandible in certain cases.
         (2) Induced by exertion, emotions, excess food.

      b. Acute myocardial infarction (coronary thrombosis, coronary occlusion).
         (1) Prolonged severe pain in the cardiac region accompanied by fall in blood pressure and other symptoms of shock; sometimes pain in abdominal region.
         (2) Cause: inadequate coronary blood supply resulting from occlusion of coronary arteries by embolism or thrombosis.

D. **Hypertension:** pathological elevation of the blood pressure secondary to an underlying disturbance of the heart or blood vessels. Symptoms for hypertensive heart disease are frequently the same as those for arteriosclerotic heart disease.

III. **APPLIED TECHNIQUES FOR DENTAL HYGIENE CARE**

A. **Characteristics Affecting Appointment Procedures**
1. Physical handicaps
   a. Diminished tolerance for exercise.
   b. Readily fatigued.
   c. Shortness of breath (dyspnea).
2. Psychological handicaps[5]
   a. Fear of sudden death; overconcern about the heart; anxiety.
   b. Depression; feelings of rejection or hostility.
   c. Unwillingness to accept limitations required by the physical condition.
   d. Attitude of family: when cooperative and understanding, may make complete difference in patient's attitude; overprotective or fearful family influences patient's attitude.

B. **Appointment Planning and Preliminary Procedures**[6]
1. Appointment planning
   a. Time: early in morning before patient becomes fatigued.
   b. Length: short, to prevent fatigue; oral prophylaxis may be performed by quadrants or even fewer teeth may be involved at a single appointment depending on the requirements of the individual mouth.
   c. Recall: frequent to avoid need for extended appointments.
2. Premedication which physician may recommend
   a. Sedative: to allay fears and prevent anxiety.
   b. Antibiotic: to prevent subacute bacterial endocarditis in patient with damaged heart valve (see page 431).
3. Discontinuance of anticoagulant drug: drugs are prescribed to prevent blood coagulation which could lead to thrombosis or embolism in susceptible patients. When dental or dental hygiene procedures are expected to produce extensive bleeding the physician may advise patient to withhold taking the anticoagulant drug for a period of time prior to the appointment.[7-9]

C. **Suggestions for Appointment Procedure**
1. Patient position: patient who has difficulty breathing may require an upright position.

2. Room temperature: should be adjusted and maintained. Sudden chilling can initiate attack of angina pectoris in the susceptible patient.
3. Avoid anxiety or undue apprehension on part of patient.
    a. Explain carefully in nontechnical language what is going to be done, how long it will take, the type of discomfort which the patient may expect and what cooperation is required of him.
    b. Plan for premedication.
4. Avoid inflicting pain: use of a topical anesthetic during scaling procedures may help (see page 159.)
5. Avoid excessive hemorrhage as a result of unnecessary trauma to the tissues: take particular care during scaling procedures.
6. Emergency care: see Table 15 on pages 470–471.

IV. PATIENT INSTRUCTION

A. Oral Physical Therapy

1. Stress the importance of meticulous care.
2. Distribute teaching over several appointments to avoid patient fatigue.
3. Instruct attendant of patient who is incapable of caring for his own mouth.

B. Diet

1. Suggestions may be limited by diet prescribed by physician: this should always be checked.
2. Example: patients with arteriosclerosis are frequently required to omit fats and other foods with high cholesterol content: substitutes frequently may be carbohydrates which are cariogenic; practical suggestions should be made accordingly.

PREVENTION OF SUBACUTE BACTERIAL ENDOCARDITIS

Subacute bacterial endocarditis is of particular importance because a transient bacteremia can follow oral prophylactic procedures.[10-12] Considerable information is available concerning the possible effect of oral surgical trauma in effecting a bacteremia which in turn can infect a damaged heart valve and produce subacute bacterial endocarditis. A routine of prophylactic antibiotic therapy has therefore been established.

Subacute bacterial endocarditis is a serious disease and the prognosis depends on the degree of cardiac damage, the valves involved, the duration of the infection, and the treatment. Patients are prone to develop heart failure leading to death unless the infection is promptly controlled.

I. ETIOLOGY[13]

A. **Causative Agent:** a nonhemolytic streptococcus in 60 to 80 per cent of the cases.

B. **Predisposing Factors:** previous cardiac damage particularly valvular abnormalities resulting from rheumatic fever or congenital malformations of the valves, or defects in the wall of the heart.

C. **Exciting Factors**

1. Trauma: general or oral surgery, scaling, curettage.
2. Upper respiratory infections.

D. **Disease Process**[14]

1. Trauma from oral surgery, scaling and curettage ruptures blood vessels in gingival sulcus.
2. Pressure from trauma forces oral microorganisms into blood stream thereby initiating a bacteremia.
   a. Ease of bacterial entry directly relates to amount of trauma.
   b. The greater the trauma, the greater the ease of bacterial entry.
3. Circulating microorganisms attach to endocardium of defective heart valve.
4. Microorganisms proliferate to form bacterial masses.
5. Heart valve becomes inflamed and cannot function properly.
6. Clumps of bacteria may break off, get into the systemic circulation, and be spread throughout the body.

II. **APPLIED TECHNIQUES FOR DENTAL HYGIENE CARE**[11]

A. **Patient's Medical History**

1. Contact physician when patient history indicates previous rheumatic fever, congenital heart disease or other cardiovascular involvement to inform him of required dental and dental hygiene procedures.
2. Determine from physician the nature of the heart defect and the recommendation for premedication.

B. **Preoperative Procedure:** Arrange for prophylactic antibiotic medication in accord with advice of physician and dentist.[6,14-17]

C. **Oral Prophylaxis**

1. Postpone oral prophylaxis appointment if gingival inflammation is present.
   a. Instruct patient in oral care procedures to aid in reduction of inflammation.
   b. Reappoint patient for oral prophylaxis when inflammation has subsided.
2. Complete oral prophylaxis following prophylactic antibiotic medication.
3. Use extreme care in all instrumentation procedures to prevent unnecessary trauma.
4. Schedule frequent recall appointments.
   a. To maintain optimum oral health.
   b. To prevent periodontal involvements.
   c. To prevent need for extensive, traumatic oral prophylactic techniques.

D. **Patient Instruction**

1. Observe patient's demonstration of toothbrushing to ascertain absence of toothbrush abrasion; when gingival inflammation is present even slight trauma may lead to initiation of bacteremia.

2. Emphasize necessity of personal oral care procedures in preventing periodontal involvements.
3. Emphasize inclusion of elements in diet necessary for maintenance of health of oral tissues.
    a. Nutritive elements necessary for tissue health: particularly
vitamins A, B complex, C.
    b. Detergent foods necessary for gingival stimulation, tissue
keratinization, cleansing of teeth.

BLOOD DISEASES

Oral tissue changes, lowered resistance to infection, and tendencies to
hemorrhage are the major factors to be considered for patients with blood
disorders. Oral symptoms of blood diseases are exaggerated as a result of
neglect of health of the mouth. Routine care and instruction in personal oral
physical therapy are indicated to aid in the prevention of the need for complicated dental and periodontal treatments.

I. FINDINGS OF ORAL INSPECTION WHICH INDICATE POSSIBLE BLOOD DISORDER

The patient's medical history may not reveal the existence of a blood
disorder. Oral manifestations which may be indicative of a blood
disease should be called to the dentist's attention. The oral findings
are not conclusive evidence that a disease exists and reference for
medical study and blood tests is necessary. The findings listed below
are important indications for recommending further clinical study for
the patient.[18]

A. Spontaneous hemorrhage from the gingiva or mucous membranes.
B. Numerous petechiæ.
C. History of difficulty in controlling postoperative hemorrhage by
usual procedures.
D. Marked pallor of the mucous membranes.
E. Chronic oral infections which do not respond to treatment.
F. Atrophy of the papillæ of the tongue without apparent cause.
G. Persistently sore tongue and mouth without evidence of local
irritation.
H. History of prolonged bleeding episodes or ready bruising.
I. Severe ulcerations in the mouth associated with signs of severe
illness or not responding to treatment.
J. Acute infections of the oral mucosa which do not respond promptly
to treatment.

II. DISEASES INVOLVING THE RED BLOOD CELLS[19–21]

A. Types

1. *Anemias:* reduction in number of red blood cells, hemoglobin,
or both.
    a. Due to blood loss: hemorrhage.
    b. Due to defective blood production.
        (1) Deficiencies in required nutrients

      (a) Iron-deficiency anemia: caused chiefly by faulty intake of iron, chronic blood loss, or pregnancy.

      (b) Pernicious anemia: caused by deficiency in vitamin B_{12}.

    (2) Depression of bone marrow activity: caused by x-ray, radium, toxic chemicals, tumor invasion, or chronic infection.

  c. Due to increased blood destruction: hemolytic anemias.

  2. *Polycythemias:* increase in hemoglobin concentration due to increase in number of red blood cells.

B. Oral Characteristics[22–24]

1. Anemias

    Anemia is most frequently a symptom of a systemic disease remote from the tissues of blood formation or destruction. Because of reduced oxygen-carrying capacity of the blood, the patient exhibits signs of fatigue, weakness, lethargy and shortness of breath.

  a. General characteristics: all anemias

    (1) Prolonged healing time.

    (2) Lowered resistance to infection.

    (3) Pale mucous membranes.

  b. Iron-deficiency anemia

    (1) Interdental papillæ and free gingiva: purplish-red when inflammation is present.

    (2) Tongue: atrophic, hypersensitive, loss of muscle tone.

    (3) Lips: angular cheilosis.

    (4) Black stain of teeth and tongue: related to taking liquid preparation of iron.

  c. Pernicious anemia

    (1) Glossitis: atrophy of papillæ leaves smooth, red tongue, manifestations of vitamin B complex deficiency.

    (2) Mucosa and lips: susceptible to ulceration by minor trauma: may be yellowish in advanced case.

2. Polycythemias

  a. Mucous membranes: reddish-blue.

  b. Tendency to bleed on slight trauma.

C. Dental Hygiene Care and Instruction

1. Appointment planning

  a. Short appointments: for patients with physical symptoms of weakness.

  b. Recall: frequent enough to prevent complications of oral diseases which require extensive, traumatic dental or periodontal treatment.

2. Oral prophylaxis

  a. Instrumentation: apply unusual care to prevent trauma to delicate tissues.

  b. Apply petroleum jelly or cream for protection of angles of lips particularly when there is evidence of cheilosis.

3. Patient instruction

  a. Emphasize personal oral care to promote healthy gingival tissues to minimize hemorrhage and infection.

b. Describe need for diet containing a variety of foods representing all of the basic food groups to compensate for nutritional deficiencies.

c. Recommend that liquid iron preparations be taken through a straw and that the mouth be rinsed with water immediately following to prevent stains.

III. DISEASES INVOLVING THE WHITE BLOOD CELLS[25,26]

A. Types

1. *Leukopenia:* reduction in white blood cells due to depression of bone marrow activity by infections, drugs, or radiation.
2. *Leukemia:* a fatal disease characterized by excessive and abnormal proliferation of white blood cells; generally considered neoplastic.

B. Oral Characteristics of Acute and Subacute Leukemia[27,28]

Gingival changes are present in response to local irritation in acute and subacute leukemia, but rarely in chronic. Gingivitis and stomatitis are frequently among the earliest symptoms to be observed at the onset of acute leukemia. The marked tissue changes listed below may not be present in the absence of local irritation.

1. Gingiva: bluish-red, with rounded gingival margins and blunted interdental papillæ.
2. Tissue friable and spongy; bleeds with slight trauma.
3. Areas of necrosis and ulceration: unpleasant odor associated with necrosis.
4. Gingival enlargement which tends to obscure the teeth as the disease progresses; interference with mastication.
5. Marked susceptibility to bacterial infection.

C. Dental Hygiene Care and Instruction

Because local irritation causes severe tissue reaction, dental hygiene care is directed at the removal of deposits for alleviation of symptoms. Techniques are performed only after the dentist and physician determine required precautionary measures against infection and hemorrhage.

1. Appointment planning
   a. Short appointments: techniques limited to a few teeth at a time.
   b. Recall: frequent to attempt to maintain tissues in best possible condition.
2. Antibiotic premedication: arranged at advice of dentist and physician to minimize possibility of postoperative infection.
3. Oral prophylaxis
   a. Superficial scaling of a few teeth at a time followed by deep scaling at successive appointments.[29]
   b. Topical anesthetic may be used to aid patient comfort.
   c. Techniques adapted to enlarged tissue with extreme care to prevent unnecessary trauma.
   d. Sterile technique: use of antiseptic solution on tissue; unusual care in sterilization of instruments.

   e. Polishing frequently contraindicated to avoid gingival irritation by abrasive polishing agent.
4. Patient instruction
   a. Toothbrushing: soft multitufted brush recommended; routine care emphasized when tissues are not too tender for brushing.
   b. Mouth wash: to combat unpleasant taste and odor from necrotic tissues.

IV. HEMORRHAGIC DISEASES: Abnormalities in Coagulating Ability of the Blood

A. Types[30,31]

1. *Prothrombin deficiency:* lack of vitamin K or faulty utilization of vitamin K as in liver damage.
2. *Hemophilia:* a hereditary disease characterized by delayed clotting of the blood. It is inherited by males through the mother as a sex-linked character.
3. *Purpura:* extravasation of blood into the skin, subcutaneous tissues and mucous membranes resulting from increased permeability of capillary walls.

B. Oral Characteristics[32]

1. Hemophilia: prolonged hemorrhage from even slight wounds; spontaneous bleeding into skin but not the oral mucous membranes.
2. Purpura: spontaneous bleeding from skin and mucous membranes; petechiæ in oral mucous membranes.

C. Dental Hygiene Care for Patients with Hemorrhagic Tendency

Periodontal care is given only with extreme precautions advised by the physician and frequently only under hospital routines.[33] Advice to the patient for prevention of periodontal diseases which would require extensive treatment is of particular significance. Specific instruction in personal oral care procedures will aid the patient in maintaining the gingival tissues in a healthy condition and therefore limit the amount of hemorrhage which would result. When extreme care is taken during instrumentation and precautions are taken to prevent postoperative infection, problems are reduced.[34]

REFERENCES

1. Beeson, P. B. and McDermott, Walsh: *Cecil-Loeb Textbook of Medicine,* 11th ed. Philadelphia, Saunders, 1963, pp. 618–798.
2. Anderson, W. A. D.: *Synopsis of Pathology,* 5th ed. St. Louis, Mosby, 1960, pp. 270–309.
3. Vander Veer, J. B.: Coronary Heart Disease, Am. Dent. A. J., *66,* 348, March, 1963.
4. Burket, L. W.: *Oral Medicine,* 4th ed. Philadelphia, Lippincott, 1961, pp. 209–224.
5. Lee, P. R.: Rehabilitation of the Cardiac, Pub. Health Rep., *73,* 475, June, 1958.
6. American Dental Association and American Heart Association: Management of Dental Problems in Patients with Cardiovascular Disease, Am. Dent. A. J., *68,* 333, March, 1964.
7. Dinon, L. R. and Strang, J. E.: The Dental Patient with Heart Disease, in Burket, L. W.: Interrelationship of Oral and Systemic Disease. Dental Clinics of North America, July, 1958, p. 335.

8. BEHRMAN, S. J. and WRIGHT, I. S.: Dental Surgery During Continuous Anticoagulant Therapy, Am. Dent. A. J., *62*, 172, February, 1961.
9. KWAPIS, B. W.: Anticoagulant Therapy and Dental Practice, Am. Dent. A. J., *66*, 172, February, 1963.
10. WINSLOW, M. B. and KOBERNICK, S. D.: Bacteremia after Prophylaxis, Am. Dent. A. J., *61*, 69, July, 1960.
11. BENDER, I. B., SELTZER, S., TASHMAN, S., and MELOFF, G.: Dental Procedures in Patients with Rheumatic Heart Disease, Oral Surg., Oral Med. & Oral Path., *16*, 466, April, 1963.
12. BANDT, C. L., KORN, N. A., and SCHAFFER, E. M.: Bacteremias from Ultrasonic and Hand Instrumentation, J. Periodont., *35*, 214, May-June, 1964.
13. BEESON and McDERMOTT: op. cit., pp. 761-765.
14. BENDER, I. B., PRESSMAN, R. S., and TASHMAN, S. G.: Comparative Effects of Local and Systemic Antibiotic Therapy in the Prevention of Postextraction Bacteremia, Am. Dent. A. J., *57*, 54, July, 1958.
15. American Heart Association, Committee on Prevention of Rheumatic Fever and Congenital Heart Disease: Prevention of Rheumatic Fever and Bacterial Endocarditis Through Control of Streptococcal Infections. New York, American Heart Association, 1955. 7 pp. (Reprint from Circulation, *11*, 317, February, 1955.)
16. PRESSMAN, R. S.: Transient Bacteremias Associated with Dental Operative Procedures and Their Prophylactic Treatment, in Burket, L. W.: Interrelationship of Oral and Systemic Disease. Dental Clinics of North America, July, 1958, p. 351.
17. BENDER, I. B.: Premedication in Valvular or Congenital Heart Disease for the Prevention of Subacute Bacterial Endocarditis, in Ostrander, F. D.: Practical Oral Therapeutics. Dental Clinics of North America, March, 1958, p. 119.
18. COLLINS, L. H. and CRANE, M. P.: *Internal Medicine in Dental Practice*, 5th ed. Philadelphia, Lea & Febiger, 1960, p. 367.
19. BEESON and McDERMOTT: pp. 1071-1120.
20. ANDERSON: op. cit., pp. 504-517.
21. SHAFER, W. G., HINE, M. K., and LEVY, B. M.: *Textbook of Oral Pathology*, 2nd ed. Philadelphia, Saunders, 1963, pp. 600-613.
22. GLICKMAN, IRVING: *Clinical Periodontology*, 2nd ed. Philadelphia, Saunders, 1958, pp. 410-412.
23. ORBAN, B. J. and WENTZ, F. M.: *Atlas of Clinical Pathology of the Oral Mucous Membrane*, 2nd ed. St. Louis, Mosby, 1960, pp. 137-138.
24. VOGEL, PETER: Oral Manifestations in Hematologic Disorders, Oral Surg., Oral Med., & Oral Path., *16*, 21, January, 1963.
25. BEESON and McDERMOTT: op. cit., 1121-1140.
26. ANDERSON: op. cit., pp. 517-522.
27. GLICKMAN: op. cit., pp. 404-409.
28. ORBAN and WENTZ: op. cit., p. 140.
29. GLICKMAN: op. cit., p. 914.
30. BEESON and McDERMOTT: op. cit., 1172-1186.
31. ANDERSON: op. cit., pp. 522-524.
32. ORBAN and WENTZ: op. cit., pp. 142-143.
33. GLICKMAN: op. cit., p. 915.
34. RUBIN, B., LEVINE, P., and ROSENTHAL, M. C.: Complete Dental Care of the Hemophiliac, Oral Surg., Oral Med., & Oral Path., *12*, 665, June, 1959.

SUGGESTED READINGS

Cardiovascular

American Dental Association, Council on Dental Therapeutics: *Accepted Dental Remedies*, 29th ed. Chicago, American Dental Association, 1964, pp. 2-4.
Committee on Child Care, American Public Health Association and American Heart Association: *Services for Children with Heart Disease and Rheumatic Fever.* New York, American Public Health Association, 1960.
EISEMAN, B., SPENCER, F., and DACHI, S. F.: Role of the Dentist in the Diagnosis and Prevention of Cerebrovascular Accidents, Oral Surg., Oral Med., & Oral Path., *16*, 1174, October, 1963.
HEAP, B.: Diet Care and Services for Patients with Cardiovascular Disease, Pub. Health Rep., *74*, 1086, December, 1959.
KOGAN, STANLEY: Medical Emergencies for Dentists, Oral Surg., Oral Med., & Oral Path., *11*, 246, March, 1958; *11*, 359, April, 1958.
LEWIS, T. M.: Reduce Stress for Your Congenital Heart Patient, J. Dent. Child., *30*, 74, 2nd Quarter, 1963.

OLSEN, N. H.:   Dental Patients with Rheumatic Heart Disease, Dent. Prog., *1*, 115, January, 1961.

TOLNICK, B.:   Evaluation and Management of Cardiac Disease Complicating Dental Therapy, J. Dent. Med., *15*, 14, January, 1960.

Blood Diseases

ANTIOCH, R. J.:   Hemorrhage in Oral Surgery, Oral Surg., Oral Med., & Oral Path., *12*, 265, March, 1959.

DREIZEN, S.:   Oral Manifestations of Human Nutritional Anemias, Arch. Environ. Health, *5*, 66, July, 1962. (Abstract: D. Abs. *8*, 122, February, 1963.)

DUFFY, J. H. and DRISCOLL, E. J.:   Oral Manifestations of Leukemia, Oral Surg., Oral Med., & Oral Path., *11*, 484, May, 1958.

KERR, D. A.:   Oral Manifestations of Blood Dyscrasias, J. Canad. D. A., *27*, 149, March, 1961.

SHAFER, W. G., HINE, M. K., and LEVY, B. M.:   *A Textbook of Oral Pathology*, 2nd ed. Philadelphia, Saunders, 1963, pp. 613–634.

SINROD, H. S.:   Leukemia As a Dental Problem, Am. Dent. A. J., *55*, 809, December, 1957.

Chapter 38

PATIENTS WITH DIABETES MELLITUS

ENDOCRINE GLANDS

ENDOCRINE (ductless) glands secrete their products, called hormones, directly into the circulatory system. In contrast, the exocrine glands may release their products by way of ducts. Hormones are chemical compounds that act as catalysts to exercise control over the functions of every cell in the body. Some hormones influence the secretion of hormones by other endocrine glands. The balance of hormonal secretion is a delicate one and small imbalances may cause dramatic body responses.

Persons with severe untreated hormonal imbalances are seldom seen. The most outstanding physical results of hormonal imbalance appear when excessive or deficient secretions occur during childhood or puberty. Severe prepubertal imbalances may result in exaggerated or retarded growth and development. An adult afflicted with hormonal disturbances of sufficient degree may exhibit signs of overgrowth, atrophy of mature tissues, or other metabolic disturbances.

The most important of the endocrine glands are the pituitary (hypophysis), thyroid, parathyroids, adrenals (cortex and medulla), gonads, and the islets of Langerhans in the pancreas. Until the last decade, relatively little was known about the structure of hormones and about their specific functions. With refined methods of biochemical investigation, discoveries in this field continue to advance.

Because of the complex nature of hormonal functions, and because of the relative rarity of severe disorders of the pituitary, thyroid, parathyroid and adrenal glands, only a brief description of general characteristics of patients with hypo- or hyperactivity of glandular function is included here. For a more detailed description, the reader is referred to the "Suggested Readings" at the end of this Chapter.

The functions of the gonads are explained in Chapter 39. Diabetes mellitus, a condition resulting from an underfunction of the islets of Langerhans, occurs frequently and is included in this Chapter.

HORMONAL IMBALANCES

Hyperactivity (overfunction) of a gland causes oversecretion of its hormones, with accelerated metabolism. Conversely, hypoactivity (underfunction) of a gland results in undersecretion of its hormone or other hormones, and is accompanied by reduced metabolism.

Whether patients have hypo- or hyperactive endocrine glands, they are usually susceptible to headaches and fatigue. Because these patients have less stamina than normal individuals, they require shorter, more frequent appointments.

Hypoactive glands may give rise to a lowered basal metabolic rate and lowered blood pressure. Generally, these patients are less active than normal individuals, and are subject to fainting and dizziness. Hypoactive patients have subnormal temperatures and are oversensitive to external cold. When they are in the dental chair, the room temperature can be raised, or drafts can be eliminated to provide a greater measure of comfort. Warm air or water, rather than cold, must be used to prevent discomfort.

Patients with hyperactive thyroid or adrenocortical function tend to be irritable, nervous, and over-react to emotional disturbances. Every effort should be made to help them remain calm in the dental situation. Endocrine hyperactivity may give rise to an increased basal metabolic rate and an elevated blood pressure, with a concomitant sensitivity to external heat. When possible, the room temperature should be lowered to provide greater comfort.

DIABETES MELLITUS

Diabetes mellitus is a chronic metabolic disorder caused by an inability of the cells to utilize glucose, probably as a result of deficient insulin production by beta cells of the islet tissue of the pancreas. It has been estimated that one of eighty persons in the United States has diabetes, and that one-half of the cases of this disease are undiagnosed.[1] The onset of diabetes is insidious, and oral disturbances may be early indications of the disorder. Because of its prevalence, and because serious complications may result, particularly in uncontrolled cases, its early signs and symptoms should be recognized and called to the dentist's attention.

Diabetes means "pass through" (increased urination), and mellitus means "honey" (sweet urine), thus the disorder was named for two of its cardinal symptoms.[2] Diabetes has been recognized as a disease entity for almost 2000 years, but until the discovery and administration of insulin, the pancreatic hormone, the diabetic had a very short life span. However, with modern medical supervision, the life expectancy of a diabetic who is diagnosed early and who follows instructions to control his condition approaches that of a nondiabetic individual.[3]

All diabetics do not require insulin therapy. The milder form of the disease can be controlled by regulation of carbohydrate intake. Regardless of the measures taken to control diabetes mellitus, the patient must remain under fairly close medical supervision from the time the disease is diagnosed. The diabetic is instructed to inform his dentist, surgeon and other health personnel of his condition, but often forgets to do this, so it is a responsibility of health workers to question a patient to ascertain the presence of the disease.

Individual requirements of diet and insulin (when necessary) are prescribed for each patient. These requirements undergo constant change. Insulin and carbohydrate intake must be balanced carefully, since an excess as well as a deficiency of insulin can produce severe consequences. It is imperative that the patient's physician be consulted with respect to precautions that can be taken to protect the diabetic from undesirable complications which may result from dental operative procedures.

Brief descriptions of the etiology and characteristics of deficient and excessive insulin states are given in this Chapter. Diabetes mellitus is under extensive study, and new discoveries are reported constantly from various branches of research.   Perusal of these reports, especially in the dental literature, will assist the professional to provide maximum preventive care for the diabetic patient.

ETIOLOGY

Carbohydrate metabolism is regulated by hormones from the islet tissue of the pancreas, the anterior lobe of the pituitary, the adrenal medulla and the cortex, and the thyroid.   Insulin is believed responsible for the transport of glucose through the cell wall and for the promotion of glycogenesis. Other hormones that regulate carbohydrate metabolism are antagonistic to insulin and promote the release of glycogen as glucose from the liver. Fasting blood glucose levels normally are maintained at between 70 and 100 mg. per 100 ml. of blood.[4] If there is a breakdown in the regulatory mechanism, the usual reaction is an excess of blood sugar, and the organism can operate for a time as the excess sugar is removed from the blood by the kidney and excreted in the urine.   If the blood sugar level is below normal, no natural mechanism exists to compensate and the brain and nerve cells fail to metabolize, with a resultant loss of consciousness.

The diabetic condition is a result of an underproduction of insulin due to breakdown or exhausted activity of the beta cells of the pancreas islet tissue. In the nondiabetic, the blood sugar level rises after the ingestion of carbohydrates, then returns to normal in one or two hours.   The diabetic's blood glucose concentration remains elevated because he has insufficient insulin, and sugar that is in excess of his renal threshold is excreted in the urine.   Although every cell in the diabetic's body is surrounded by a high concentration of glucose, this principal source of energy for cellular metabolism cannot be delivered, thus the cells literally are starved for energy.

I. PREDISPOSING FACTORS

A. **Heredity:** Diabetes mellitus is inherited with the Mendelian recessive pattern and a modified sex linkage.   Since the discovery of insulin, diabetics have been able to live and raise children. These offspring are either diabetic or carry the tendency to develop diabetes which has caused the incidence of the disease to rise.[5]

B. **Obesity:** Excess weight causes continued overproduction of insulin and eventual breakdown of glands, which may precipitate disease in susceptible individuals.   In adults, the higher the weight above normal, the lower the glucose tolerance level.[6]   In children, overweight has no significant relationship to the development of the disease.[7]

C. **Race:** Individuals of Jewish origin show an increased incidence.[8]

II. PRECIPITATING FACTORS[9]

A. **Chronic Systemic Infection** (adults): may increase the insulin requirement, decrease insulin output, or both.

B. **Anxiety, Stress:** as result of extended illness which reduces the patient's working capacity.   These factors may cause an increased metabolic rate and increased production of insulin, that, together, exhaust the cells that produce insulin.

C. **Acute Infection:** may disclose pre-existing decreased glucose tolerance (latent diabetes mellitus).

D. **Excessive Ingestion of Carbohydrates with Too Little Exercise:** often precipitates onset of disease in middle life in the patient with an inherited tendency.[8]

CHARACTERISTICS, COMPLICATIONS AND CONTROL OF DIABETES MELLITUS

Individual reactions to diabetes mellitus vary with respect to the severity of the disease, length of time the condition has existed, age of the patient at onset, and the presence or absence of complications that accompany the condition.

Diabetes mellitus usually develops more rapidly and presents more severe symptoms in children and young adults than in later life. The growth rate may be retarded seriously, but diabetic children usually grow at an accelerated rate before the onset of the disease. Generally, individuals are not born with diabetes, but symptoms become apparent sooner in those individuals who are more susceptible to the degeneration of cells that produce insulin. The onset of childhood diabetes mellitus occurs most frequently around the ages of three, six and twelve years, while the incidence of adult diabetes increases with age, the highest percentage occurring between 65 and 74 years. Some patients exhibit only one or a few of the characteristics listed below.

I. GENERAL CHARACTERISTICS

A. Metabolic Disturbances

1. Physical efficiency: general weakness, lack of energy, tiredness.
2. Blood sugar level raised; sugar in excess of renal threshold is excreted in urine and volume of urine excretion is increased.
3. Thirst greatly increased because of dehydration of body tissues from excess urination.
4. Dietary carbohydrate utilization is diminished by lack of insulin; body protein and fat are broken down by glyconeogenesis to provide adequate energy supply for nervous system.
5. Increased appetite does not compensate for excessive breakdown of body protein and fat, so patient loses weight.

B. Sensory Disturbances

1. Pain: may have muscular pain, headache, backache.
2. Vision: may be disturbed if diabetes is uncontrolled; weakness of accommodation; sudden changes in refraction.

C. Physical Appearance

1. Weight
   a. Undiagnosed or uncontrolled case: usually obese in early stages; may become underweight later.
   b. Controlled case: usually try to maintain ideal weight, which is slightly below normal for age, height and build.

2. Skin
   a. Dry, with frequent, intense itching.
   b. Susceptible to recurrent infections.
3. Complexion: often flushed if patient is obese.

II. COMPLICATIONS THAT MAY ACCOMPANY DIABETES MELLITUS

Complications that may accompany this disturbed metabolic state arise when the condition has existed undiagnosed for a long period, when the condition has been of long duration, or, most frequently, when the patient has failed to follow the prescribed therapeutic regimen. Acute complications of diabetes are insulin shock and diabetic acidosis or coma, which result from too much or too little insulin, respectively. Either of these conditions may occur while the patient is in the dental office, thus the professional must be prepared to recognize and differentiate between them and to give immediate attention to the patient's needs.

Each diabetic patient taking insulin therapy is advised to carry a card provided by the American Diabetes Association. On the card is the warning: "I am a diabetic! If found in a dazed condition, administer a sweet drink, orange juice, or sugar if possible, and call a physician immediately." Pertinent information including the patient's name, address and telephone number, and the prescribed insulin therapy is also on the card.

Chronic complications of diabetes mellitus involve the acceleration of the patient's normal physiological degenerative changes, especially within the vascular system. Lowered resistance to infection, metabolic imbalance, and disturbance of the vascular system contribute to delayed wound healing. Even mild coronary and peripheral arterial diseases constitute a hazard to the diabetic. Generally, when an individual is afflicted in later life, his life expectancy is less affected and, with improved methods for control, other diseases may be responsible for death.

A. **Insulin Shock:** occurs when blood sugar falls below 60 mg. per 100 ml. of blood.[10]

1. Causes: insufficient food intake, as a missed meal or regurgitation after insulin therapy; overdose of insulin; strenuous exercise with insufficient food intake.
2. Characteristics
   a. Onset: may be sudden if patient uses regular or short-acting insulin, and symptoms are more difficult to recognize. Slower-acting insulin is used for most patients, and most attacks occur in the morning or early in the evening.
   b. Progress: with sudden onset, patient may progress almost without warning to epileptiform convulsions or diabetic coma; with gradual onset, patient develops general muscular weakness, mental confusion, restlessness, profuse perspiration, vertigo, pale or flushed face, numbness of tongue, mucosa or lips, trembling, and occasionally experiences hunger pangs.

3. First aid (see page 471).
   a. Conscious patient: immediately administer sugar cubes, orange juice, or any food sweetened with sucrose.
   b. Unconscious patient: call physician immediately, then prepare sugar cubes, orange juice or sweet food for administration as soon as consciousness returns.

B. Diabetic Acidosis and Coma

1. Causes: insufficient insulin or an insensitivity to insulin therapy; presence of infections; surgical procedures or trauma; dietary indiscretions.[10]
2. Characteristics[11]
   a. Onset: gradual in older diabetic; may be acute in undiagnosed juvenile.[12]
   b. Progress: increasing weakness, malaise, headache, insatiable thirst; pain in abdomen and muscular cramps; drowsiness precedes coma.
   c. Physical findings
      (1) Skin: red, dry.
      (2) Mucous membranes: dry.
      (3) Eyes: sunken with "soft" eyeballs.
      (4) Breath: characteristic fruity or acetone odor.
      (5) Breathing: labored, increased rate and depth.
3. First aid
   a. Immediately call physician who will provide therapeutic first aid; coma and death can result if treatment is delayed.
   b. Provide fluid intake for conscious patient.
   c. Prevent injury to unconscious patient.

III. DEGENERATIVE CHANGES ACCELERATED BY DIABETES MELLITUS

Although improved therapy has reduced the rate of degenerative changes in the diabetic, these changes cannot be prevented until their true etiology has been discovered. The rate of change is dependent upon the degree of control maintained over the blood sugar level, the length of duration of the disease, and the occurrence of complications. Consequently, poor control, long duration, and/or the presence of infection will accelerate degenerative changes.

Early signs of chronic degeneration are often observed in the eyes. Chronic changes are vascular degeneration of the retina, edema, or cyst formation. Cataracts occur infrequently in cases of severe diabetes.

Diabetic degeneration of the nervous system may be characterized by numbness, tingling and abnormal burning or itching. Muscular cramps, tenderness, aches and occasional sharp pains also may be observed.

IV. CONTROL OF DIABETES MELLITUS

An individual who excretes sugar in the urine may not have diabetes, and a diabetic does not always excrete sugar, but, if a patient exhibits this condition, and, in addition, has a typical low blood glucose tolerance level as determined by a laboratory test, he is presumed to have diabetes. When the diagnosis is established, the physician attempts to regulate the condition through dietary control, and, in the more severe form of the disease, with insulin therapy. The objectives of control are to keep the urine almost sugar free but to avoid either insulin shock or diabetic coma. Constant control is required to achieve these objectives. The patient sees the physician occasionally, but he is taught to supervise his own care and to accept responsibility for his own routine treatment. The diabetic's educational program includes nine basic elements of treatment as suggested by the American Diabetes Association, Inc.: diet, urine testing, action of insulin and other hypoglycemic agents, technic of insulin injection and sites for it, care of syringe and of insulin, symptoms of hypoglycemia, symptoms of uncontrolled diabetes, care of the feet, and what to do in case of acute complications.[13]

A. **Dietary Control**[14]

1. Purposes: may be adequate to prevent the rise of blood sugar level, yet provide sufficient nutritional requirements for maintenance of body function at patient's ideal weight for his age, height, build, and degree of activity; when inadequate to prevent rise in blood sugar, this method is supplemented by administration of insulin.
2. Dietary
   a. Carbohydrate, fat, and protein intake are regulated in accord with the patient's ideal weight, insulin requirement, age and physical condition.
   b. Mineral and vitamin intake is usually adequate if patient is on regulated normal caloric intake, but must be supplemented if caloric intake is restricted.

B. **Insulin Therapy**

1. Indications for insulin therapy: excess blood sugar over normal fasting level (hyperglycemia); urinary excretion of glucose over 10 per cent of daily intake (glycosuria); or presence of ketone bodies in blood (ketonemia) or urine (ketonuria).[15]
2. Forms of insulin administration[14]
   a. Oral: for patient who needs insulin but who is not obese, one who has mild diabetes, or one who experienced onset after adulthood had been reached.
   b. Hypodermic injection: for a diabetic child, a diabetic adult who experienced excessive weight loss, one with acute complications, or one who has a severe form of the disease.
3. Conditions that modify requirements[15]
   a. Increased requirement: for a diabetic who ingests excess carbohydrates, has restricted activity, cannot exercise moderately, is under mental or emotional tension, or undergoes surgery.
   b. Decreased requirement: for diabetic with decreased carbohydrate intake or for one who exercises strenuously.

V. PSYCHOLOGICAL CHARACTERISTICS

When diabetes with its serious potential complications occurs during childhood, the child's and his parents' daily routines will be somewhat

abnormal. Parents may fear the complications of blood sugar imbalance, and the child may become fearful or submissive as a result of
overprotection, or belligerent as a reaction to constant supervision. His
behavioral attitudes will be carried into his adult life, and he should
be assisted as early as possible to develop a positive, optimistic attitude
toward the maintenance of his oral health.

Typical backgrounds of children with emotional and mental problems are listed below to help the professional assess the patient and to
plan preventive services and instruction. A child may not fit into any
of the categories listed because of his individual personality, because
he had other environmental influences, or because his parents possess
traits other than those listed.

A. Associated with Child Diabetic[16]

1. Overprotected child may be fearful, anxious, or nervous as result
   of parental attitudes toward his condition.
2. Child with behavioral problems may have used physical condition as threat to gain own way from overindulgent parents.
3. Shy, submissive, timid child may be dominated by authoritative
   parents with regard to his illness and behavior.
4. Resentful, rebellious child may feel resentment toward parental
   attitude of indifference; may show overt, delinquent behavior.

B. Associated with Adult Diabetic: loss of ability to concentrate; slight depression.

VI. ORAL CHARACTERISTICS[17,18]

The patient with controlled diabetes mellitus does not present soft
tissue lesions characteristic for the disease. His gingiva and mucosa are
less resistant to infection and trauma.

A rather high incidence of gingival disturbances has been observed
in patients with untreated diabetes mellitus. If the diabetes remains
untreated, periodontal damage becomes progressively severe. The
gingival and mucosal symptoms in uncontrolled diabetes are those of
Vitamin B and C deficiencies that tend to occur with the disturbed
carbohydrate metabolism. No conclusive evidence has been presented
to show that the attack rate from dental caries is altered either when
diabetes is controlled or uncontrolled, although it seems reasonable
to assume that decreased ingestion of fermentable carbohydrates would
be followed by decreased caries incidence, at least in children. The
characteristics listed below may be seen in the patient with undiagnosed
or uncontrolled diabetes mellitus.

A. Breath: advanced uncontrolled cases may have acetone odor.

B. Saliva: decreased flow.

C. Calculus Deposits: increased.

D. Tongue: coated; swollen with marginal indentations; fissured; pa-
tient may notice dry, burning or metallic sensations.

E. Oral Mucous Membranes

1. Dry, generalized redness, lowered tone.
2. Decreased resistance to infection; delayed healing rate.
3. Soft tissue under denture may be enlarged or hemorrhagic.

F. **Gingiva:** deep red in color; edematous, sometimes slightly enlarged; tendency toward recurrent periodontal abscess formation.

G. **Bone:** vertical and horizontal resorption (may be arrested with adequate control of diabetes); dry sockets may develop after extractions.

H. **Teeth:** may be loosened due to bone resorption; may be sensitive to percussion.

APPLIED TECHNIQUES FOR PROFESSIONAL CARE AND INSTRUCTION

Frequent and thorough dental hygiene and dental care, coupled with thorough personal oral care by the patient, are of particular importance in prevention of unnecessary periodontal complications for the diabetic patient who is susceptible to infection and whose tissues heal at a slow rate. Chronic infection intensifies diabetic symptoms, so the oral cavity must be maintained in a healthy state.

I. APPOINTMENT PLANNING

A. **Time**
1. Morning hours better because patient is more refreshed and has less time to anticipate appointment, hence anxiety is reduced.
2. Mid-morning best for patients on insulin therapy because blood sugar level is under better control at this time.

B. **Length:** shorter periods of time preferred because patient may fatigue easily.

C. **Number of Appointments**
1. Reappoint patient with extensive calculus deposits.
2. Second appointment desirable to check gingival response after deposit removal.
3. Elderly patient or patient with cardiovascular disease should have oral prophylaxis completed in several short appointments.[19]

D. **Recall Intervals:** The diabetic patient should receive an oral prophylaxis frequently since he is highly susceptible to infection and gingival disturbances from even slight local irritations. Routine, thorough oral prophylaxes will reduce local irritation to the minimum, thus aid in the prevention of unnecessary complications.

II. PATIENT'S MEDICAL HISTORY

A. **Diabetes Mellitus Under Therapeutic Control:** When patient's diabetic condition is known, consult physician for instructions with regard to preventive measures such as antibiotic or sedative administration.

B. **Suspected Diabetes Mellitus:** call to dentist's attention; dentist may wish to consult patient's physician before extensive dental and dental hygiene care is instituted.

III. ORAL RADIOGRAPHY

A. **Number and Frequency of Exposures:** dependent upon dentist's requirement for continued observation of vertical and horizontal bone levels.

B. **Findings:** note alveolar bone level and compare with possible mobility of teeth which have decreased bone support.

IV. ORAL PROPHYLAXIS

A. **Plan for Premedication**
   1. Sedative: may be prescribed by physician or dentist to relieve apprehension.
   2. Antibiotic: may be prescribed by physician or dentist to prevent infections.
   3. Vitamins B, C: may be prescribed to increase healing, reduce potential for infection.[20]

B. **Avoid Use of Iodine Solutions, Phenol and Salicylic Acid Compounds:** soft tissue may slough, and healing may be delayed.[17]

V. PATIENT INSTRUCTION

The diabetic patient usually has received thorough instructions with regard to his responsibilities in the control of his disease. Because he has been made conscious of other health procedures, he is potentially receptive to dental health instruction.

A. **Oral Physical Therapy**
   1. Toothbrushing: stress that thorough toothbrushing after food ingestion will reduce calculus deposition and will massage the gingiva to maintain its normal tone.
   2. Modified Stillman's or Charters' Method of toothbrushing may be recommended to massage gingiva that is of lowered tone or that has a tendency for enlargement or hemorrhage.

B. **Dietary Habits and Dental Caries**
   1. The restriction of fermentable carbohydrate ingestion in the diabetic's dietary may contribute to a reduced rate of dental caries incidence.
   2. The relationship of fermentable carbohydrates to dental caries should be stressed as this may serve as a further stimulus for the patient to follow his therapeutic diet.

REFERENCES

1. BRUNNER, L. S., EMERSON, C. P., JR., FERGUSON, L. K., and SUDDARTH, D. S.: *Textbook of Medical-Surgical Nursing.* Philadelphia, Lippincott, 1964, p. 826.

2. CHERASKIN, E. and LANGLEY, L. L.:　*Dynamics of Oral Diagnosis.* Chicago, Year Book, 1956, p. 202.
3. BRUNNER, EMERSON, FERGUSON, and SUDDARTH:　op. cit., p. 836.
4. FOSDICK, L. S.:　Carbohydrate Metabolism, in Muhler, J. C. ed., *Textbook of Biochemistry for Students of Dentistry.* St. Louis, Mosby, 1959, p. 244.
5. FORSHAM, P. H. and THORN, G. W.:　The Pancreas, in Williams, R. H.:　*Textbook of Endocrinology,* 2nd ed. Philadelphia, Saunders, 1955, p. 423.
6. Ibid., pp. 424–425.
7. PASCHKIS, K. E., RAKOFF, A. E., and CANTAROW, ABRAHAM: *Clinical Endocrinology,* 2nd ed. New York, Hoeber-Harper, 1958, p. 723.
8. BRUNNER, EMERSON, FERGUSON, and SUDDARTH:　op. cit., p. 827.
9. FORSHAM and THORN:　op. cit., pp. 428–429.
10. BRUNNER, EMERSON, FERGUSON, and SUDDARTH:　op. cit., p. 830.
11. FORSHAM and THORN:　op. cit., pp. 444–448.
12. DAUGHADAY, W. H.:　Diabetic Acidosis, in Williams, R. H.:　*Diabetes.* New York, Paul Hoeber, 1960, p. 527.
13. American Diabetes Association, Inc., 1 East 45th St., New York 17, N. Y., Checklist, cited in Brunner, Emerson, Ferguson and Suddarth: op. cit., p. 836.
14. BRUNNER, EMERSON, FERGUSON, and SUDDARTH:　op. cit., p. 828.
15. FORSHAM and THORN:　op. cit.: p. 440.
16. Ibid., pp. 450–451.
17. BURKET, L. W.:　*Oral Medicine,* 4th ed. Philadelphia, Lippincott, 1961, pp. 390–391.
18. BURKET, L. W. and SINDONI, ANTHONY, JR.:　Diabetes and the Dental Patient, Am. Dent. A. J., *58*, 81, February, 1959.
19. GLICKMAN, IRVING: *Clinical Periodontology,* 2nd ed. Philadelphia, Saunders, 1958, p. 916.
20. BURKET: op. cit., p. 395.

SUGGESTED READINGS

ADELSON, J. J.:　Dental Treatment of the Diabetic Child, J. Dent. Child., *27*, 55, First Quarter, 1960.
CHERASKIN, E.:　The Problem of Diabetes Mellitus in Dental Practice, J. Dent. Med., *15*, 67, April, 1960.
COHEN, M. M.:　*Pediatric Dentistry,* 2nd ed. St. Louis, Mosby, 1961, pp. 476–478.
COLLINS, L. H., JR. and CRANE, M. P.:　*Internal Medicine in Dental Practice,* 5th ed. Philadelphia, Lea & Febiger, 1960, pp. 263–279.
GOTTSEGEN, ROBERT:　Dental Considerations in Diabetes Mellitus, New York State J. Med., *62*, 389, February, 1962 (abstracted in Dent. Abstr., *8*, 278, May, 1963).
HOWARD, E. E. and MARLETTE, R. H.:　Rationale of Management in Oral Surgery Procedures on Diabetics, Oral Surg., Oral Med., & Oral Path., *9*, 1032, October, 1956.
JOOS, T. H. and JOHNSTON, J. A.:　A Long-Term Evaluation of the Juvenile Diabetic, J. Pediat., *50*, 133, February, 1957.
KNAPP, R. G., NATHANSON, I. G., and MALLETT, S. P.:　Acute Dental Infection in Diabetes, Oral Surg., Oral Med., & Oral Path., *4*, 1369, November, 1951.
LANGLEY, L. L. and CHERASKIN, E.:　*The Physiological Foundation of Dental Practice,* 2nd ed. St. Louis, Mosby, 1956, pp. 526–531.
MacKENZIE, R. S. and MILLARD, H. D.:　Interrelated Effects of Diabetes, Arteriosclerosis and Calculus on Alveolar Bone Loss, Am. Dent. A. J., *66*, 191, February, 1963.
SHERIDAN, R. C., CHERASKIN, E., FLYNN, F. H. and HUTTO, A. C.:　Epidemiology of Diabetes Mellitus. I. Review of the Literature, J. Periodont., *30*, 242, July, 1959; II. A Study of 100 Dental Patients, J. Periodont., *30*, 298, October, 1959.
SINDONI, ANTHONY, JR.:　The Diabetic Dental Patient, in Burket, L. W., ed.: *Symposium on the Interrelationship of Oral and Systemic Disease, Dental Clinics of No. America.* Philadelphia, Saunders, July, 1958, pp. 459–469.
SINDONI, A. M.:　The Role of the Dentist in Diabetes Mellitus, J. Dent. Med., *9*, 203, October, 1954.
SWENSON, H. M.:　Alveolar Bone Resorption Associated with Diabetes, J. Periodont., *25*, 52, January, 1954.
WILKINS, E. M.:　The Diabetic Dental Hygiene Patient, Am. Dent. Hygienists' A. J., *36*, 111, Third Quarter, 1962.
WILLIAMS, R. C., JR. and MAHAN, C. J.:　Periodontal Disease and Diabetes in Young Adults, Am. Med. A. J., *172*, 776, February 20, 1960.
WOLF, WILLIAM:　Oral Manifestations of Endocrine Dysfunctions, in Miller, S. C.: *Oral Diagnosis and Treatment,* 3rd ed. New York, Blakiston Division, McGraw-Hill, 1957, pp. 762–765.

Chapter 39

PATIENTS DURING PUBERTY, MENSTRUATION AND MENOPAUSE

Hormonal influences may cause physiological and emotional changes in the human organism during the development, maturation and cessation of the reproductive period. Disturbances of the oral soft tissues sometimes occur during puberty, menstruation, pregnancy and the climacteric (menopause). When the period of major change in an individual's reproductive life has been completed, oral symptoms usually recede, although untreated conditions do not return to their previously normal states.

Routine, thorough oral prophylaxes, dental care, and oral physical therapy measures combined with a protective diet will aid the patient to maintain oral health throughout periods of major change in the reproductive system.

THE GONADS

The ovaries are two grayish-pink nodular glands, one located on each side of the uterus. Their main functions are the production of ova and the secretion of female sex hormones.

The testes, also two in number, are ovoid glandular bodies suspended from the inguinal region by the spermatic cord and enclosed by the scrotal sac. Their major functions are the production of sperm and the secretion of male sex hormones.

I. FEMALE GONADAL HORMONES (OVARIAN HORMONES)

A. **Estrogen** (*estrone*);
  1. Sources and control
    a. Produced by the ripening Graafian follicle under the stimulation of the follicle-stimulating hormone (FSH) of the anterior lobe of the hypophysis.
    b. Secreted in very small amounts by the adrenal cortex (both male and female).
  2. Actions
    a. Causes development of primary female reproductive organs.
    b. Prepares uterus to receive fertilized ovum.
    c. Stimulates growth and development of mammary glands.
    d. Influences development of female secondary sex characteristics.
    e. Inhibits secretion of FSH and stimulates production of ICSH (interstitial cell-stimulating hormone).

29   (449)

B. **Progesterone**
1. Sources and control
   a. Produced from the corpus luteum after collapse of the Graafian follicle, under stimulation of the interstitial-cell-stimulating hormone (ICSH) of the anterior lobe of the hypophysis.
   b. Secreted in very small amounts by the adrenal cortex (both male and female).
2. Actions: prepares mucosa of uterus to receive fertilized ovum and maintain embryo; inhibits maturation of Graafian follicle, ovulation and secretion of estrone, thus prevents menstruation during pregnancy; and stimulates further growth of mammary glands if these have been stimulated previously by estrone.

II. MALE GONADAL HORMONES (ANDROGENS)

Hormones which induce male characteristics are called androgens. Many androgens have been isolated and synthesized, but the most active is testosterone, the testicular hormone.

A. Sources and Control

1. Testosterone: formed by the Leydig cells of the testes under the stimulation of the interstitial-cell-stimulating hormone (ICSH) of the anterior lobe of the hypophysis.
2. Androgens are secreted in very small amounts by the adrenal cortex (both male and female.)

B. Actions

1. Stimulates growth and development of primary male reproductive organs.
2. Influences development of male secondary sex characteristics.
3. Stimulates growth of body hair of male distribution.
4. Causes epiphyseal cartilage to age.
5. Promotes cell growth.
6. Assists in production of the "adolescent growth spurt."
   a. Males: growth due to testicular and adrenocortical growth hormone stimulation.
   b. Females: growth due to adrenocortical and possibly ovarian hormone stimulation.

PUBERTY

Puberty is that developmental period when sex glands mature, reproductive organs become functional, and secondary sex characteristics appear. In comparison, adolescence is that period of life that begins with the appearance of secondary sex characteristics and terminates with the fulfillment of body growth.

The normal pubertal period for both sexes may begin at any time within the broad range of 9 and 17 years of age. Secondary sex characteristics usually begin to appear in the female between the ages of 11 and 13, and in the male between 13 and 14 years.

I. NORMAL PUBERTAL CHANGES

A. Reproductive System

1. Female: ovaries mature and produce hormones under FSH stimulation; secondary sex organs mature under ovarian estrogenic stimulation; menarche (onset of menstruation) occurs.
2. Male: testes mature and produce testosterone under FSH stimulation; accessory organs and glands develop; mature spermatozoa are produced.

B. Secondary Sex Characteristics

1. Female: fat is distributed in characteristic locations, body hair grows, and breasts enlarge.
2. Male: voice timbre deepens due to enlargement of larynx, voice cracks until development is completed, and body and facial hair grows.

C. Linear Growth (height)

1. Female: increases before body changes occur and continues to increase at reduced rate 2 or 3 years after menarche until epiphyses unite.
2. Male: increases before body changes occur and continues at a reduced rate for 2 or 3 years longer than female, until epiphyses unite.

D. Skin: acne vulgaris frequently occurs; urticaria, signs of allergy, pallor or blushing may occur.

II. EMOTIONAL CHARACTERISTICS

The sex drive is awakened with the onset of puberty. At this time, personality and emotional changes are marked.

A. Emotional Disturbances[1]

Moodiness, increased secretiveness, or lack of emotional control may be caused by a hypersensitivity to the manner in which the adolescent reacts to other people, or the way they react to him. His self-consciousness stems from a desire to adjust to social situations. Overt disturbances and some of their causes are listed below.

1. Embarrassment: when he is teased, ridiculed, mistaken or praised; his social status is lowered; or his appearance and/or physical development are deficient.
2. Depression: when he is disappointed, slighted or humiliated, or has failed in social situations.
3. Anger: when he is treated unjustly or as a child; his rights are encroached; a privilege is refused; or his accomplishments are frustrated.
4. Fear: when he must speak in public; he anticipates embarrassment; he is pushed beyond capabilities; or he is subjected to sarcasm or ridicule.
5. Worry: when he experiences pubertal changes and/or anticipates abnormal development; family relationships are disturbed, for example by quarrels or illnesses.

B. **Signs of Psychological Disturbances:** Restlessness, insomnia, irritability or other signs of instability or lack of emotional control may result from hyperstimulation caused by hormonal imbalance.

III. ORAL CHARACTERISTICS

A. **Dental Caries:** The growth spurt and emotional tension of puberty and adolescence intensify hunger and the desire to eat. Frequently the hunger drive is satiated by the consumption of an excess of foods containing fermentable carbohydrates. Dental caries incidence is higher in the teen-age group than at any other age.

B. **Gingival Conditions:** Gingival enlargement and/or an unusual sensitivity to local irritants may be observed in the adolescent. The enlargement is marginal, tends to occur on the facial surfaces only, and may involve one or more papillae. The disturbed tissue is bluish-red and, in severe cases, edema may be extensive. In addition to hormonal imbalance, a number of contributory factors may be involved, including crowded teeth, pronounced overbite, mouth breathing, diet imbalance, and inadequate personal oral care. As adulthood is reached, gingival conditions approach normal, but untreated cases do not always return completely to normal.[2]

IV. APPLIED TECHNIQUES FOR DENTAL HYGIENE CARE

A. **Appointment Planning**
1. Number: more than one appointment may be indicated for patients with extensive gingival disturbances to allow observation of tissue response and instruction.
2. Recall intervals: frequent for patients with a high rate of dental caries incidence or lowered gingival tone.

B. **Oral Prophylaxis**
1. Importance: essential to remove local irritants because gingiva may be hypersensitive to slight trauma.
2. Instrumentation: may be hampered by enlarged and hemorrhagic gingiva or by extensive carious lesions.

V. PATIENT INSTRUCTION

Although parents should be aware of the adolescent's oral health problems and requirements, responsibility for good personal oral care habits and diet should be placed with the adolescent. The development of good habits can be fostered by the professional who assumes a positive attitude toward the individual's abilities and desires to maintain oral health, and who avoids situations that may embarrass or disturb the patient. Suggested procedures for patient instruction are outlined in Chapter 25. A dental caries control study may aid the patient who exhibits rampant dental caries (see Chapter 31). General instructions that should be stressed to the adolescent patient are listed below.

A. **Oral Physical Therapy**

1. Regular, effective use of the toothbrush immediately after food ingestion will help to prevent dental caries incidence and to maintain normal, healthy gingiva.
2. Gingival massage, applied with the toothbrush and other devices if indicated, will stimulate and improve the tone of hypersensitive or enlarged gingiva.

B. **Dietary Habits**

1. Use of adequate quantities of basic foods will promote general as well as oral health.
2. Use of detergent foods will help cleanse teeth and massage the gingiva.
3. Avoidance of fermentable carbohydrates, especially between meals, and substitution of noncariogenic snacks and party foods will help reduce incidence of dental caries; the relationship of fermentable carbohydrates to dental caries should be stressed.

C. **Dental Care:** frequent dental examinations and treatment will prevent unnecessary loss of tooth structure and will decrease expense.

MENSTRUATION

Menstruation is the process of normal cyclic uterine bleeding which occurs in the female at approximately 28-day intervals from menarche to menopause, except during pregnancy and lactation. Hormonal changes that occur with the menstrual cycle do not affect the oral tissues significantly, but minor emotional disturbances and physical discomforts may be experienced by the individual just before and at the onset of menstruation. Knowledge and consideration of these effects will permit the professional to adapt routine appointment procedures and thereby provide more effective care for the patient.

I. **GENERAL CHARACTERISTICS**

A. **Metabolic Disturbances**

1. Physical efficiency diminished; fatigue, insomnia, dizziness, faintness may occur.
2. Thirst usually increased.
3. Elimination
   a. Prior to onset: water retention with edema and increased weight, abdominal tension.
   b. At or after onset: frequent urination.
4. Breasts: tender, sometimes sore before onset.

B. **Physical Appearance:** skin may bruise easily; tendency for eruptions, acne.

II. **MENTAL AND EMOTIONAL CHARACTERISTICS**

A woman may exhibit signs of emotional tension from 1 to 2 weeks before and until the onset of menstruation. One or more of the signs listed below may be observed.

A. **Emotional Disturbances:** general tension, unrest, irritability.

B. **Psychological Disturbances:** moodiness, increased sexual desire (excessive for the individual), depression, anxiety, emotional outbursts.

III. ORAL CHARACTERISTICS[3]

Menstruation usually is not accompanied by clinical signs that require professional care. Capillaries dilate, gingival vascularity may increase, and therefore, hemorrhage may be prolonged after instrumentation for an occasional patient.

A nonspecific gingivitis with gingival bleeding, or recurrent aphthous ulcers of the mucous membranes may be experienced. If these conditions are present without apparent cause, interrogation of the patient may reveal a recurrence related to the menstrual cycle.

IV. APPLIED TECHNIQUES FOR DENTAL HYGIENE CARE

Unless a menstrual disorder causes extreme discomfort, professional care may be administered without unusual precautions. Extra precaution to avoid trauma of hypersensitive or enlarged gingival tissue may be indicated.

V. **PATIENT INSTRUCTION:** The use of a soft-textured toothbrush and an interdental stimulator may be recommended for hypersensitive gingiva.

MENOPAUSE

Menopause is one phase of the climacteric or "change of life" period. It occurs normally between the ages of 45 and 50 years as a result of the cessation of physiologic endometrial bleeding (menstruation). The climacteric is a gradual aging process caused by a change in gonadal function which gives rise to distinct structural and physiological changes in the individual. Males rarely experience a true climacteric. Several characteristics listed below may occur with menopause. All or most of the characteristics are seldom experienced by an individual.

I. GENERAL CHARACTERISTICS

A. **Predisposition to Other Diseases:** hyperthyroidism, and more frequently, hypothyroidism; simple goiter; diabetes mellitus; hypertension.

B. **Metabolic Disturbances**
1. Physical efficiency diminished: lack of energy, tiredness, weakness, insomnia.
2. Heart and circulation: palpitations; intermittent rapid pulse; hot flushes, excessive perspiration due to unstable vasomotor control; high blood pressure or low pulse rate.
3. Appetite: may be increased due to heightened emotional tension.
4. Respiration: shortness of breath after slight exertion.
5. Reproductive organs: atrophy due to estrogen deficiency.
6. Urination: frequent.

C. **Sensory Disturbances**

1. Pain: tendency to headaches, neuritic and joint pains.
2. Voice: virile (lower-pitched).
3. Body temperature: oversensitive to external heat.

D. **Physical Appearance**

1. Stature: tendency to gain weight; some women become more masculine in appearance.
2. Facial hair: often increases on upper lip, less often on chin.

II. EMOTIONAL AND MENTAL CHARACTERISTICS

Emotional and mental disturbances may not occur as menstruation ceases. A woman may experience a few minor disturbances, usually after menopause when she realizes her reproductive capacity is lost and she fears the aging process.

A. **Emotional Disturbances:** instability, irritability; sudden outbursts.

B. **Psychological Disturbances:** nervousness, depression, failing memory and power of concentration.

III. ORAL CHARACTERISTICS

A woman usually does not experience oral disturbances related to menopause. Infrequent mild signs that appear are related to endocrine disturbances or vitamin deficiencies. Occasionally, a condition called menopausal gingivostomatitis develops with severe symptoms comparable to chronic desquamative gingivitis.

A. **Mild Disturbances:** thinly keratinized gingiva; tendency to hemorrhage, slight edema. These characteristics may be prevented or overcome with thorough dental hygiene care and personal oral care by the patient.

B. **Menopausal Gingivostomatitis**[4,5]

1. Incidence: rare; chronic, with periods of remission and frequent acute flare-ups; mastication difficult; acute condition is aggravated by toothbrushing.[6]
2. Gingiva (facial)[7]
   a. Vesicles filled with watery fluid may appear occasionally; may recur if traumatized.
   b. In absence of vesicles, gingiva may appear smooth and cyanotic.
3. Oral mucosa: generalized edema, redness, and painful burning sensation; epithelium may desquamate; aphthous ulcers may occur before or after menstruation in early stages, if patient is susceptible.
4. Tongue: reddened; fissured, with marginal serrations; similar to vitamin B deficiency.
5. Sensory disturbances
   a. Taste sensations abnormal: described as salty, peppery, or sour.

        b. Dryness and burning sensation of tongue, buccal gingiva, and throat.

        c. Reaction to prosthetic appliances: discomfort and intolerance of even well-adapted appliances because oral tissues are covered by thin epithelial layer.

IV. **APPLIED TECHNIQUES FOR DENTAL HYGIENE CARE**

    A. **Recall Intervals:** frequent because of hypersensitivity of gingiva to local irritants.

    B. **Room Temperature:** slightly cooler than normal to accommodate patient's oversensitivity to external heat.

    C. **Oral Prophylaxis:** instrumentation may be difficult to accomplish because patient is irritable and oversensitive to pain.

V. **PATIENT INSTRUCTION**

    Instruction may be well-received and followed by the woman in menopause because she wishes to retard the aging process and to preserve oral health.

    A. **Oral Physical Therapy:** a soft-textured toothbrush may be recommended to avoid injury to hypersensitive gingiva, and supplementary measures to massage the gingiva may be employed to maintain gingival tissue tone.

    B. **Dietary Habits:**

        1. Use of adequate quantities of basic foods will promote general as well as oral health.

        2. Use of detergent foods will help cleanse teeth and massage the gingiva.

        3. Avoidance of fermentable carbohydrates, especially between meals, and substitution of noncariogenic snacks will help reduce incidence of dental caries and irritation of marginal gingiva; the relationship of fermentable carbohydrates and dental caries should be stressed to individuals who eat frequently between meals as a result of tension or heightened emotion.

REFERENCES

1. MALM, MARGUERITE and JAMISON, O. G.: *Adolescence.* New York, McGraw-Hill, 1952, pp. 220–221.
2. GLICKMAN, IRVING: *Clinical Periodontology,* 2nd ed. Philadelphia, Saunders, 1958, pp. 97, 150–151.
3. BURKET, L. W.: *Oral Medicine,* 4th ed. Philadelphia, Lippincott, 1961, p. 251.
4. Ibid., pp. 255–256.
5. MASSLER, MAURY and HENRY, J.: Oral Manifestations During the Female Climacteric, The Alpha Omegan, p. 105, September, 1950, cited by Glickman, Irving: *Clinical Periodontology,* 2nd ed. Philadelphia, Saunders, 1958, pp. 162–163.
6. ORBAN, B. J. and WENTZ, F. M.: *Atlas of Clinical Pathology of the Oral Mucous Membrane,* 2nd ed. St. Louis, Mosby, 1960, p. 66.
7. BEUBE, F. E.: *Periodontology.* New York, Macmillan, 1953, pp. 670–671.

SUGGESTED READINGS

AMADOR, F. A.:   Hormonal Gingivitis, Dent. Students' Mag., *40*, 100, November, 1961.

BERNIER, J. L.:   *The Management of Oral Disease.* St. Louis, Mosby, 1955, pp. 397–398, 401.

BOOKMILLER, M. M. and BOWEN, G. L.:   *Textbook of Obstetrics and Obstetric Nursing*, 4th ed. Philadelphia, Saunders, 1963, Ch. 6.

CHERASKIN, E. and LANGLEY, L. L.:   *Dynamics of Oral Diagnosis.* Chicago, Year Book, 1956, pp. 205–206, 210–211.

KERR, D. A., ASH, M. M., JR. and MILLARD, H. D.:   *Oral Diagnosis*, St. Louis, Mosby, 1959, pp. 96–98, 202–203.

PARFITT, G. J.:   Periodontal Diseases in Children, in Finn, S. B., ed.: *Clinical Pedodontics*, 2nd ed. Philadelphia, Saunders, 1962, p. 508.

SORRIN, SIDNEY, ed.:   *The Practice of Periodontia.* New York, Blakiston Division, McGraw-Hill, 1960, pp. 110, 134, 159–161, 400.

THOMA, K. H. and ROBINSON, H. B. G.:   *Oral and Dental Diagnosis*, 5th ed. Philadelphia, Saunders, 1960, pp. 125–126.

TUTTLE, W. W. and SCHOTTELIUS, B. A.:   *Textbook of Physiology*, 14th ed. St. Louis, Mosby, 1961, Ch. 33.

Chapter 40

PRENATAL DENTAL HYGIENE CARE

During pregnancy, attention is focused on good health practices for the mother. She is anxious and concerned for the health of her baby and for herself. This alertness to total health, of which oral health is an important part, provides an unusual opportunity to help the patient learn principles which may be applied to the future care of the child.

The term *prenatal care* refers to the supervised preparation for childbirth which helps the mother enjoy optimum health during and after her pregnancy and the reward of a healthy baby. Such a program involves the combined efforts of the obstetrician, nurse, dentist, dental hygienist and the expectant parents. Pregnancy is arbitrarily divided into 3 periods of 3 months each, referred to as the first, second and third trimesters, respectively.

Unfortunately there are still many women who do not seek care until delivery. Oral health is neglected along with general health. Some of these patients will appear for emergency dental service, and may be receptive to a program of care and instruction to prevent further emergencies. The dental hygienist in public health will participate in community educational programs with public health nurses whereby some of the less informed or less motivated women may learn of the need for professional dental care and advice during pregnancy.

Obstetricians routinely recommend dental care early in pregnancy. This brings to the dental office many women who previously would not have had a regular plan for obtaining professional service. Many of these have not known the advantages of personal habits of daily care and diet related to the health of the oral tissues. There are numerous misconceptions or "old wives' tales" to counteract in providing up-to-date information about the relationship of pregnancy and oral health.

I. ORAL MANIFESTATIONS OF PREGNANCY[1,2,3,4]

That pregnancy is a "physiological state of systemic imbalance"[1] has been widely quoted. Every organ and tissue in the mother's body are affected to some degree by the physiologic changes which occur as a result of the influences of the placental hormones.

The condition of the gingiva is related to the presence of local irritants, namely calculus and soft deposits. When the mouth is in good health and the patient practices routine personal oral care procedures, no gingival changes may be expected.

Pregnancy will tend to aggravate an existing gingival condition, and is therefore a secondary or conditioning factor. Since the principal gingival reaction in pregnancy is an inflammatory one, the pregnancy itself cannot be the cause.

Approximately one-half of the prenatal patients exhibit noticeable gingival involvement which is equally true of nonpregnant women.[2]

Usually the gingivitis is noticed during the second trimester or late in the first trimester when the patient may become more aware of her mouth than she was during the earlier emotional period. Exaggerated symptoms abate after the birth of the child, but it should not be expected that a completely healthy condition will result. Patients with a gingival disturbance during pregnancy will continue to have the disturbance somewhat lessened in degree.

A. **Gingivitis Associated with Pregnancy:** "Pregnancy Gingivitis"
  1. Clinical appearance
     Symptoms are generally limited to the free gingiva. The appearance varies as suggested by the possible characteristics of inflamed tissues listed below.
     a. Enlargement: hyperplasia, edema.
     b. Shiny, smooth surface.
     c. Hemorrhages readily with slight trauma.
     d. Color: possibly either bluish-purple or raspberry red.
     e. Loss of normal resiliency.
     f. Ulceration: when superimposed infection occurs.
  2. Predisposing factors
     a. Local irritation due to unhygienic oral condition and deposits on the teeth related to laxity in personal care procedures.
     b. Increase in estrogenic hormone during pregnancy may alter the tissue reaction.[2]

B. **"Pregnancy Tumor"** (Granulomatous Epulis)
  Isolated inflammatory lesions which are accentuations of "pregnancy gingivitis" occur in 0.5 per cent of pregnant women, approximately the occurrence in the nonpregnant.[1] Predisposing factors are the same as for gingivitis associated with pregnancy. The use of the word tumor is misleading since the lesion is not a tumor, but a hyperplasia.

  1. Clinical appearance
     a. Location: superficially on the free gingiva, usually associated with an interdental papilla.
     b. Mushroom-like, flattened mass.
     c. Smooth glistening surface.
     d. Color: purplish-red, magenta, or deep blue, sometimes dotted with red; color depends on vascularity.
  2. Symptoms
     a. Hemorrhages readily with slight trauma.
     b. Painless unless it becomes large enough to interfere with occlusion and mastication.

II. PSYCHOLOGICAL CHARACTERISTICS[5,6]

Mental hygiene of the expectant mother is influenced by her attitude toward herself, her husband, her other children, and her unborn child. Normally, in a large majority of cases, when the husband is pleased and there is security in the marriage, there will be genuine happiness and anticipation, or at least tranquil acceptance. When there is emotional instability, the mother may exhibit degrees of apprehension or even open rebellion in her rejection of the baby.

The first few months are the most difficult, and anxiety may be observed since pregnancy provides an emotional experience with many adjustments to be made. Generally these early problems resolve themselves and, if they continue throughout the pregnancy, may disappear when the baby is born. A few of the possible characteristic emotional manifestations of pregnancy are listed below with suggestions for the dental hygiene appointment.

A. **Changes in Mood from Happiness to Depression:** At times the change may be abrupt. Adapt conversation and instruction to receptiveness of patient.

B. **Hypersensitivity:** Be cautious about joking over personal matters and avoid calling attention to size or appearance.

C. **Irritability:** Minimize disturbances, interruptions or noises; make operations smooth; adjust room temperature; avoid topics of discussion which might bring patient reaction.

D. **Increased Introversion, Passivity, Dependence on Others:** Help patient to feel the responsibility for her oral health being taken by the dentist and dental hygienist, yet interest her in the need for her own personal care.

E. **Physical and Mental Indifference:** May explain lack of conscientiousness in the patient's personal oral care habits.
   1. Plan sufficient appointments for oral prophylaxis to counteract patient's own lack of care.
   2. Plan for special reminders such as telephone to help patient who is indifferent to keeping appointments.
   3. Be firm with patient instruction; take advantage of teachable moments.

F. **Impaired Judgment:** Be specific in outlining the plan for oral care, both professional and personal. Help patient visualize realistically the possible effects of neglect.

G. **Hidden Fears Not Recognized or Admitted:** Fear of the pregnancy, the child's health, her own health or of adjustments which must be made after the birth of the child. Offer reassurance. Conversation should dwell on positive factors, not morbid.

H. **Changes in Appetite; Craving for Unusual Foods:** Provide specific information concerning the use of foods other than fermentable carbohydrates, particularly as snacks.

III. INTERRELATIONSHIP OF DENTAL AND DENTAL HYGIENE CARE

The dental hygienist needs to be well informed concerning aspects of dental care since she will have the opportunity to motivate the patient and dispel fears related to certain services. The patient may consult the dental hygienist for reassurance and interpretation concerning the dentist's recommendations and procedures.

A. **Oral Examination and Treatment Planning:** Made early in pregnancy as possible, avoiding periods of nausea. Consultation with patient's physician is of particular importance in order that the total prenatal care may be integrated.

B. **Restorative Dentistry:** All required work should be completed with permanent restorations. One important contraindication for the use of temporary restorations lies in the fact that after the baby is born the mother will be much too busy to attend to appointments and may postpone them.

C. **Radiography:** There is no contraindication for routine radiographs being made since the oral cavity is sufficiently removed from the pelvic region. Ordinary precautions of ultra-speed film, extended target-film distance, and the use of an adequate diaphragm and filter should be observed as for any patient. The number of exposures should be restricted to a minimum. A lead apron placed across the patient's lap will reduce hazards of secondary radiation to that region (see page 226).

D. **Anesthesia:** Use of precautions against cardiovascular distress and anoxia prevents hazards. Oxygen should be available for administration in an emergency. Premedication is used to relieve emotional stress.[7]

E. **Removal of Local Irritants and Their Causes:** Areas of food impaction should be corrected and all overhanging restorations replaced. Occlusal adjustment may be indicated. Such procedures have a direct relationship to the success of dental hygiene care.

F. **Periodontal Treatment:** Pregnancy does not interfere with the success of periodontal treatment and such care may be performed as needed.[3,8]

IV. DENTAL HYGIENE CARE

As stated previously, severe gingival involvement need not be expected when the teeth are kept free of deposits, the surrounding tissues have no local irritants, and the patient practices conscientious habits of oral cleanliness and gingival massage. This calls for a specific recall appointment plan for oral prophylaxis and patient instruction.

A. Appointment Planning

1. Recall intervals: range from monthly appointments to three times during the 9-month period depending on the individual mouth and the patient's motivation in personal care.
2. Length of individual appointment: short, one-half hour preferably. A series of appointments is needed to complete the case with heavy calculus.
3. Recall following birth of child: for the patient who has not been on a regular recall plan prior to pregnancy, emphasis must be placed on motivating the patient to continue regular dental hygiene appointments and inspections for needed dental care.

B. **Appointment Procedures**

1. Patient's medical history: it should be remembered that the prenatal patient may require applied techniques for conditions other than pregnancy. For example, diabetes offers serious possible complications. Dental and dental hygiene care have double significance since the diabetic is more prone to infection.[9,10]

2. Procedures related to physical characteristics: techniques of the dental hygiene appointment require very little if any, special adaptation in themselves. The important considerations are related to the physical and mental condition of the patient.

   It is not within the scope of this book to review all of the physiologic changes which occur during pregnancy. There are a number of common minor disturbances which should be identified since they can affect appointment procedures. Nearly every pregnant woman is bothered by one or more minor complaints.

   Attention to small details will provide the patient with comfort and motivate her to continued oral care. Table 14 lists the more common minor physical disturbances of pregnancy and suggests a few appointment considerations.

V. PATIENT INSTRUCTION

A. **Oral Physical Therapy**

Emphasis is on the need for meticulous personal care. Toothbrushing and the use of auxiliary methods are in accord with the individual's need (see Chapters 26 and 27).

B. **Diet**

A majority of expectant mothers will base their diets on the recommendations of their physicians. However, instruction must be provided in the relationship of dental caries prevention and the health of the supporting structures of the teeth to the use of a varied diet containing the essential protective foods.

In any discussion of dietary needs, specific foods should be mentioned rather than the nutritive elements. Assistance in meal planning for use of specific foods is sometimes indicated to be certain that there is clear understanding.

1. Purposes of adequate diet during pregnancy
   a. To maintain daily strength.
   b. To prepare for labor by building up the muscle tone of the body to meet the crisis of labor and delivery.
   c. To hasten the patient's convalescence after delivery.
   d. To prepare the patient to be better able to nurse the baby.
   e. To provide the essential building materials for the developing fetus.
   f. To protect and promote the health of the oral tissues of the mother.

TABLE 14.—APPOINTMENT RELATIONSHIPS TO PHYSICAL CHARACTERISTICS
OF THE PRENATAL PATIENT

Characteristic	Dental Hygiene Implication
Fatigues easily, may even fall asleep.	Short appointments; several in series, as needed.
Discomfort of remaining in one position too long.	Interrupt in middle of appointment to change chair position. Instruction in oral physical therapy may be given in middle of oral prophylaxis so that patient may be in upright position.
Backache.	Adjust chair appropriately for comfort.
Frequent urination.	Allow long enough appointment time for interruptions. Suggest at beginning of appointment that patient mention need for interruption.
General awkwardness because of size and shape.	Move bracket table out of way when patient is rinsing or sitting up. Attend to details such as gently lowering chair and straightening it for patient to get out. Make sure rinsing facilities are convenient; provide emesis basin during third trimester as necessary.
Faintness and Dizziness.	Be prepared for first aid. Have ammonia ampule ready (See Table 15, page 470).
Nausea and Vomiting *a.* Unpleasant taste in mouth. *b.* Gagging. *c.* Reactions to odors and flavors of medicaments and other office materials. *d.* Physician's recommendations for alleviation of symptoms: frequent eating of small amounts of foods, preferably carbohydrates.	Suggest toothbrushing or rinsing. Care in instrument and radiographic film placement. Attention to cleanliness of cuspidor. Determine particularly obnoxious odors for patient and remove them. Encourage use of starches rather than more readily fermentable carbohydrates, particularly if problem continues for several months; relate to dental caries initiation.
Unusual food cravings.	If cravings are for sweets, clearly define relationship of frequent nibbling of fermentable carbohydrate to dental caries.
Constipation.	Suggestions of desirable foods for oral health are related to prevention of constipation, particularly fresh fruits and vegetables.

2. Normal dietary needs of pregnancy[11]
    a. Caloric requirement: not increased.
    b. Basic needs: well planned diet containing a variety of foods which represent all of the basic food groups.[12]
    c. Increased needs
        (1) Protein: tissue building for mother and fetus.
        (2) Iron

> > > (a) For prevention of nutritional anemia in the mother and to meet the needs of the fetus, particularly in third trimester.
> > > (b) Source: usually a diet high in animal protein contains sufficient iron.
> > (3) Calcium and phosphorus
> > > (a) For all body tissues, both mother and fetus, particularly during third trimester when calcification of the fetus' bones and teeth is occurring.
> > > (b) Source: minimum of one quart of milk daily is generally considered sufficient. Milk is considered a better source than prescribed concentrates since there is greater absorbability and utilization of naturally occurring minerals.
> > > (c) Use in diet: when a patient does not care for plain milk, suggestions should be made for the preparation of milk-containing foods as well as the use of milk products such as cheese.
> > (4) Vitamins
> > > (a) Vitamin D: important for utilization of calcium and phosphorus.
> > > (b) Relation to gingival health: Vitamins A, B complex, and C are particularly important.
> > (5) Fluids: liberal amounts; at least 2 quarts total daily to maintain mother's fluid balance.
>
> d. Decreased needs
> > (1) Fermentable carbohydrates: particularly those eaten frequently as between-meal snacks since they are most effective in the initiation of dental caries.
> > (2) Salt: because of possible relationship of excess sodium to the toxemia of pregnancy.

3. Calcium and the mother's teeth[13-15]

There has been widespread misconception concerning the withdrawal of calcium from the mother's teeth and its relationship to dental caries. It is important to review the known facts and provide references for further reading on the subject since the patient's beliefs may need clarification. When discussing the problem a summary of the process of dental caries initiation will be helpful (see pages 113–115).

a. Minerals contained in the erupted tooth enamel and dentin are not available and no removal of minerals can occur by way of the pulp.

b. Minerals contained within the alveolar bone are available as from other bones of the body. When the mother's diet does not contain sufficient calcium and phosphorus, her own reserve is utilized.

c. Majority of calcium and phosphorus of bones and teeth is added to fetus during the third trimester. Incidence of dental caries in the mother is not different during that period although the carious lesions may be larger if the teeth have been neglected throughout the pregnancy.

d. There is a definite tendency for the teeth of the fetus to develop and calcify normally in spite of the diet of the mother since the reserve in her bones is used.

C. Dental Caries Prevention

Certain patients believe that they have more dental caries due to pregnancy. Research has shown that this is not true, and that any relationship is an indirect one. Factors which produce dental caries are the same during pregnancy as at other times.[16]

1. Incidence: normal increment related to the usual effects of fermentable carbohydrates and the acid-forming bacteria of the dental plaque.
2. Factors which may contribute to apparent increase in dental caries rate
   a. Previous neglect: patient may not have kept regular appointment plan so that the existing dental caries during pregnancy represents an accumulation, possibly even of years.
   b. Diet during pregnancy: possible increase in intake of fermentable carbohydrates.
   (1) Unusual cravings may be for sweet foods.
   (2) Frequency of eating: patient may be eating every few hours for prevention of nausea and these foods may be cariogenic.
   c. Neglect of personal oral care procedures: lack of interest or laxity in toothbrushing or rinsing immediately following intake of fermentable carbohydrates.
3. Relationship of fluoride: there is no evidence to show that prenatal fluoride intake will influence the dental caries rate in the child.[17,18] When the community water supply is not fluoridated, dietary fluoride by prescription is advised for the baby after birth (see pages 197–198).

REFERENCES

1. MAIER, A. W. and ORBAN, B. J.: Gingivitis in Pregnancy, Oral Surg., Oral Med., & Oral Path., *2*, 334, March, 1949.
2. ORBAN, B. J. and WENTZ, F. M.: *Atlas of Clinical Pathology of the Oral Mucous Membrane.* 2nd ed., St. Louis, Mosby, 1960, pp. 110–111.
3. GLICKMAN, IRVING: *Clinical Periodontology*, 2nd ed. Philadelphia, Saunders, 1958, pp. 94–96, 153–157.
4. GRANT, D., STERN, I. B., and EVERETT, F. G.: *Orban's Periodontics*, 2nd ed. St. Louis, Mosby, 1963, pp. 124–125.
5. FITZPATRICK, E. and EASTMAN, N. J.: *Zabriskie's Obstetrics for Nurses*, 10th ed. Philadelphia, Lippincott, 1960, pp. 187–193.
6. CAPLAN, GERALD: Psychological Aspects of Maternity Care, Am. J. Pub. Health, *47*, 25, January, 1957.
7. SELDIN, H. M., SELDIN, S. D., and RAKOWER, WILLIAM: The Management of Pregnant Patients in Dental Practice, in Cameron, J. R.: Emergencies in Dental Practice. Dental Clinics of North America, July, 1957, pp. 417–429.
8. GLICKMAN: op. cit., pp. 763–764, 924–926.
9. ROUSE, G. P.: Pregnancy and Diabetes, Am. J. Nurs., *58*, 100, January, 1958.
10. CROASMUN, RUTH: Nursing Care of the Pregnant Diabetic, Am. J. Nurs., *58*, 101, January, 1958.
11. FITZPATRICK and EASTMAN: op. cit., pp. 146–151.
12. United States Department of Agriculture, Agricultural Research Service: *Essentials of an Adequate Diet.* Home Economics Research Report No. 3. Washington, D. C., United States Government Printing Office, November, 1957. 21 pp.
13. SCHOUR, ISAAC: Calcium Metabolism, Pregnancy, and Caries, J. Dent. Child., *12*, 22, 1st Quarter, 1945.
14. BURKET, L. W.: *Oral Medicine*, 4th ed. Philadelphia, Lippincott, 1961, pp. 251–253.
15. BAWDEN, J. W.: Calcium Metabolism During Pregnancy, J. Dent. Child., *30*, 93, 2nd Quarter, 1963.

16. SHAFER, W. G., HINE, M. K., and LEVY, B. M.: *Textbook of Oral Pathology*, 2nd ed. Philadelphia, Saunders, 1963, pp. 332–334.
17. STOOKEY, G. K., OSBORNE, J., and MUHLER, J. C.: Effects of Pre- and Postnatal Fluorides on Caries, Dent. Prog., *2*, 137, January, 1962.
18. DALE, P. P.: Prenatal Fluorides: the Value of Fluoride During Pregnancy, Am. Dent. A. J., *68*, 530, April, 1964.

SUGGESTED READINGS

COOLIDGE, E. D. and HINE, M. K.: *Periodontology*, 3rd ed. Philadelphia, Lea & Febiger, 1958, pp. 225–230.
KRESHOVER, S. J.: Prenatal Factors in Oral Pathologic Conditions, Oral Surg., Oral Med., & Oral Path., *13*, 569, May, 1960.
MACY, I. G., MOYER, E. Z., KELLY, H. J., MACK, H. C., DiLORETO, P. C., and PRATT, J. P.: Physiological Adaptation and Nutritional Status During and After Pregnancy, J. Nutrit., *52* (Supplement 1): 1–92, April, 1954.
MASTON, J. H.: The Dental Hygienist's Role in the Management of Pregnant Patients, Am. Dent. Hygienists' A. J., *32*, 57, April, 1958.

Chapter 41

FIRST AID

It is relatively easy to be skillful in techniques which are repeated each day. Emergency care through first aid measures is performed only occasionally, and in instances which involve lifesaving measures, may be performed once in many years. To be prepared for that rare moment is difficult, but the public expects an individual trained in a health profession to be able to act in an emergency. Periodic review of procedures is necessary if application is to be effective.

Emergencies may occur within or in the vicinity of the dental office or clinic. Readiness involves not only having knowledge of proper procedures but equipment kept in a convenient place. A quick, handy reference of first aid measures is important, preferably in the form of a posted chart which gives characteristic symptoms and related treatment.

The information included in this chapter is general and basic and no attempt is made to mention all types of emergencies which may arise, particularly those of involved traumatic injuries. The principle objectives are to list the symptoms and treatment of the more common emergencies which can occur and to provide a list of the equipment which should be readily available in every dental office. It is assumed that other references will be kept in the dental office and that all dental personnel will familiarize themselves with such sources of information.

As an auxiliary to the dentist, the dental hygienist needs to be familiar with all procedures required in emergencies. Resuscitation involving techniques such as oxygen administration, drug injection, or tracheotomy ordinarily would be carried out by the dentist. Knowledge of procedures and required equipment or materials is necessary in order that the dentist may have immediate and efficient assistance.

I. PREVENTION OF EMERGENCIES

A. Understanding the Patient's Needs

The carefully prepared medical and personal history with adequate follow-up consultation with the patient's physician for integration of dental and medical care can prevent many emergencies by alerting dental personnel to the individual patient's needs and idiosyncrasies. Factors which should be included in the patient's history have been listed in Tables 2 and 3 on pages 73 to 76.

1. Knowledge of specific physical conditions which may require first aid.
2. Knowledge of diseases for which the patient is or has been under the care of his physician and the type of treatment, particularly drugs currently being prescribed.
3. Information concerning allergies or drug reactions.

4. Reference to records of previous appointment experiences with the particular patient.
5. Observation of the patient's present physical and mental state.

B. **Preparation of the Patient for the Appointment**
1. Prevention of excess exertion on the part of a patient.
   a. Arrange time of appointment in accord with personal health requirements.
   b. Limit length of appointment.
2 Establishment of rapport; aid in allaying fears.
3. Use of premedication when indicated and recommended by physician and dentist.

II. **GENERAL PROCEDURES**[1]

A. **Seek Assistance** as required by the nature of the emergency.
1. When alone: judgment must be used to determine the proper moment to leave the patient to telephone the physician.
   a. Leave patient in a safe position.
   b. Perform immediate first aid when hemorrhage is present.
2. When summoning dentist from another part of the dental office care should be taken not to alarm other patients who may be present in the waiting room or other operatory.

B. **Lie Patient Flat** with head on level with rest of body when nature of emergency is not known; loosen tight clothing.

C. **Determine Most Urgent Problem** and attend to conditions in the order listed below.
1. Stop bleeding.
   a. Apply pressure to area with compress.
   b. Apply pressure to pressure point.
   c. Apply tourniquet only when other methods are inadequate.
2. Start artificial respiration when breathing has stopped.
3. Treat for shock (see Table 15).

D. **Keep Patient Warm:** eliminate drafts.

E. **Do Not Attempt to Give Liquids** to an unconscious patient or one with breathing difficulties until the nature of the problem is known.

F. **Keep Calm; Act Promptly** but not hastily; the incorrect procedure may be more harmful than none at all.

G. **Reassure the Patient.**

III. **FIRST AID FOR SPECIFIC CONDITIONS**

A. **Summary of Procedures:** Table 15 lists the symptoms and general procedures for treatment of common emergencies.

B. **Artificial Respiration**[2]
Some form of artificial respiration should be started immediately when it is determined that the patient has stopped breathing. The

mouth-to-mouth technique has been established as the most practical emergency ventilation of an individual of any age.

The objectives in any technique are to obtain and maintain an open air passageway from the lungs to the mouth and to provide for an alternate increase and decrease in the size of the chest, internally or externally, to move air in and out.

Mouth-to-mouth, Chest Pressure-arm Lift, and Back Pressure-arm Lift techniques are outlined below. In any method, when there is foreign matter in the mouth, it should be wiped out with the fingers or with a cloth wrapped around the fingers, before artificial respiration procedures are started.

1. *Mouth-to-mouth (or Mouth-to-nose) Method*
    a. Tilt the head back so the chin is pointing upward. Pull or push the mandible into a jutting position. This aids to move the base of the tongue away from the back of the throat.
    b. Open mouth wide and place it tightly over the patient's mouth. At the same time pinch the patient's nostrils closed. The patient's mouth may be closed and the operator's mouth may be placed tightly over the nose.
    c. Blow into the patient's mouth or nose. Determine immediately whether or not there is obstruction. Clear by rechecking patient's position, wiping the mouth, or otherwise attempting to dislodge foreign matter.
    d. Remove mouth, turn head to one side to listen for the return rush of air that indicates air exchange.
    e. Repeat blowing at a rate of approximately 12 breaths per minute.
    f. Child: take relatively shallow breaths depending on the size of the child, at a rate of approximately 20 per minute.
    g. Plastic airway: commercial device which may be kept in the dental office. It is inserted posterior to the patient's tongue. Blowing is at the same rate as by the direct method.

2. *Chest Pressure-arm Lift (Silvester) Method*
    a. Place patient in a face-up position and place something under the shoulders to allow the head to drop backward.
    b. Kneel at the patient's head, grasp his wrists, cross them, and press them over the lower chest. This should cause air to flow out.
    c. Immediately release the pressure and pull the arms outward and upward over his head and backward as far as possible. This should cause air to rush in.
    d. Repeat the cycle at a steady rate, approximately 12 per minute. Check the mouth frequently for obstructions. Turning the patient's head to one side may aid to prevent aspiration of foreign materials.

3. *Back Pressure-arm Lift Method*
    a. Place the patient face-down, bend his elbows and place his hands one over the other. Turn his head slightly to one side and extend it as far as possible. Be sure the chin is jutting out.
    b. Kneel at the head of the patient. Place hands on the flat of the patient's back so that the palms lie just below an imaginary line drawn between the armpits.

    c. Rock forward until the arms are approximately vertical and allow weight of body to exert steady, even pressure downward upon the hands.

    d. Immediately draw the patient's arms upward. Apply enough lift to feel resistance and tension at the patient's shoulders. Lower the arms to the ground.

    e. Repeat the cycle at a steady rate, approximately 12 per minute. Check the mouth frequently for obstructions.

TABLE 15.—FIRST AID REFERENCE CHART

Emergency	Symptoms	First Aid Procedures

HEMORRHAGE	Prolonged bleeding
	  a. Spurting blood: artery.
	  b. Oozing blood: vein.
		Compression over bleeding area
		  a. Apply gauze pack with pressure.
		  b. Bandage pack into place firmly where possible.
		Severe bleeding: digital pressure on pressure point of supplying vessel.

	Bleeding from tooth socket.	Pack with gauze. Have patient bite down firmly.
	Bleeding of an extremity.	Elevate the part: support with pillows or substitute. Apply tourniquet only in extreme case.
	Nosebleed.	Tell patient to breathe through mouth. Apply cold application to nose. Press nostril on bleeding side for a few minutes. Plug nostril with gauze (not cotton); leave end hanging out. Advise patient not to blow the nose for an hour or more.
RESPIRATORY FAILURE	Cessation of breathing. Cyanosis.	Lay patient down flat: turn head to one side. Check for and remove any foreign bodies or obstruction in mouth. Pull tongue forward. Perform artificial respiration. May require tracheotomy. May need oxygen administration.
SHOCK	Pale skin, sometimes cyanotic. Moist skin: cold, clammy. Restless; sometimes unconscious. Dilated pupils. Rapid and shallow breathing. Rapid pulse.	Place patient in recumbent position: head lower than rest of body. Turn head to one side. Keep warm and dry. Give fluids unless patient is nauseated or unconscious. Use stimulants unless patient has hemorrhage.
SYNCOPE (fainting)	Pale, gray face. Weakness, giddiness, dizziness, faintness. Profuse cold perspiration. Rapid pulse at first, followed by slow pulse. Shallow breathing. Loss of consciousness.	Place in recumbent position: lower back of dental chair so head is lower than feet. Loosen tight clothing. Place cold wet towel on forehead. Have patient inhale aromatic spirits of ammonia (ampule). Check room temperature; check drafts.

TABLE 15.—FIRST AID REFERENCE CHART (*Continued*)

Emergency	Symptoms	First Aid Procedures
HEART FAILURE[3]	Symptoms vary depending on cause (see pages 428–429).	*For all Cases* Be calm and reassure patient. Keep patient warm and quiet; restrict effort. Call physician.
	A. *With symptoms of fainting* Weak pulse. Pale face. May be unconscious. May have pain in heart region. Fails to recover rapidly as from fainting.	Place patient in recumbent position with legs raised. Have patient inhale aromatic spirits of ammonia (capsule). Administer oxygen.
	B. *With chest pain* Pain may radiate to arms, neck, jaw. Anxiety; fear.	Place patient in sitting position. Administer oxygen. Administer (or help patient to take) nitroglycerin tablet: place under tongue.
	C. *With shortness of breath* Red face. Conscious. Cannot breathe easily unless sitting or standing.	Place patient in sitting position. Administer oxygen.
	D. *When unconscious*	Place patient in recumbent position with legs raised. Make sure airway is open; administer oxygen. Administer artificial respiration for patient who is not breathing. May require closed chest cardiac resuscitation.
DIABETIC: INSULIN SHOCK	Hunger. Nervousness; trembling. Weakness. Abdominal pain; nausea. Sweating; possible drooling. Transient period of unconsciousness. Dizziness.	When conscious: feed patient sugar cubes, orange juice, or candy. When unconscious: call physician. No first aid procedures (see page 442).
EPILEPTIC SEIZURE	A. *Grand Mal* (see page 399). Pale face; may become cyanotic. Dilated pupils. Muscular contractions. Loss of consciousness. May bite tongue.	Prevent injury: move patient to open area on floor. Insert rubber mouth prop or instrument wrapped in towel between teeth. Place pad or pillow under head. Loosen tight belt or collar. Allow patient to sleep during post-convulsive period.
	B. *Petit mal* (see page 400) Brief loss of consciousness. Fixed posture. Rhythmic twitching of eyelids, eyebrows, or head. May be pale.	Take objects from patient's hands to prevent dropping.

TABLE 15.—FIRST AID REFERENCE CHART (*Continued*)

Emergency	Symptoms	First Aid Procedures
DISLOCATED JAW	Mouth is open: patient is unable to close.	Stand in front of seated patient. Wrap thumbs in towels and place on occlusal surfaces of mandibular posterior teeth. Curve fingers and place under body of the mandible. Press down and back with thumbs and at same time pull up and forward with fingers. As joint slips into place, quickly move thumbs outward. Place bandage around head to support jaw.
BURNS	*First degree:* skin reddened. *Second degree:* blisters. *Third degree:* severe damage, skin burned off.	*Minor burn* Apply sterile petroleum jelly or burn ointment. Cover with sterile gauze pack. Chemical: wash with water; where possible hold under running water. *Serious burn* Do not apply petroleum jelly or ointment. Cover loosely with nonadherent dressing to permit comfort and protect from air and dust. Seek medical attention.
	Chemical burn of oral mucous membrane.	Have patient rinse with solution of bicarbonate of soda immediately.
INTERNAL POISONING	Nausea. Evidence from empty container or information from patient.	Give fluid in large amounts to dilute the substance. Have patient swallow strong bicarbonate of soda solution to induce vomiting. Administer universal antidote.
FOREIGN BODY IN EYE	Tears. Blinking.	Wash hands. Ask patient to look down. Bring upper lid down over lower lid for a moment; move it upward. Turn down lower lid and examine: if particle is visible remove with moistened cotton applicator. Use eye cup: wash out eye with mild boric acid solution. When unsuccessful, seek medical attention: prevent patient from rubbing eye by placing gauze pack over eye and stabilizing with adhesive tape.

IV. FIRST AID MATERIALS FOR THE DENTAL OFFICE

A. Reference Materials

1. Books: examples:
   a. American Red Cross, *First Aid Textbook*.[4]
   b. American Dental Association, *Accepted Dental Remedies*.[5]
   c. Equitable Life Assurance Society of the United States, *Home Health Emergencies*.[6]
2. Telephone numbers
   a. Number for each patient's physician in convenient reference place in permanent record.
   b. Numbers available at dental office telephone.
      (1) Physicians who may be called when patient's physician is not available or distance is too great for immediate assistance.
      (2) Fire department.
      (3) Police department.
      (4) Ambulance service.
      (5) Nearest hospital.
   c. For clinic or specialized dental practice: telephone number for each patient's dentist.

B. Contents of First Aid Kit

Every dental office should have a first aid kit and everyone in the office must be familiar with its contents and know where the kit is kept. The kit should be in order and its contents replenished and old materials replaced as needed.

The first aid equipment should be kept in a place readily accessible to the dental and dental hygiene operating rooms. Materials are kept separate from other office supplies and the kit plainly marked. Materials listed below are considered standard first aid equipment.[7,8]

1. Assorted bandages and dressings
   a. Adhesive compresses.
   b. Two and 3-inch bandage compresses.
   c. One and 2-inch bandage gauze.
   d. Two and 3-inch sterile compresses.
   e. Triangular bandages.
   f. Absorbent gauze: one-half square yard, 18 by 36 and 24 by 72 inches.
2. General equipment
   a. Blanket and pillow (not be kept in the kit, but should be readily available).
   b. Scissors.
   c. Cotton pliers.
   d. Sterile suture and needle holder.
   e. Rubber bite block (mouth prop).
   f. Eye rinsing cup.
   g. Tongue depressors.
   h. Safety pins.
   i. Hemostat.
   j. Plastic airway.
   k. Tourniquet.

3. Drugs and related substances
   a. Antiseptic solution.
   b. Bicarbonate of soda.
   c. Table salt.
   d. Sugar cubes or canned fruit juice.
   e. Ammonia ampules.
   f. Aromatic spirits of ammonia.
   g. Boric acid.
   h. Tube of burn ointment.
   i. Universal antidote.

C. **Oxygen Administration Equipment:** tank of oxygen, regulator valve, mask, breathing bag.

D. **Sterile Syringes:** 2, 5, 10 ml. capacity with sterile needles for intravenous, intramuscular, and subcutaneous injections.

REFERENCES

1. American National Red Cross: *First Aid Textbook*, 4th ed. New York, Doubleday, 1957, pp. 5–10.
2. American Red Cross: *Supplement on Artificial Respiration.* American Red Cross, 1086B, May, 1959 (January, 1962 printing). 14 pp.
3. American Dental Association and American Heart Association: Management of Dental Problems in Patients with Cardiovascular Disease, Am. Dent. A. J., *68*, 333, March, 1964.
4. American National Red Cross: op. cit. 241 pp.
5. American Dental Association, Council on Dental Therapeutics: *Accepted Dental Remedies*, current edition.
6. LARIMORE, G. W.: *Home Health Emergencies.* New York, Equitable Life Assurance Society, 1956. (Rev. and ed. by the Bureau of Public Health of the Medical Dept. of the Equitable Life Assurance Society.) 256 pp.
7. MacLEAN, D. G. and KIDWELL, M. K.: Seattle, University of Washington, Department of Physical Education for Women, personal communication.
8. American National Red Cross: op. cit., pp. 186–189.

SUGGESTED READINGS

BERLOVE, I. J.: *Dental-Medical Emergencies and Complications*, 2nd ed. Chicago, Year Book, 1963, 491 pp.
DOBBS, E. C.: Prevention and Treatment of Dental Office Emergencies, Am. Dent. Hygienists' A. J., *36*, 107, 3rd Quarter, 1962.
DOBKIN, A. B. and BROOK, M.: Management of Sudden Collapse in the Dental Chair, J. Oral Surg., Anes., and Hosp. D. Serv., *19*, 122, March, 1961.
ERICKSON, R. I. and HALE, M. L.: Effective and Simplified Method for Cardiac Resuscitation, J. Oral Surg., Anes., and Hosp. D. Serv., *19*, 322, July, 1961.
EVON, W. J.: Resuscitation in the Dental Office, Canad. Dent. A. J., *29*, 1, January, 1963.
FREEDMAN, S. O.: Medical Emergencies in Dental Practice, Dental Clinics of North America, July, 1963, p. 513.
GEHRIG, J. D.: Dental Emergencies, in Dille, J. M.: *Drug Therapy for Dentists.* Chicago, Year Book, 1963, pp. 185–218.
GORDON, A. S., *et al*: Mouth-to-mouth Versus Manual Artificial Respiration for Children and Adults, J.A.M.A., *167*, 320, May 17, 1958.
KOGAN, STANLEY: Medical Emergencies for Dentists, Oral Surg., Oral Med., & Oral Path., *11*, 246, March, 1958; *11*, 359, April, 1958.
LITWIN, R. I. and SNEDDON, E. A.: Simplified Approach to Cardiac Arrest, Oral Surg., Oral Med., & Oral Path., *14*, 1283, November, 1961.
MONHEIM, L. M.: Emergencies in the Dental Office, P.D.M., July, 1963, 46 pp.
ROSENCRANS, M. and MALKIN, M.: Chart to Aid in the Management of Dental Office Emergencies, Dent. Digest, *68*, 65, February, 1962.
RYAN, M. M.: First Aid in the Dental Office, Am. Dent. Hygienists' A. J., *31*, 104, July, 1957.
SADOVE, M. S. and WYANT, G. M.: Principles of Resuscitation in the Dental Office, Am. Dent. A. J., *53*, 168, August, 1956.

DENTAL TERMINOLOGY: IMPORTANT PREFIXES, SUFFIXES AND COMBINING FORMS

IT has been estimated that 75 per cent of the medical and dental terminology in current use is derived from either the Latin or Greek language.* A knowledge of fundamental vocabulary principles will aid in the interpretation of new scientific terms in the literature.

a-, an- Absence of, not, without.
ab- From, away, off.
ac-, ad- To, toward.
-algia Pain.
ante- Before.
anti- Against, opposite.
auto- Self, same.
aux- Increase.

bi- Two, twice.
-bio- Life.
brady- Slow.
bucc- Cheek.

-cardi- Heart.
cata- Down, negative.
-cele- Distention, swelling; tumor.
-cephal- Head.
cervic- Neck.
cheil- Lip.
-chlor- Green.
-chrom- Color.
-cide Cut, kill.
co- With, together.
-coma- Sleep.
contra- Against, opposite.
cut- Skin.
cyan- Blue.
-cyt- Cell.

dactyl- Finger, toe.
de- Down, away.
dent- Tooth.
-derma- Skin.
di- Two, twice.
dia- Through, across, between.
digit- Finger, toe.
dis- Apart, away from.
dur- Hard.

dys- Painful, bad, improper.

ec-, ect- Out of, outside.
-ectomy Cutting out.
em-, en-, end- Inside, within, on.
-emia (-aemia) Blood.
-encephal- Brain.
epi- On, above, after, in addition.
-erythr- Red.
ex-, extra- Outside, beyond.

faci- Face.

-galact- Milk.
-gastr- Stomach, abdomen.
-gen-, -genic Producing, originate.
germ- Bud, a growing thing in its early stages.
-gloss- Tongue.
glyc- Glucose, sugar.
-gnath- Jaw.
-gnosis Knowledge.
-gram, -graph- Write, record.
gran- Grain, particle.
-gyn- Woman, wife.

hem- (haem-) Blood.
hemi- One-half.
-hepat- Liver.
heter- Other, different.
-hist- Tissue.
hom- Same, common.
hydr- Water.
hyper- Over, excessive, above.
hypn- Sleep.
hypo- Beneath, under, less than.

-ia Pertaining to disease.

*DALY, L. W.: Fundamentals of Medical Etymology, in Arey, L. B., Burrows, William, Greenhill J. P., and Hewitt, R. M., Eds.: *Dorland's Illustrated Medical Dictionary*, 23rd ed. Philadelphia, Saunders, 1957, p. 1583.

(475)

-ic Pertaining to or belonging to.
idio- One's own, separate and distinct.
im-, in- In, on; not, without.
infra- Beneath.
inter- Between, together, among.
intra- Within, inside.
is- Equal, alike, same.
-ist One who does.
-itis Inflammation.

-kerat- Horny.
-kyanos- Blue.

labio- Lip.
-lact- Milk.
-laryng- Windpipe.
later- Side.
leuco-, leuko- White.
lingu- Tongue.
-lip- Fat.
-logy Science or study of.
lymph- Water; pertaining to lymph.
-lysis Breaking down, decomposition.

macr- Large.
mal- Bad, abnormal.
medi- Middle.
mega- Large, great, multiple.
-melan- Black.
mes- Middle.
-meter-, metr- Measure.
micr- Small.
mon- One, alone.
morph- Form, shape.
-my- Muscle.

nas- Nose.
ne- New, young.
-necr- Death, corpse.
-nephr- Kidney.
neur- Pertaining to nerves.

-odont- Tooth.
-oid Like or resembling, form.
-ology A science or branch of knowledge.
-oma Tumor, neoplasm, swelling.
-opia Sight.
or- Mouth.
-orth- Straight.
-osis Production, condition, process.
-oss-, -oste- Bone.
-otic Suffering from.

path- Sickness, disease.
ped- Child; feet.
peri- Around.
-phag Eat.
-phi- Like, have affinity for, loving.
-phleb- Vein.
-phob- Fear, dread.
-plasia Formation.
-pleg-, -plex- Strike.
-pne- Breathing, trauma to.
-pneum- Breath, air; lung.
pont- Bridge.
pre- Before, in front of.
pro- Giving rise to, before.
pseud- False.
-psych- Soul, mind.
pulmo- Lung.
pur-, pyo- Pus.

-renal Kidney.
retro- Backward.
-rhag- Break, burst forth.
-rhe, -rhea Flow.
-rhin- Nose.

sarc- Flesh, muscle.
-scler- Hard.
semi- Half.
sial- Saliva.
-soma, -some Body.
squam- Scale.
-stasis Position; halt of flow.
-sthen- Strength.
-stom- Mouth, orifice.
sub- Under, below.
super- Above, beyond, extreme.
syn- With, together.

tachy- Fast.
tact- Touch.
-tax-, -taxis Order, arrangement.
therm- Heat.
-thromb- Clot, coagulation.
-tome, -tomy Cutting.
-trophy Nourishment.

-ule Small.
ulo- Scar.

-vas- Vessel.

-xanth- Yellow, blond.

GLOSSARY

THIS brief glossary includes primarily the words which have been used but not defined in the text. Those defined in the text may be located through the Index. The meaning of words from the basic medical and dental sciences frequently can be determined from the list of word prefixes, suffixes and combining forms of the previous pages. A medical dictionary should be an important adjunct to guide professional reading.

Abrasion:
    of tooth: progressive loss of tooth structure by mechanical wear other than mastication, for example, abrasive dentifrice or habits of grinding hard objects with the teeth.
    of soft tissue: a spot rubbed bare of skin or mucous membrane.
Abrasive: material or substance used for grinding, polishing; tending to produce abrasion.
Abscess: a localized collection of pus in a cavity formed by the disintegration of tissues.
Absorption: taking up of fluids or other substances by the skin or mucous surfaces; passage of substances to the blood, lymph, and cells from the alimentary canal after digestion.
Abutment: a supporting structure to sustain lateral pressure; in dentistry, a terminal tooth which retains or supports a partial denture; for a fixed partial denture, it is attached to the denture proper by means of the retainer.
Accessory: subordinate, attached or added for convenience; contributing to a general effect.
Acid: compound having a sour taste and capable of neutralizing alkalis; pH below 7.0.
Acidogenic: acid forming or producing.
Acne vulgaris: a chronic inflammatory disease of the sebaceous glands which appears on the face, back, and chest in the form of eruptions.
Acquired characteristics: those obtained after birth, as a result of environment, use or disuse.
Acuity: sharpness or clearness, especially of the vision.
Acute: having rapid onset, short, severe course, and pronounced symptoms; opposite of chronic.
Adsorption: the attachment of one substance to the surface of another.
Aerobe: a microorganism that requires free oxygen to exist.
Agar: gelatin extracted from various seaweeds used as a nutrient solidifying agent in bacteriologic culture media.
Agglutination: state of being united; adhesion of parts; clumping, as bacteria or other cells.
Alkali: compound which reacts with acids to form salts, saponifies fat, and forms soluble carbonates; pH above 7.0.
Allergy: a hypersensitive state gained from exposure to a specific substance, re-exposure causes an altered capacity to react.
Alloy: a substance composed of two or more metals fused or melted together.
Amalgam: an alloy of two or more metals, one of which is mercury.
    Dental Amalgam: an alloy of silver, tin, copper, zinc, and mercury, used for dental restorations.
Ameloblast: epithelial cell of the enamel organ which functions in the formation of enamel.
Amorphous: lacking specific form or shape; unorganized.
Ampere: unit of quantity of electric current.
Amylase: an enzyme which converts starch into sugar.
Anaerobe: a microorganism that requires complete, or almost complete, absence of free oxygen to exist.
    Facultative anaerobe: microorganism that can exist under either aerobic or anaerobic conditions.
    Obligative anaerobe: microorganism that can exist only in the complete, absence of free oxygen because oxygen is toxic to it.

Analgesia: absence of sensibility to pain; loss of sensibility to pain without loss of consciousness; first stage of general anesthesia.

Anemia, nutritional: deficiency anemia; caused by some deficiency or fault in the diet or in nutrition.

Anesthesia: loss of feeling or sensation.

    General anesthesia: depressed state of consciousness.

    Local anesthesia: loss of sensibility to pain in a circumscribed area, not accompanied by loss of consciousness.

Ankylosis: union or consolidation of two similar or dissimilar hard tissues previously adjacent but not attached, as a tooth and its surrounding bone.

Anodontia: congenital absence of teeth; failure of teeth to form; may be partial or complete.

Anodyne: any agent which neutralizes or relieves pain.

Anomaly: deviation from the normal.

Anoxia: oxygen deficiency; a condition in which the cells of the body do not have or cannot utilize sufficient oxygen to perform normal function.

Antibiotic: a chemical substance produced by microorganisms, which, in dilute solutions, can destroy or inhibit the growth of bacteria and other microorganisms; used in the treatment of infectious diseases of man, animals and plants.

Antidote: a medicine or other remedy for counteracting the effects of poison.

    Universal antidote: a specifically prepared antidote sometimes containing tannic acid, magnesium oxide, and charcoal; used in counteracting poisoning by acids, alkaloids, glycosides, and heavy metals.

Antiseptic: a substance that will inhibit the growth and development of microorganisms without necessarily destroying them; term is applied to human tissue.

Apatite: inorganic compound with a complex formula containing calcium and phosphate; makes up the inorganic portion of bones and teeth; **fluorapatite,** containing fluoride radical, **hydroxyapatite,** containing hydroxyl radical.

Aphasia: defect of loss of the power of expression by speech, writing or signs, or of comprehending spoken or written language, due to injury or disease of the brain centers.

Aphtha: a little ulcer.

Aphthous ulcer: aphthous stomatitis; canker sore, vesicle which ruptures after one or two days and forms depressed, spherical, painful ulcer with elevated rim.

Aqueous: watery; prepared with water.

Armamentarium: the equipment, such as books, medicines, instruments, with which a practitioner supplies himself.

    Dental Hygiene Armamentarium: all the instruments and equipment used during a dental hygiene procedure.

    Dental Hygiene Instrumentarium: set of instruments used for a particular operation by the dental hygienist.

Articulation: the place where two or more bones of the skeleton join or unite; the contact relationship of the moving occlusal surfaces of opposing arches.

Artifact: in radiography, a substance or structure not naturally present in living tissues, but of which an authentic image appears in a radiograph.

Asepsis: condition in which septic, infective, putrefactive material is absent; prevention of admittance of microorganisms.

Asphyxia: suffocation or a temporary state of lifelessness as a result of cessation of breathing.

Aspirator: an apparatus employing suction.

Astringent: a substance which causes contraction or shrinkage and arrests discharges.

Atom: the smallest particle of an element which is capable of entering into a chemical reaction.

Atrophy: a defect or failure of nutrition manifested as a wasting or gradual reduction in the size of a cell, tissue or organ; usually applied to wasting that is secondary to some known cause.

Attenuation: the process by which a beam of radiation is reduced in energy when passing through some material.

Attrition: gradual, physiologic wearing away of tooth structure resulting from mastication.

Autoclave: an apparatus for effecting sterilization by high temperature obtained from steam under pressure.

Autonomic (involuntary) nervous system: division of the nervous system which supplies the sensory innervation for the glands, heart and smooth muscles. It is divided into the parasympathetic (craniosacral) and the sympathetic (thoracolumbar) systems.

Auxiliary: giving support; helping; aiding; assisting.

Backscatter: radiation deflected by scattering processes at angles greater than 90 degrees to the original direction of the beam of radiation.

Bacteremia: presence of bacteria in the blood stream. It may be transient, intermittent or continuous.

Bacterial spore: a resistant form of bacteria encapsulated by a thick cell wall which enables the cell to survive in environments unfavorable to immediate growth and division; not a reproductive mechanism.

Bactericidal: capable of destroying bacteria.

Bacteriostatic: capable of inhibiting the growth and multiplication of bacteria.

Basal metabolism: the least amount of energy utilized by the body in as nearly a completely resting condition as possible.

Base: a compound which reacts with an acid to form a salt; pH above 7.0.

Benign: as applied to tumors: grow slowly, are not recurrent or malignant, and do not metastasize.

Bevel: the inclination one line or surface makes with another when they are not at right angles.

Bifid: cleft into two parts or branches.

Biopsy: the removal and examination, usually microscopic, of a section of tissue or other material from the living body for the purposes of diagnosis.

Bite-wing radiographic survey: dental radiographs which show the coronal portions of maxillary and mandibular teeth, used for detecting deviations in the structure or form of the proximal surfaces of teeth or interseptal bone.

Body mechanics: proper balance of the skeleton by muscular alignment which favors function with the least amount of expended energy; refers to a dynamic position as opposed to **posture** which is alignment in a rigid position.

Bruxism: grinding of the teeth in other than chewing movements of the mandible; nocturnal grinding.

Buffer: any substance in a fluid which tends to lessen the change in hydrogen ion concentration (reaction) which otherwise would be produced by adding acids or alkalis.

Bulla: large blister or cutaneous vesicle filled with serous fluid.

Burnish: to make smooth and bright; to polish by friction.

Calcification: the process by which organic tissue becomes hardened by a deposit of calcium and other inorganic salts within its substance.

Cancer: malignant and invasive growth or tumor.

Canker sore: see **Aphthous ulcer.**

Carbohydrate: organic compound of carbon, hydrogen and oxygen; includes starches, sugars, cellulose; formed by plants and used for growth and source of energy.

Carcinoma: a malignant, new, epithelial growth which tends to metastasize; cancer.

Caries: see **Dental caries.**

Cariogenic: caries producing; conducive to caries.

Carious: affected with caries or decay; in dentistry, a carious lesion is a cavity in a tooth which is the result of dental caries.

Carrier: an individual who harbors in his body the organisms of a specific disease without observable symptoms and who transmits the infection to others.

Cartilage: firm, elastic, flexible connective tissue which is attached to articular bone surfaces and which forms certain parts of the skeleton.

Cassette: light-tight container in which x-ray films are placed for exposure to x-radiation; usually backed with lead to eliminate the effect of backscattered radiation.

Cataract: a clouding or opacity of the lens of the eye which leads to blurring of vision and eventual loss of sight.

Caustic: an agent which burns or corrodes; destroys living tissue; having a burning taste.

Cauterize: to burn, corrode, or destroy living tissue by means of a caustic substance, heated metal, or an electric current.

Central Ray: a hypothetical *x*-ray whose direction of travel corresponds to the geometric center of a useful beam of *x*-radiation.

Cephalometer: an orienting device for positioning the head for radiographic examination and measurement.

Cephalometrics: scientific study of the measurements of the head.

Cheilosis: a condition marked by fissuring and dry scaling of the surface of the lips and angles of the mouth; characteristic of riboflavin deficiency.

Chronic: long continued; opposite of acute.

Clinic: an establishment where patients are admitted for study and treatment by a group of practitioners.

Clinical: pertaining to a clinic or to the actual observation and treatment of patients, as distinguished from theoretical or experimental.

Coagulation: changing of a soluble into an insoluble protein; process of changing into a clot.

Col: concavity of the interdental gingiva; ridge-shaped depression between two peaks formed by the buccal and lingual papillae.

Communicable: capable of being transmitted from one person to another.

Compatible: capable of existing together in harmony; with medications, suitable for simultaneous administration.

Concentration: a solution which has been strengthened by the evaporation of its nonactive parts.

Conduction: the transfer of sound waves, heat, nerve influences or electricity.

Cone: an accessory device on a dental *x*-ray machine designed to indicate the direction of the central axis of its *x*-ray beam and to serve as a guide in establishing a desired source-to-film distance. Such "cones" may be conical or tubular in form; provision for beam collimation and/or added filtration is often incorporated in the construction of the "cone."

Congenital: existing at or before birth.

Contracture: shortening or distortion; permanent as from shrinkage of muscles, or temporary from sudden stimulus.

Contaminate: to render impure by contact or mixture; in sterile technique, to introduce microorganisms.

Convalescence: the gradual recovery of health and strength after illness.

Coronary: encircling in the manner of a crown; a term applied to vessels, nerves, ligaments.

Corrode: to eat away or wear away, as by rust, causing deterioration of a substance.

Crepitation: a crackling sound; noise made by rubbing together the ends of a broken bone.

Cryptogenic: of obscure, doubtful or undeterminable origin.

Curet (Fr. curette): spoon-shaped instrument with its peripheral edges sharpened to facilitate removal of material.

Curettage: application of a curet to a tissue in order to remove debris or a portion of the tissue; a surgical procedure; in periodontics, the technique is applied to the tissues comprising the periodontal pocket, primarily the lining of the gingival sulcus and the cementum.

Current: the number of electrons per second passing a given point on a conductor. Electrons are negatively charged and move toward the positive.

Cuticle, primary: a delicate membrane covering the crown of a newly erupted tooth; produced by the ameloblasts after they produce the enamel rods.

Cuticle, secondary: appears on both enamel and cementum, is formed in the course of eruption, is keratinous, homogenous, and occurs external to the primary cuticle on the enamel. On the cementum it appears as a thin homogenous, noncellular keratinous structure.

Cyanosis: blueness of the skin often due to insufficient oxygenation of the blood.

Cyst: a sac, normal or pathologic, containing fluid or other material.

Dentigerous cyst: formed by a dental follicle, containing one or more well-formed teeth.

Radicular cyst: an epithelial lined sac, formed at the apex of a pulpless tooth, containing cystic fluid.

Debridement: removal of debris, foreign material, or devitalized tissue.

Decalcification: process by which calcium salts and other inorganic substances are removed.

Degeneration: change from a higher to a lower form; especially change of tissue to a less functional form.

Dehydration: removal of water; the condition which results from undue loss of water.

Dental Caries: a disease of the calcified structures of the teeth, characterized by decalcification of the mineral components and dissolution of the organic matrix. The word has no plural.

Denticle: a pulp stone; relatively large body of calcified substance in the pulp chamber of a tooth.

Dentition: the kind, size, and arrangement of the teeth.

    Primary (deciduous) dentition: the first teeth; normally will be shed and replaced by permanent teeth.

    Mixed dentition: combination of both primary and permanent teeth present in the oral cavity; state occurs when the first permanent molars erupt and extends until the last primary tooth is exfoliated.

    Permanent dentition: teeth which must function throughout the adult life.

    Succedaneous dentition: permanent teeth that erupt in positions of exfoliated primary teeth.

Denture, complete: an appliance which restores all of the natural teeth and their associated parts in a dental arch.

Denture, fixed partial (bridge): a structure which restores one or more but fewer than all the natural teeth in a dental arch, and is held in position by permanent attachments to the adjacent teeth which furnish the support.

Denture, removable partial: an appliance which restores one or more but fewer than all the natural teeth in a dental arch, and which depends on the oral mucosa for its support and on the natural teeth for retention and secondary support; can be removed readily by the patient.

Denudation: laying bare; surgical or pathologic removal of epithelial covering.

Depressant: a substance which reduces functional activity and the vital energies in general by producing muscular relaxation and perspiration.

Desensitization: process of removing the reactivity or sensitivity.

Desquamation: the shedding of epithelial elements, chiefly of the skin, in scales or sheets.

Detergent: agent which cleanses, purifies.

Detritus: debris which adheres to tooth surfaces.

Devitalize: to deprive of vitality or of life; in dentistry, to destroy the vitality of the dental pulp.

Diagnosis: the process of determining by examination the nature and circumstances of a diseased condition; the decision reached as to the nature of a disease.

    Differential diagnosis: the art of distinguishing one disease from another.

Diastema: a space or cleft; in dentistry, a space between teeth.

Diet: the customary allowance of food and drink taken by a person from day to day.

Dietary: a regular or systematic scheme of diet.

Diffuse: widely spread; not definitely limited or localized.

Digital: of, pertaining to, or performed with a finger.

Dilate: to make wider or larger; cause to expand.

Dilution: a form of something which has been made weaker or thinner by the addition of water or the like.

Discrete: separate, not together; characterized by lesions which do not become blended.

Distilled water: water which has been subjected to a process of vaporization and subsequent condensation for purification.

Distortion: (radiographic) deviation of a radiographic image from the true outline or shape of an object or structure.

Dorsum: the back surface or a part similar to the back in position.

Duct: a passage with well-defined walls; especially a tube for the passage of excretions or secretions.

Dyscrasia: abnormal composition of the blood.

Dysplasia: disharmony between component parts; developmental abnormality.

Dystrophy: defective or faulty nutrition within a tissue or organ manifested by wasting and atrophy.

Ecchymosis: black and blue discoloration of the skin caused by the escape of blood from the vessels into the tissues; bleeding into the subcutaneous tissues.

Edema: collection of abnormally large amounts of fluid in the intercellular spaces, causing swelling.

Pitting edema: pressure on edematous area causes pits which remain for prolonged period after pressure is released.

Edentulous: without teeth.

Electron: a negatively charged elementary particle constituent in every neutral atom.

Emaciation: condition of excessive leanness or wasted body tissues.

Embolism: sudden blocking of an artery or vein by a clot or obstruction which has been brought to its place by the blood current.

Embryo: the fetus in its earlier stages of development, especially before the end of the second month.

Emesis basin: a basin, usually kidney shaped, used for receiving material expectorated or vomited.

Emollient: softening or soothing; an agent used to soften the skin or other body surface.

Endemic: present in a community or among a group of people; the continuing prevalence of a disease as distinguished from an epidemic.

Endocardium: the endothelial lining membrane of the heart.

Endodontics: that branch of dentistry concerned with the etiology, diagnosis, and treatment of diseases of the dental pulp and their sequelæ.

Enzyme: an organic compound, frequently protein in nature, which can accelerate or produce by catalytic action some change in a specific substance.

Epidemic: affecting at the same time a large number of persons in a locality; usually applied to a disease which spreads from person to person which is not prevalent permanently in the area.

Epiphysis: a piece of bone which is separated from a long bone in early life by cartilage, but later becomes a part of the long bone; the site of growth of long bones.

Epithelization: growth of epithelium over a raw surface.

Epithelize, epithelialize: to cover or become covered with epithelium.

Erosion: progressive loss of tooth structure by a chemical process without the aid of bacteria which appears as a sharply defined wedge-shaped depression in the cervical area of the facial surface; area is smooth, hard and polished.

Eruption: the act of breaking out, appearing or becoming visible; a visible pathologic lesion of the skin, marked by redness, swelling, or both.

Erythema: abnormal redness of the skin due to local congestion; may result from inflammation or excess exposure to x-ray.

Escharotic: corrosive; capable of producing sloughing.

Ethics: the science of right conduct; a system of rules or principles governing the conduct of a professional group planned by them for the common good of man; the principles of morality.

Etiology: the science or study of the cause of disease; that which is known about the causes of a disease.

Euphoria: well-being; absence of pain or distress; in psychiatry, an abnormal or exaggerated sense of well-being.

Exfoliate: to fall off in scales or layers; in dentistry, to shed primary teeth.

Exodontics: that branch of dentistry concerned with the extraction of teeth.

Exudate: the material composed of serum, fibrin, and white blood cells in variable amounts that escapes from blood vessels into a superficial lesion of an area of inflammation.

Extirpation: complete removal or eradication of a part; in dentistry, the removal of the dental pulp from the pulp chamber and root canal.

Extrusion: the condition of a tooth which has erupted beyond the plane of occlusion.

Febrile: pertaining to fever; feverish.

Fermentable: term applied to a substance which is capable of undergoing chemical change as a result of the influence of an enzyme; usually applied to substances which break down to an acid or an alcohol; applied to carbohydrate breakdown to form acid in the dental plaque.

Fetus: the unborn offspring in the uterus after the second month.

Fibrosis: the formation of fibrous connective tissue.

Film badge: a pack containing a radiographic film or films to be used for the detection and measurement of radiation exposure in personnel monitoring.

Fistula: a narrow passage or duct leading from one cavity to another, as from a periapical abscess to the oral cavity.

Flash point: lowest temperature at which a volatile oil will give off explosive or ignitable vapors.

Flora: bacterial content of a given region or locality.

Oral flora: the bacterial content of the oral cavity.

Fluorescence: emission of radiation of a particular wave length by certain substances as the result of absorption of radiation of shorter wave length. The emission occurs only during the irradiation as contrasted to phosphorescence.

Fluoroscope: a fluorescent screen suitably mounted with respect to an x-ray tube for ease of observation and protection, used for the indirect visualization by means of x-rays of internal structures in living organisms or inanimate objects.

Focal infection: the metastasis from a focus of infection of organisms or their toxins that is capable of injuring tissue.

Focus of infection: a circumscribed area of tissue which is infected with pathogenic micro-organisms and which is usually located near a mucous or cutaneous surface.

Fog: darkening of the whole or part of a developed radiograph from sources other than the radiation of the primary beam to which the film was exposed.

Chemical fog: darkening due to imbalance or deterioration of processing solutions.

Light fog: darkening due to unintentional exposure to light to which the emulsion is sensitive, either before or during the processing.

Radiation fog: darkening due to radiation from sources other than intentional exposure to the primary beam, for example, scatter radiation, film storage not protected from radiation.

Follicle (dental): the sac that encloses the developing tooth before its eruption.

Forceps: a two-bladed instrument with handles for pulling, compressing, or grasping.

Friable: easily broken or crumbled.

Friction: the rubbing of one surface against another; the resistance to sliding or rolling motion of surfaces in contact.

Furcation: area or region lying between and at the base of two or more normal anatomically divided roots.

Germicide: anything that destroys bacteria; applied especially to chemical agents that kill disease germs, but not necessarily bacterial spores: applied to both living tissue and in-animate objects.

Gerodontics: that branch of dentistry which treats all problems peculiar to the oral cavity in old age and aging including clinical problems of senescence and senility.

Glaucoma: a disease of the eye marked by intense intraocular pressure, resulting in hardness of the eye, atrophy of the retina, cupping of the optic disk and blindness.

Glossitis: inflammation of the tongue.

Glucose tolerance test: based upon the ability of the normal liver to absorb and store excessive amounts of glucose as glycogen. Following ingestion of 100 gm. of glucose, the fasting blood sugar promptly rises, then falls to normal within 2 hours. In a diabetic the increase is greater and the return to normal usually prolonged.

Grit: the size of abrasive particles, determined by the number of particles which, end to end, equals one inch; fine, stony, hard particles used for grinding.

Habilitation: application of measures which will assist a person in obtaining a state of health, efficiency and independent action; make over in an improved form.

Half value layer (HVL): the thickness, or surface density, of a layer of a specified material which attenuates the beam to such an extent that the exposure rate is reduced to one-half, under narrow beam conditions.

Halitosis: offensive or bad breath, may be related to systemic disease or uncleanliness of the oral cavity.

Health: state of complete physical, mental and social well-being, not merely the absence of disease.

Hemangioma: a benign tumor consisting chiefly of blood vessels.

Hematoma: a tumor containing effused blood.

Hemoglobin: the protein coloring matter of the red blood cells which conveys oxygen to the tissues; occurs as oxyhemoglobin in arterial blood and reduced hemoglobin in venous blood.

Hemorrhage: an escape of blood from the blood vessels.

Hemostat: an instrument or other agent used to arrest the escape or flow of blood.

Hepatitis: inflammation of the liver.

  Serum hepatitis: caused by a virus transmitted by human blood.

  Infectious hepatitis: caused by a virus transmitted by fecal contamination.

Heredity: physical or mental qualities inherited by offspring from their ancestry.

Homeostasis: equilibrium or harmony of cellular metabolism in relationship to cellular environment.

Hone: a fine grit stone used for sharpening a cutting instrument (noun); to sharpen (verb).

Hydrogen peroxide: clear, colorless liquid which is a strong oxidizing and bleaching agent.

Hydrolysis: a chemical process of decomposition involving addition of the elements of water.

Hygiene: the science which deals with the preservation of health.

Hygroscopic: readily absorbs moisture.

Hyperkeratosis: excessive formation of keratin on the superficial layers of the epithelium.

Hyperplasia: increase in size of a tissue or organ caused by the increase in number of cells in normal arrangement.

Hypertension: Pathologic elevation of the blood pressure.

Hypertonic: having excessive tone, tonicity or activity.

  Hypertonic solution: one which has a higher molecular concentration than another to which it is compared; of greater concentration than isotonic.

Hypertrophy: increase in size of a tissue or organ caused by the increase in size of its cells.

Hypnotic: inducing sleep.

Hypocalcification: deficiency in the mineral content of the enamel resulting from disturbance in the maturation phase during development; may be due to systemic, local or hereditary factors; dental fluorosis is an example of a systemic cause.

Hypoplasia: defective or incomplete development; enamel hypoplasia results when the enamel matrix formation is disturbed.

Hypotonic: having diminished tone, tonicity or activity.

  Hypotonic solution: one which has a lesser molecular concentration than another to which it is compared; of less concentration than isotonic.

Idiopathic: self-originated; of unknown cause.

Idiosyncrasy: any tendency, characteristic or the like, peculiar to an individual.

Immunity: ability to resist the development of a specific disease.

  Acquired immunity: that possessed as a result of having and recovering from a disease or from building up resistance against vaccines, toxins, or toxoids.

  Natural immunity: that which is inherited by the child from the mother or from the race.

  Passive immunity: that possessed as a result of injection of antibodies or antitoxins in serum from an immune individual or lower animal.

Incipient: beginning to exist; coming into existence.

Incubation: the keeping of a culture of bacteria in an incubator to facilitate development; **incubation period** used to denote the time between exposure to a communicable disease and the appearance of clinical symptoms.

Inert: without intrinsic active properties; no inherent power of action, motion, or resistance.

Infarct: a circumscribed portion of tissue which has suddenly been deprived of its blood supply by embolism or thrombosis and which results in necrosis of the tissue.

Infection: invasion of the body by pathogenic microorganisms and the body's response to the microorganisms and their toxic products; transfer of disease from one part to another or one person to another.

Inflammation: reaction of living tissue to trauma; reaction is characterized by heat, redness, swelling, pain, and loss of function.

Inhibitor: a chemical substance which arrests or restrains the action of a tissue organizer or the growth of microorganisms.

Inoculation: introduction of microorganisms or some substance into living tissues or culture media; introduction of a disease agent into a healthy individual to induce immunity.

Inorganic: not characterized by organization of living bodies or vital processes; also, pertaining to compounds not containing carbon, except cyanides and carbonates.

Insidious: stealthy, treacherous; having a more serious effect than is apparent.

Intensifying screen: a card or plastic sheet coated with fluorescent material, positioned in a cassette to contact the film in radiography, so that the visible light from its fluorescent image, when exposed to x-radiation, will add to the latent image being produced directly by x-radiation, on a film sensitive to both visible light and x-rays.

In vitro: outside the living body: in a test tube or other artificial environment.

In vivo: in the living body of a plant or animal.

Ion: an electrically charged atom or group of atoms.

  Anion: negatively charged ion which passes to the positive pole in electrolysis.

  Cation: positively charged ion which passes to the negative pole in electrolysis.

I.Q.: Intelligence Quotient; the relationship between intelligence and chronological age.

Irrigation: the covering or washing out of anything with water or other liquid for the purpose of making it moist, diluting another substance present, or cleaning the area.

Isotonic: having a uniform tonicity or tension.

  Isotonic solution: one which has the same molecular concentration as another to which it is compared.

Isotope: atom having the same atomic number but different atomic weight; isotopes of a particular element have virtually identical chemical properties.

Jaundice: condition in which there are bile pigments in the blood and deposition of bile pigments in the skin and mucous membranes with resulting yellowish appearance.

Kaolin: a fine white clay; used in pharmacy in ointments and for coating pills.

Keratinization: process of formation of a horny protective layer on the surface of stratified squamous epithelium of certain body surfaces including the epidermis and masticatory oral mucosa; **keratin,** a protein material, is formed as a transformation product of the cellular proteins of the flat cells on the surface of the epithelium; form of protective adaptation to function.

Kilovoltage: in x-ray machines, the potential difference between the anode and cathode of an x-ray tube.

Laceration: a wound produced by tearing or irregular cutting.

Latent: concealed, not apparent, hidden.

Lesion: any pathological hurt, wound, degeneration of structure or of functional capacity.

Lethargy: condition of drowsiness or sleepiness of mental origin.

Leukocyte: white or colorless blood cell concerned in the destruction of disease-producing microorganisms.

Leukoplakia: white plaque formed upon the oral mucous membrane from surface epithelial cells; premalignant surface lesion characterized by hyperkeratosis of the stratified squamous epithelium.

Lipid: one of a group of organic compounds which makes up the fats.

Local: restricted to one spot; not generalized.

Macroglossia: enlargement of the tongue.

Malaise: any vague feeling of illness, uneasiness or discomfort.

Malignant: as applied to tumors, rapidly growing, infiltrate into normal structures, metastasize, and if untreated invariably lead to death.

Malnutrition: imperfect assimilation and nutrition.

Mandrel: a spindle, axel, or shaft designed to fit a dental handpiece for the purpose of supporting a revolving instrument.

Manifestation: that which is made evident, especially to the sight and understanding.

Manikin: model of human body or a part used for teaching purposes.

Massage: manipulation of tissues for remedial or hygienic purposes with the hand or other instrument; the systematic application of frictional rubbing and stroking to the gingival tissues for cleansing purposes, for increasing the circulation of blood through the tissues and for increasing the keratinization of the surface epithelium.

Mastication: a series of highly coordinated functions involving the teeth, tongue, muscles of mastication, lips, cheeks and saliva, in the preparation of food for swallowing and digestion.

Matrix: the place or substance within which something originates, takes form, or develops.
>   **Amalgam matrix:**   thin piece of metal fastened around a tooth to support amalgam as it is placed in a cavity preparation.

Medication: use of medicine or medicaments for treatment of a disease.

Metabolism: alteration of food elements into tissue and tissue into energy.
>   **Anabolism:**   the total physical and chemical processes by which living organized substance is produced and maintained.
>   **Catabolism:**   the transformation by which energy is made available for the uses of the organism.

Micron: unit of linear measurement; one-thousandth of a millimeter.

Milliliter: one-thousandth part of a liter, usually abbreviated **ml.** It is approximately equal to 1 cubic centimeter.

Miscible: capable of being mixed.

Morphology: the science which deals with form and structure without regard to function.

Mucin: secretion of the mucous or goblet cell; a polysaccharide protein which, combined with water, forms a lubricating solution called mucus; contained in saliva.

Myocardium: heart muscle; muscular substance of the heart.

Nasmyth's membrane: see **Cuticle, primary.**

Necrosis: cell or tissue death within the living body.

Necrotizing ulcerative gingivitis: an acute, inflammatory, painful process with ulceration of the interdental papillæ; the tissues bleed easily, a pseudomembrane may be present, and an offensive mouth odor is usually associated with the necrosis.

Neoplasm: a new growth of different or abnormal tissue; tumor.

Neuromuscular: condition involving nerves and muscles.

Nidus: the point of origin or focus of a process.

Node: a swelling or protuberance which is solid and can be detected by palpation.

Nostrum: a quack, patent, or secret remedy.

Nutrition: sum of processes by which an animal or plant absorbs, or takes in and utilizes, food substances; ingestion, digestion, absorption (of products of digestion) of food materials through mucous membranes of the alimentary tract, transportation by blood and lymph to body cells where they are used or stored.

Obese: excessively fat.

Obstetrician: a physician who specializes in the management of pregnancy, labor, and the period of confinement after labor.

Obtundent: having the power to dull sensibility or soothe pain; a soothing or partially anesthetic medicine.

Odontalgia: toothache; pain in a tooth.

Odontoblast: connective tissue cell which functions in the formation of dentin.

Olfactory: pertaining to the sense of smell.

Ophthalmologist: physician with specialized training and experience who specializes in the diagnosis and treatment of eye diseases; one versed in **ophthalmology,** the sum of knowledge concerning the eye and its diseases. (obsolete term: oculist).

Optician: technician who grinds and fits lenses; a maker of optical instruments or glasses.

Optometrist: one who practices **optometry,** the measurement of visual acuity and the fitting of glasses to correct visual defects; a term adopted by opticians who prescribe and fit glasses.

Oral surgery: the dental specialty encompassing all of the surgical diseases, injuries, and developmental abnormalities of the oral cavity, teeth, jaws and adjacent structures.

Orthodontics: the clinical science that has for its objective the prevention and correction of dental and oral anomalies; that branch of dentistry concerned with the etiology, diagnosis, prevention, and correction of malocclusion of the teeth and associated dento-facial disharmonies.

Osmosis: the passage of a solvent through a semipermeable membrane into a solution of higher molecular concentration thus equalizing the concentrations on either side of the membrane.

Osteoblast: cell whose activity initiates the formation of new bone.

Osteoclast: large multinucleated cell which brings about the resorption of bone; found only during the process of active bone or root resorption.

Osteomyelitis: inflammation of the bone caused by a pyogenic microorganism. It may remain localized or spread through the bone.

Osteoporosis: abnormal decrease in density of bone by the enlargement of its canals or the formation of abnormal spaces.

Otolaryngologist: medical specialist who treats the ears, throat, pharynx, larynx, nasopharynx, and tracheobronchial tree.

Palliative: affording relief but not cure.

Pallor: paleness; absence of skin coloring.

Palpation: the act of applying fingers lightly to the surface of the body to determine the consistency of the parts beneath in physical diagnosis.

Palpitation: rapid beating of the heart.

Parasympathetic nervous system: craniosacral division of the autonomic nervous system; composed of the ocular, bulbar, and sacral divisions.

Pedodontics: that branch of dentistry concerned with the etiology, diagnosis, and treatment of diseases of children's teeth.

Percussion: a diagnostic aid which consists of striking a part with short, sharp blows and listening to the vibrations produced to determine the condition of the parts below.

Periapical: around the apex of a tooth.

Periapical tissues: the tissues surrounding the apex of a tooth, including the periodontal ligament (membrane), and the alveolar bone.

Pericardium: the membranous sac which contains the heart.

Periodontal care: for the patient with periodontal disease: consists of effective treatment for the elimination of disease and the creation of conditions conducive to the maintenance of periodontal health.

Periodontal care, maintenance phase: after or between phases of active therapy; requires close supervision to prevent recurrence of periodontal disease; includes control of calculus formation, diet and oral physical therapy supervision, follow-up radiographs, complete operative care.

Periodontics: the practice of periodontology.

Periodontium: the tissues which surround, support, and are attached to the teeth; includes gingiva, cementum, periodontal ligament (membrane), and alveolar bone.

Periodontology: the clinical science that deals with the periodontium in health and disease; that branch of dentistry concerned with the etiology, diagnosis, and treatment of diseases of the supporting structures of the teeth.

Petechia: small spot formed by the escape of blood into the tissue.

Petri plate: a small shallow dish of thin glass with a loosely fitting, overlapping cover, used for plate cultures in microbiology.

pH: symbol commonly used to express hydrogen ion concentration, the measure of alkalinity and acidity. Normal (neutral) pH is 7.0. Above 7.0 the solution is alkaline; below, acid.

Phosphorescence: emission of radiation by a substance as a result of previous absorption of radiation of shorter wave length; contrasts with fluorescence in that the emission may continue for a time after cessation of the ionizing radiation.

Physiologic saline solution: a 0.9 per cent sodium chloride solution which exerts an osmotic pressure equal to that exerted by the blood, thus is compatible with blood.

Pipette: a slender graduated tube for measuring and transferring liquids from one vessel to another.

Plasma: fluid portion of the blood (serum and fibrinogen) without formed elements; fluid portion of the lymph without its corpuscles or cells.

Pocket: a gingival sulcus pathologically deepened by periodontal disease.

Polyethylene: a synthetic plastic material.

Pontic: the suspended member of a fixed partial denture; it replaces the lost natural tooth, restores its functions, and usually occupies the space previously filled by the natural crown.

Precipitate: to cause a substance in solution to settle down in solid particles.

Predisposition: a concealed but present susceptibility to disease which may be activated under certain conditions.

Premaxilla: the intermaxillary bone situated in front of the maxilla proper; carries the incisor teeth.

Premedication: preliminary treatment usually with a drug, to prevent untoward results which may be affected by the operation to be performed.

Prescribe: to designate or recommend a remedy for administration; to direct in writing the dosage, preparation and dispensing of a remedy or drug.

Primate space: diastema or gap in tooth row occasionally observed in primary dentition. Characteristic of almost all species of Primate except Man. Maxillary primate spaces accommodate mandibular cuspids and mandibular primate spaces accommodate maxillary cuspids when teeth are in occlusion. Reduced length of cuspids accompanied Man's evolution so cuspids no longer protruded beyond occlusal level and diastema was no longer functional.

Prognosis: a forecasting of the probable course and termination of a disease; the prospect as to recovery from a disease as indicated by the nature and symptoms of the case.

Proliferation: reproduction or multiplication of similar forms.

Prone: flat, prostrate; **prone position,** lying flat.

Prosthodontics: that branch of dentistry concerned with the replacement of missing teeth or other oral tissues by artificial means.

Protective Barrier: barriers of radiation-absorbing material such as lead, concrete or plaster which serve to reduce radiation hazards.

Protein: any one of a group of complex organic nitrogenous compounds widely distributed in plants and animals and which form the principle constituents of cell protoplasm. They are essentially combinations of alpha amino acids and their derivatives.

Proteolytic: effecting the digestion of proteins.

Protoplasm: the only known form of matter in which life is apparent; it composes the essential material of all plant and animal cells.

Protrusion: condition of being thrust forward as the protrusion of the anterior teeth.

Psychiatry: that branch of medicine which deals with disorders of the mind.

Psychosomatic: pertaining to the mind-body relationship; having body symptoms of a psychic, emotional or mental origin.

Ptyalin: an enzyme occurring in the saliva which converts starch into maltose and dextrose.

Pulp stone: see **Denticle.**

Pyorrhea: a purulent discharge; discharge of pus.

Quadrant: any one of the four parts or quarters of the dentition with the dividing line of the maxillary or mandibular teeth at the midline between the central incisors.

Radiation, ionizing: any electromagnetic or particulate radiation capable of producing ions, directly or indirectly, in its passage through matter.

Radiology: the science of the study and use of radiant energy, including x-rays, radium, and radioactive isotopes, as applied to dentistry and medicine.

Radiolucent: a substance, which because of its lack of density, permits the passage of x-rays with only very slight resistance; radiolucent objects appear dark on radiographs.

Radiopaque: a substance, which because of its density, resists the passage of x-rays; radiopaque objects appear light on radiographs.

Radioresistant: relatively resistant to injury by ionizing radiation.

Radiosensitive: relatively susceptible to injury by ionizing radiation.

Raphe: a ridge, furrow, or seam-like union between two parts or halves of an organ or structure.

Rarefaction: being or becoming less dense.

Recession: gradual drawing away of a tissue or part from its normal position, as the progressive exposure of the root surface by an apical shift of the gingiva following loss of the alveolar crest and loss of the corresponding part of the periodontal ligament (membrane).

Rectification: conversion of alternating current to direct current.

Recurrent: returning after intermissions.

Rehabilitation: restoration to former state of health, efficiency, and independent action; regeneration.

Relative Biological Effectiveness (R.B.E.): a factor used to compare the biological effects of absorbed doses of differing types of ionizing radiation in a particular organism or tissue. The standard of comparison is medium voltage x-rays delivered at about 10 rads/minute. The unit of R.B.E. is the **rem.**

Remission: a decrease or arrest of the symptoms of a disease; also the period during which such decrease occurs.

Resorption: removal of bone or tooth structure by osteoclasts effected by pressure; gradual destruction of dentin and cementum of the root, as the primary teeth prior to shedding; in orthodontic tooth movement, bone formation on one side compensates for resorption of bone on the other side.

Resuscitation: the restoration to life of one apparently dead.

Retromolar area: that area distal to the most posterior mandibular molar.

Rh factor: agglutinogens of red blood cells responsible for isoimmune reactions such as occur in erythroblastosis fetalis and incompatible blood transfusions; erythroblastosis fetalis results when a mother is Rh negative and develops antibodies against the fetus which is Rh positive.

Rheostat: an appliance for regulating the resistance and thus controlling the amount of current entering an electric circuit; the dental unit control is located in a device operated by the foot.

Rheumatic: pertaining to or affected with **rheumatism** a disease marked by inflammation of the connective tissue structures of the body, especially the muscles and joints.

Roentgen (R): an international unit based on the ability of radiation to ionize air.

Root planing: instrumentation applied to the root surface to divest it of deposits and softened or rough cementum.

Rubefacient: reddening the skin; an agent that reddens the skin by producing active or passive hyperemia.

Ruga: ridge, wrinkle, fold.

Saddle: a ridge connecting two higher elevations; in dentistry, a partial denture base that fits over the edentulous area.

Sarcoma: a tumor, frequently malignant, which originates in the connective tissue.

Sclerosis: abnormal hardening or thickening of tissue, especially as a result of inflammation or disease of the interstitial substance.

Sedative: a remedy that allays activity, excitement, apprehension.

Senescence: process or condition of growing old; physiologic aging not necessarily related to chronologic age.

Senile: of or pertaining to old age; characteristic of old age.

Senility: old age; feebleness of body and mind occurring with old age.

Septum: a dividing wall, partition, or membrane.

Sequestrum: a piece of dead bone that has become separated from living bone during the process of necrosis.

Serrated: having a sawlike edge.

Serum: the clear, liquid part of blood separated from its more solid elements after clotting; the blood plasma from which fibrinogen has been removed in the process of clotting.

Shelf-life: the length of time a substance or preparation can be kept without changing its chemical structure or other properties.

Slough: a mass of dead tissue in, or cast out of, living tissue.

Sorbitol: a proprietary sugar solution which will mix with water and glycerin and is slightly soluble in alcohol; used as a moistener, softener, and binder in dental preparations.

Space maintainer: a fixed or removable appliance used to replace missing primary teeth to prevent drifting of surrounding teeth until eruption of permanent teeth.

Spore: see **Bacterial spore.**

Stabile: not moving, stationary, resistant; opposite of labile.

    Heat stabile (thermostabile): resistant to moderate degrees of temperature.

Stannous: compound containing tin.

Sterile: aseptic, free from microorganisms.

Stomatitis: inflammation of the oral mucosa, due to local or systemic factors; inflammation may involve entire oral soft tissues.

Subclinical: without clinical manifestations; said of early stages of, or slight degree of, a disease.

Submerged tooth: one which is below the line of occlusion and may be ankylosed; intrusion; infraocclusion.

Supernumerary tooth: extra tooth; one which is in excess of the normal number.

Suppuration: formation of, conversion into, or act of discharging pus.

Susceptibility: tendency to be affected easily.

Suture: a surgical stitch or seam; line of junction of adjacent cranial or facial bones.

Sympathetic nervous system: that part of the autonomic (involuntary) nervous system which arises in the thoracic and the first three lumbar segments of the spinal cord.

Systemic: pertaining to or affecting the whole body.

Tactile: pertaining to the touch; perceptible to the touch.

Tarnish: to dull or alter the luster of a metallic surface by oxidation; discolor, stain, blemish.

Tensile strength: the load necessary to break a given material that is stretched lengthwise.

Therapeutic: pertaining to the treating or curing of disease; curative.

Therapy: the treatment of disease.

Threshold: that amount of stimulus which just produces a perceptible sensation.

  Pain threshold: that amount of stimulus which just produces a sensation of pain.

Threshold exposure: the minimum exposure that will produce a detectable degree of any given effect.

Thrombosis: the formation, development or presence of a thrombus.

Thrombus: a plug or clot in a blood vessel or in one of the cavities of the heart formed by coagulation of the blood and remaining at the point of its formation.

Tic: quick, sudden spasm occurring usually in persons with neurotic tendency.

  Motor tic: any spasmodic movement or twitching, as of the face, not related to neurotic tendency.

Tincture: an alcoholic solution of a drug or other chemical substance.

Tone: the normal degree of vigor and tension; a healthy state of a part.

Tonguetie: abnormal shortness of the frenum of the tongue resulting in limitation of the motion of that organ.

Tonus: the slight, continuous contraction of muscle, which in skeletal muscles aids in the maintenance of posture and the return of blood to the heart. See **Tone.**

Topical: on the surface; pertaining to a particular spot; local.

Topography: the detailed description and analysis of the features of an anatomical region or of a special part.

Torus: a swelling; bulging projection; protuberance.

  Torus mandibularis: a bony prominence or protuberance on the lingual surface of the mandible.

  Torus palatinus: a bony prominence or protuberance of the hard palate.

Toxin: any poisonous substance of microbic, vegetable or animal origin which causes poisonous symptoms only after a period of incubation; can induce the elaboration of specific antitoxins in suitable animals.

Toxoplasmosis: infection with or a condition produced by protozoa of the genus *Toxoplasma.*

Tracheotomy: surgical operation to provide an artificial opening into the trachea.

Transformer: an electrical device which increases or reduces the voltage of an alternating current by mutual induction between primary and secondary coils or windings.

Trauma: an injury; damage; impairment; external violence producing body injury or degeneration.

Traumatic occlusion: abnormal occlusal stress which may injure the dental or periodontal tissues; a condition of imbalance between the force applied to teeth during mastication and the tissue resistance to the force.

Treatment: the management and care of a patient for the purpose of curing a disease or disorder.

Tremor: involuntary trembling or quivering.

Trismus: motor disturbance of the trigeminal nerve, especially spasm of the masticatory muscles, which causes difficulty in opening the mouth.

Triturate: to pulverize by rubbing, grinding.

Tumor: a swelling of tissue; an overgrowth of cells which are independent of normal growth controls, serve no useful purpose, and are often injurious to normal tissues.

Ulcer: a loss of substance on a cutaneous or mucous surface, causing gradual disintegration and necrosis of the tissues.

Urticaria: smooth, slightly raised patches of the skin which are redder or paler than the surrounding skin and accompanied by intense itching; may be caused by systemic disturbance, allergy to certain foods, menstruation, or emotion.

Vehicle: a substance, usually fluid, possessing little or no medicinal action, used as a medium to confer a suitable consistency or form to a drug.

Vesicle: a small sac containing liquid; a small elevation of the epidermis containing serous liquid.

Vincent's disease: trench mouth.   See **Necrotizing Ulcerative Gingivitis.**

Virulent: capable of causing infection or disease.

Viscosity: stickiness; ability of a fluid to resist change in shape or arrangement during flow.

Volatile: tending to evaporate readily.

Volt: unit of electromotive force or potential difference, sufficient to cause a current of one ampere to flow through a resistance of one ohm.

Voltage: the potential or electromotive force of an electric charge, expressed in volts.

Vulcanite: a hard rubber prepared by vulcanizing India rubber with sulfur; formerly used for making artificial dentures.

Xerostomia: dryness of the mouth due to functional or organic disturbances of the salivary glands.

INDEX

A

Gingiva, menopausal gingivostomatitis, 455
  menstruation and, 454
  mucogingival junction, 86
  normal, defined, 85
  oral inspection and, 84
  oral prophylaxis, appearance after, 192, 193
    effect, 102
  parts, described, 86–88
  porte polishing, effects, 173
Gingiva, pregnancy and, 458–459
  puberty and, 452
  recession. See *Gingival recession.*
  scaling procedures and, 152
    ultrasonic, 156, 158
  self-cleansing mechanisms and, 104
  stannous fluoride and, 205
  Stillman's cleft, 261
  stimulation, natural, 271
  topical anesthetic and, 159
  trauma. See *Trauma, gingival.*
Gingival crest, described, 86, 87
  irritation by dental plaque, 113
    by materia alba, 116
  porte polisher and, 173, 176
  scaling and, 152, 155
  wood point width and, 175
Gingival disease. See also *Periodontal disease.*
  diabetes mellitus and, 446
Gingival enlargement, classified and defined, 261
  dilantin hyperplasia, 401–402
  leukemia and, 434
  puberty and, 452
Gingival hemorrhage. See also *Hemorrhage.*
  dilantin hyperplasia and, 402
  green stain formation and, 131
  leukemia and, 434
  massage and, 273
  menstruation and, 454
  patient history and, 75
  pregnancy and 459
  scaling and, 162
    ultrasonic, 158
  symptoms, blood disease, 432
Gingival hyperplasia. See *Gingival enlargement.*
Gingival inflammation. See also *Inflammation.*
  calculus, effect, 125
  dilantin hyperplasia and, 402
  pregnancy and, 458–459
  puberty and, 452
  stannous fluoride and, 205
  subacute bacterial endocarditis and, 431
Gingival margin. See *Gingival crest.*
Gingival massage. See *Massage, gingival.*
Gingival recession, aging and, 338
  defined, 261
  factor in exposure of cementum, 209
  hypersensitive teeth and, 209
  physiological, and deposit retention, 109
  recession, defined, 488
  toothbrushing, cause of, 293, 294, 295–296
    method for, 283, 286, 289
Gingival sulcus. See *Sulcus, gingival.*
Gingival trauma. See *Trauma, gingival.*

Gingivitis, diabetes mellitus and, 446
  fractured jaw and, 375
  necrotizing ulcerative. See *Necrotizing ulcerative gingivitis.*
Glands, endocrine. See *Endocrine glands.*
  exocrine, 438
  salivary, secretion, aging and, 338
Glaucoma, 483
Glossitis, anemia and, 433
  defined, 483
  gerodontic patient and, 338
Glucose tolerance test, 483
Glycerin, in dentifrice, 309
  in desensitizing paste, 210
  in polishing agent, 171
Glycol, in dentifrice, 309
  in polishing agent, 171
  in topical anesthetic, 160
Glycosuria, 444
Gonads, 438, 449–450. See also *Menopause, Menstruation, Pregnancy, Puberty.*
Graafian follicle, 449, 450
Grand mal, 399–400, 404, 471. See also *Epilepsy.*
Granulomatous epulis, 459
Grasp, denture, during cleaning, 182
Grasp, instrument, 140
    dental tape and floss, 187
    exercises for development, 143–146
    fulcrum for, 141
    palm, defined, 140
    porte polisher and, 175
  pen, defined, 140
    effects, correct, 140
    fulcrum for, 141
    porte polisher, 175
    prophylaxis angle, 180, 182
    scaler, 154, 155, 156
    sharpening instruments, 33, 39, 40
    ultrasonic scaler, 157
  polishing strips, 189
  purposes of, 140
Grasp, toothbrush, 276, 280
Green stain, 130–131
  decalcification and, 162
  removal, iodine disclosing solution, 176
Grit, defined, 483
  grades of abrasives, 168
  polishing abrasive, rubber cup and, 181
  rate of abrasion and, 168
Groove, free gingival, 86

H

HABILITATION, 483
Habits, change of, 193, 272, 363
  dietary, adolescence and, 453
    cerebral palsy and, 417–418
    deposit retention and, 107–108
    dietary survey to show, 356–361
    gerodontic patient, 341–342
    mastication and, 98
    patient history and, 74
    pregnancy and, 463, 465